Design for Critical Care

Design for Critical Care: An Evidence-Based Approach

D. Kirk Hamilton and
Mardelle McCuskey Shepley

Routledge
Taylor & Francis Group
LONDON AND NEW YORK

Architectural Press

Architectural Press is an imprint of Routledge
2 Park Square, Milton Park, Abingdon, Oxon, OX14 4RN

711 Third Avenue, New York, NY 10017

Routledge is an imprint of the Taylor & Francis Group, an informa business

First edition 2010

British Library Cataloguing in Publication Data
A catalogue record for this book is available from the British Library

Library of Congress Cataloging-in-Publication Data
A catalog record for this book is available from the Library of Congress

ISBN: 978-0-7506-6530-8

Contents

Acknowledgements

In addition to our guest bar authors, we would like to express our thanks to the many individuals and organizations without which this book would not have been possible. Each of the following design firms supplied photographs and/or plans: ARRAY Healthcare Facilities Solutions; Artekna; BSA LifeStructures; Cannon Design; Christner, Inc.; Columbia St Mary's; Cromwell Architects and Engineers; Design Partnership; Earl Swensson and Associates; H&L Architecture; HOK in association with SLAM Collaborative; Hasenstab Architects; HGA Architects and Engineers; HDR Architecture, Inc.; KMD Architects; JJCA; Loebl, Schossman & Hackl; Karlsberger Companies; Lee, Burkhart, Liu, Inc.; Morris-Switzer Environments for Health; NBBJ; Odell; Orcutt/Winslow; RTKL; Shepley Bulfinch Abbott and Richardson; Strollo Architects & Moody-Nolan; TAYLOR and Questar Construction; and WHR Architects.

This book is better for the contribution of expert guest authors who offered the sidebars included in the main text or helped review and edit portions of our text. We are grateful for the generosity of Jennifer Aliber, Diana Anderson, Phil Astley, Knut Bergsland, Paula Buick, Charles Cadenhead, Romano Del Nord, Jim Diaz, Lari Diaz, Jennie Evans, Susan Frampton, Neil Halpern, Jim Harrell, Debra Harris, Maurene Harvey, Ann Hendrich, Connie Jastremski, Joy Kalt, Jain Malkin, Sarah Markovitz, Peter McGinity, Yasushi Nagasawa, Upali Nanda, Phillip Jin Gyu Park, Ray Pentecost, Peter Pronovost, Roger Resar, Terry Ritchey, Neal Rinnela, Joan Saba, Gerri Staffileno, Owen Samuels, Nancy Silva, Bob Uhlenhake, Roger Ulrich, David Vincent, Angela Watson, and Craig Zimring.

We would especially like to thank several people for their administrative assistance and hard work supporting our writing effort: Nancy Crowley, Samira Pasha, Judy Pruitt, Anoop Gulati, and Avery Kennedy. We are grateful for the understanding of our faculty colleagues and Joyce Langenegger while we have labored to complete the manuscript. And finally, we are grateful for the confidence Elsevier has shown in trusting us to complete a long overdue book we hope will be important for the field.

Kirk Hamilton & Mardelle Shepley
College Station

About the Authors

D. Kirk Hamilton, FAIA, FACHA, is an associate professor and associate director of the Center for Health Systems & Design at Texas A&M University. Hamilton's academic credentials include a professional Bachelor of Architecture from the University of Texas at Austin, and a Master of Science in Organization Development from Pepperdine University. The focus of his academic research is the relationship of evidence-based health facility design to measurable organizational performance. Hamilton is a board certified healthcare architect with 30 years of active practice and is a founding principal emeritus of WHR Architects. He is the co-author of *Evidence-Based Design for Multiple Building Types*. He serves on the board of The Center for Health Design and is co-editor of the peer-reviewed, interdisciplinary *Health Environments Research & Design Journal* (HERD). Hamilton is a past president of the American College of Healthcare Architects and the AIA Academy of Architecture for Health. He has served as chair of the ICU Design Committee of the Society of Critical Care Medicine, of which he is one of only three architect members.

Dr. Mardelle McCuskey Shepley, AIA, ACHA, LEED AP, is a professor and director of the Center for Health Systems & Design at Texas A&M University. Dr. Shepley's academic credentials include a B.A. and Master of Architecture from Columbia University, and an M.A. (psychology) and Doctor of Architecture from the University of Michigan. A registered architect with 25 years of experience in professional practice, she is the founder of ART + Science, a firm specializing in applied design research. Mardelle has conducted research and published extensively on the topic of healthcare facility design. Co-author of *Healthcare Environments for Children and their Families*, and a specialist in building evaluation and programming, she is the William Peña endowed professor at the College of Architecture at Texas A&M.

Introduction

The critical care unit of a hospital is where life can hang in the balance every day and where skillful and timely intervention literally saves lives. The critical care setting, frequently known as the intensive care unit, the ICU, or the CCU, is where some of the hospital's most difficult and demanding work takes place. The ICU is the stage for many of life's most extraordinary dramas. Design of the setting in which this vitally important work is done will be increasingly important to physicians, nurses, pharmacists, respiratory therapists, patients, families, and hospital executives, to name only a few of those affected.

This book attempts to make the case for effective and supportive facility design that enhances rather than hinders the work of clinicians. It endorses the approach that design informed by the findings of credible research is likely to be more successful than design based on unsupported concepts. This book explores key issues in the design of facilities for critical care and provides examples of credible evidence relevant to those issues. It includes suggestions for a collaborative method in which designers and clinicians can work together to achieve improved results. We hope that design of future critical care units will be powerfully influenced by strong visions of better, more effective care, and innovative settings, rather than hollow reproductions of what has been built in the past.

We hope the book will find an audience in the world of architects and designers as well as in the medical world of intensivists, physicians, nurses, pharmacists, therapists, members of the critical care staff, and hospital executives.

Need for effective design in critical care

A facility design that supports the crucially important work of critical care must serve the minimum functional needs of physicians, staff, patients, and their families. If the physical facility can be either an enabler of high performance, or a barrier to effective performance, then appropriate design is vitally important. A good facility design will efficiently support functional requirements and will also effectively serve the physical, psychological, and emotional needs of those who use it. The best facility designs make it more likely that optimum performance can be achieved.

When time is of the essence, needed equipment and supplies should be at the fingertips of the clinicians and should be found in familiar locations. The most appropriate technologies and information systems should be present, accessible, and simple to use. Staff in one room should be able to find things intuitively based on their familiarity with other standardized rooms.

Under non-emergency conditions the space should support routine functions such as the washing of hands, best-practice care models, communication, and documentation. It should directly address the psychosocial needs of the patient and family members while serving as a pleasant, stress-free work environment for the staff.

A good facility design may be nearly invisible in the sense that it often goes unnoticed, but a poor design can be frustrating to the occupants and will make its deficiencies known time and time again. With the stakes so high, it seems there can be few settings more important than the critical care environments of our hospitals. These are settings that deserve the very best of our facility designs to support the extraordinary efforts of our hard-working clinicians, as well as the hopes and prayers of the patients at grave risk and their anxious families.

Context of continuous change

Heraclitus said, "There is nothing permanent except change." Nowhere is this adage more true than in medicine. Numerous factors contribute to medicine's state of continuous change, and change is often more evident in critical care—the frequent front line in the battle against illness and disease. There are certainly nearly continuous technological and procedural changes or upgrades as critical care medicine advances.

A dramatic shift in patient acuity is taking place (Coile, 2003). It has been said, both in the lounges of ICU units and in the halls of hospital administration, that today's critical care patients would not have survived a decade ago. Similarly, today's step-down patient may be as ill as the critical care patient of the past, and today's patients on typical acute units are those who might have gotten step-down care in the past. The former acute patient may be found at home today, recuperating from an outpatient procedure (Conly & Johnston, 2001). The inevitable result of this progression is an escalation of acuity, with caregivers responsible for patients who are sicker than ever before.

It has been possible to treat these increasingly ill patients, because there have been concurrent advances in medicine and technology. Yet these same advances in medical protocols and new technologies can at times be in conflict with the physical configuration of the ICU space. The best location for a new heart pump may be at the foot of the bed, but the room might have been designed in such a way that there isn't enough space for this unanticipated technology to be placed in the ideal location. A good facility design will have the flexibility to adapt to changing conditions.

The so-called Baby Boom generation born just after World War II, with its enormous cohort of the population, is reaching an age (the oldest members of the group are entering their 60s) at which its members will begin to consume healthcare in much larger numbers (Administration on Aging, 1997). This predictable change will produce unprecedented numbers of patients for hospitals and their critical care units.

At the same time that the population is aging and creating greater demand for critical care, the workforce is also aging (Buerhaus, Staiger, & Auerbach, 2002; Pierce, 2001), and there is a serious question about the future availability of qualified professionals in critical care (AHA Commission on Workforce for Hospitals and Health Systems, 2002). The prospect of fewer specially trained staff to care for larger numbers of seriously ill patients is a potentially serious problem (Pierce, 2001). It is not just a problem of intensivist physicians or critical care nurses; there will not be enough pharmacists, respiratory therapists, and many other clinical professionals.

Effective use of scarce resources

Resources available to healthcare organizations are limited. No healthcare organization in any part of the world has sufficient financial resources to do everything it could possibly do, everything it wishes it could do, or everything its physicians might be capable of doing. A case can be made that critical care must be funded at levels commensurate with the needs of each community, but this portion of such a scarce resource too often will be less than ideal. There is a clear obligation, then, to make every investment a wise one, including investments in facilities.

One element of the mission to ensure the wise investment of resources is to derive the maximum value for every dollar, pound, yuan, or euro spent on healthcare facilities. Design of these costly facilities should aim to maximize the productivity of nurses, physicians, and staff of each hospital. Prized facilities will be those that are efficient and that allow fewer staff to perform more tasks.

While this need for effective design to support the important work done in critical care settings is impacted by scarce resources at any one hospital or system, and in some cases national health organizations, there is an extraordinary situation. Many of today's healthcare facilities may have been constructed in the 1960s or earlier—much earlier in many cases (Carpenter, 2006). In the United States, many hospitals were built with Hill-Burton funding shortly after World War II. Europe also underwent rebuilding after the war. These increasingly obsolete facilities will need to be updated to keep up with advances in technology and medical practice. In underdeveloped nations, there is a push to develop modern medical facilities. Huge amounts of funding, therefore, will be allocated to hospital construction and replacement in the next two decades, and it will occur all across the globe.

Great Britain's National Health Service, for instance, has committed billions of pounds to replace large numbers of hospitals through a huge privatization initiative (Sussex, 2001). Significant projects in Canada, including major undertakings in Quebec, Ontario, and British Columbia, will replace multiple hospitals with new and larger consolidated ones (Aubin, 2005). In The Netherlands, teaching hospitals are being replaced, and many other nations anticipate large investments in their healthcare infrastructure (Wessels & Verweij, 2002). In addition, hospitals located around the perimeter of the Indian Ocean are being repaired or replaced as a result of the tsunamis of 2004 while others have been developed as locations for so-called destination medicine. Estimates made early in the decade regarding spending on healthcare construction in the United States exceeded $20 billion per year for each of the next 10 years, or more than $200 billion in the next decade (Babwin, 2002; Coile, 2003). More recently, the pace of healthcare facility planning has slowed, although projects under construction continue at an intense pace (Carpenter & Hoppszallern, 2009). Assuming the economic turmoil subsides by the end of 2009, the slowdown may be temporary.

The current economic situation makes a compelling case that the funds should be spent carefully (Berry et al., 2004). If some of the most critical work of the hospital occurs in the ICU, then effective design of these environments is even more important. It is the premise of this book that making evidence-based design decisions is a way to assure that the huge investment made in renovation or construction of critical care settings is appropriate. There should be a commitment to measure the results of these design decisions as they are implemented to determine those that are most effective, and the resulting data should in turn be used for subsequent plans.

Moral responsibility to improve

The performance improvement movement in healthcare accelerated with the publication of the Institute of Medicine's reports *To Err Is Human* (Kohn, Corrigan, & Donaldson, 2000) and *Crossing the Quality Chasm* (Institute of Medicine Committee on Quality of Health Care in America, 2001). The authors made the call for needed improvements based on evidence that there are significant deaths and deplorable adverse effects associated with preventable error in the healthcare system of the United States.

Organizations like the Leapfrog Group of corporate payors have called for improvement to reduce costs, and in the area of critical care they have specifically called for hospitals to make use of intensivists to guide the care in the ICU (Birkmeyer et al., 2000). They did so on the basis of evidence that intensivist-directed care appears to be more effective than traditional practice led by attending physicians. The Institute for Healthcare Improvement has initiated collaborations between hospitals to work on improving care (Rainey et al., 1998). Their efforts to improve performance in critical care as well as patient flow within hospitals are examples of ways in which data can be gathered to diagnose problems, and how structured tests of change can show the way toward solution.

In the same way that medical professionals feel obligated to continuously improve, healthcare architects and design professionals have a moral responsibility to continuously improve the performance of the buildings they design. This is especially so in healthcare, where health outcomes for patients can be at stake. Architects have long had a sacred responsibility for the life safety of building occupants. In the arena of evidence-based design for hospitals, the responsibility for the health, safety, and welfare of the building's occupants can be extended beyond the traditional role of the architect. Some might consider it a higher calling.

Guide for design: how to use this book

This book offers an overview of critical care design, provides a review of relevant categories of research that can inform design, and points the reader toward a new future. It will offer no prescriptive guidelines or formulas to apply as answers to the questions designers and their clients must ask. New research is produced continuously, so rigid prescriptions for design are soon outdated. The reader will instead find listings of important research findings and observations from completed projects. The list is not exhaustive. There will be areas where little research is available and the content is a partial record of "best practice" in North America as understood by the authors. Some recommendations for designers as examples of the types of design implications that can be elicited by research findings are included. These recommendations will be based on performance criteria, allowing for multiple interpretations of design responses. It is the task of each design team to use critical thinking to interpret research findings in the context of their own unique situation.

The material in this book is organized into four parts. Part One introduces the hypothesis that better design will lead to better outcomes, based on the concept of evidence-based design and its specific role in design for critical care. There is a brief history of design for critical care; some exemplary projects are described; international comparisons are made; and the foundations of environmental research in healthcare, which suggest a theory of supportive design, are reported.

Part Two follows with discussion of the physical aspects and design issues associated with the critical care unit, the patient room, family accommodations, and the spaces which support staff activities. Many will find it a useful review of the basic design choices which must be made to plan a critical care unit.

Part Three contains material readers can use as they begin to work with a specific design. The three chapters in Part Three are organized around the way in which social scientists have traditionally viewed research about humans and the environment: they focus on places, people, and the behaviors of people in those places. Specific research findings may be relevant to multiple sections, so some appear more than once. The authors have tried not to repeat each and every study that might be relevant for every example given. The reader should be prepared to use the major findings of various studies wherever they may be applicable.

Part Four focuses on the future, with a discussion of research methods, promising areas for research, a discussion of organizational performance as it relates to design, and a vision of the potential for critical care environments whose design has been informed by research findings.

The lengthy list of references is only the beginning of the potential citations for this important topic. They cover the basics and an introduction to many of the issues in critical care design, but the reader is advised to go to the original sources and to follow the references in the cited books, articles, and papers. Searching for references in the listed references will easily more than double the relevant sources.

The authors hope this book will help both medical professionals and design professionals in their efforts to improve the designs of critical care facilities. This book intends to point to the many types of research findings that could be relevant to designers, in the hope that many will be influenced to design and construct better units, which will produce better outcomes for many patients. The authors hope such new designs will be great places for dedicated medical professionals to be productive and to enjoy their important work.

Part One: Better Design for Better Outcomes

Evidence-based design and applied research

1

Persons associated with the world of medicine should have no trouble understanding the concept of evidence-based design. In the realm of evidence-based medicine, where physicians base best practices on the results of research studies, and in which healthcare executives have long since adopted data-driven decision-making, it is easy to understand the idea of making facility design decisions on the basis of research. Is there sufficient research about design and healthcare environments on which to base important decisions?

1.1 Hypothesis: better design will lead to better outcomes

Research findings have demonstrated the link between the design of healthcare environments and patient outcomes (Rubin, Owens, & Golden, 1998; Ulrich et al., 2004; Ulrich et al., 2008; NACHRI, 2008). It is possible to hypothesize that better design will lead to better outcomes. This can be nowhere more important than in the critical care environment, where the most ill and susceptible patients are cared for and where the difference between life and death can be attributed to any of many complicating factors associated with the intensive interventions of the caregivers.

1.2 What is evidence-based design?

Hamilton has written that evidence-based designers "make decisions, together with an informed client, on the basis of the best available information from research and project evaluations" (2003, p. 20). The belief is that in healthcare, especially in intensive care settings where the stakes are so high, one cannot consistently rely on subjective judgment to make expensive and nearly permanent design decisions. The Center for Health Design offered another definition: "Evidence-based design is the process of basing decisions about the built environment on credible research to achieve the best possible outcomes" (Levin, 2008, p. 8). The goal of evidence-based design is to use reliable information to support more effective design decisions and, in the case of this book, to examine the current state of that information as it applies to critical care.

Healthcare design practitioners find it comfortable to think of parallels with the evidence-based medicine familiar to their clinical clients. While the types of evidence in the two fields are not the same (Viets, 2009), there are a number of things in common. A prominent definition of evidence-based medicine comes from Sackett and his colleagues:

> Evidence-based medicine is the conscientious, explicit and judicious use of current best evidence in making decisions about the care of individual patients.
>
> (Sackett et al., 1996, p. 71)

Hamilton admired the clarity of this definition. He first wrote the second half of his definition for evidence-based design, about critical decisions made with clients on the basis of the best available information, in 2003. He added the language of "conscientious, explicit, and judicious use" (Hamilton, 2006) after examining definitions in evidence-based medicine, and choosing to build upon David Sackett, sometimes described as the father of evidence-based medicine (Sackett et al., 1996). Defining evidence-based design as a *process* came last, in response to the many who expected a product—the ready-made answer to their most difficult design questions. Here is the result:

> Evidence-based design is a process for the conscientious, explicit and judicious use of current best evidence from research and practice in making critical decisions, together with an informed client, about the design of each individual and unique project.
>
> (Hamilton & Watkins, 2009, p. 9)

There is growing interest in evidence-based design, as demonstrated by the increase in published articles and books on the topic, as well as by participation in related organizations and events (Hamilton, 2003, 2004b, 2004c, 2005; Hamilton & Watkins, 2009; Cama, 2009). The Center for Health Design (www.healthdesign.org) has for more than two decade promoted evidence-based design with an interdisciplinary audience. Its current focus is on the Pebble Project, in which healthcare organizations document patient outcomes associated with design projects (Joseph & Hamilton, 2008). The Center for Health Design has worked together with the Robert Wood Johnson Foundation (www.rwjf.org) and the Institute for Healthcare Improvement (www.ihi.org) to introduce evidence-based design to broader audiences of healthcare practitioners and executives. The Center for Health Design's association with *HealthCareDesign* magazine as well as an annual interdisciplinary conference helps to spread the message.

The American Institute of Architects' Academy of Architecture for Health (AIA/AAH), the American College of Healthcare Architects (ACHA), the American Society of Interior Designers (ASID), the International Interior Design Association (IIDA), and the American Academy of Healthcare Interior Designers (AAHID) all endorse the evidence-based process. There is now an interdisciplinary, peer-reviewed journal, *Health Environments Research & Design* (HERD), which publishes scholarly papers on a broad range of topics relating to design and research associated with healthcare settings.

There are an almost endless number of potential sources of information that are useful for evidence-based planning. Many of the early mentions of evidence-based design have focused on the environmental psychology aspects of the field (Malkin, 1992, 2008; Ulrich, 1991, 1997). One of the pioneering studies that brought widespread attention to the role of the environment in clinical outcomes was conducted by a behavioral scientist who demonstrated a relationship between views of nature and clinical outcomes among cholocystectomy patients (Ulrich, 1984). While these types of studies form the foundation of important theories of supportive design for healthcare, it should be understood that the research that might be used by designers and their clients is not limited to one field. There is potentially relevant research from fields as varied as management, information technology, logistics, food service, and performance improvement, to name only a few.

The scientific foundation

Roger S. Ulrich, Ph.D.

"The scientific foundation for evidence-based healthcare design is already large and surprisingly strong. A joint project at Texas A&M University and the Georgia Institute of Technology in the USA indentified nearly 700 rigorous studies, most published in international medical journals, about how the architecture of acute care hospitals affects health. A collaborative of more than 30 healthcare organizations set up by the Center for Health Design has done several multi-year clinical and safety evaluations of specific design interventions and new buildings. Much credible evidence now shows that good design of a hospital's physical environment promotes better clinical outcomes, increases safety, and reduces stress for both patients and staff" (Ulrich, 2006).

Dr. Roger Ulrich is a professor at Texas A&M University where he is a Fellow in the Center for Health Systems & Design.

Designers have used research from medicine, nursing, management, industrial design, engineering, and technology. Relevant sources also include the literature of psychology, sociology, anthropology, and economics. The journals of science may be a useful source, along with the popular press, newspapers and magazines, and documentary films and television programs. Industry data guides, guidelines from speciality boards, quality review data, infection control data, manufacturers' testing information, association reports, and the documents of accreditation agencies and code authorities provide helpful information. Practitioners can gather new information from conference presentations, workshops, continuing education programs, and benchmarking tours of exemplary facilities. The Internet has also become a rich source of information for designers. The possible sources of relevant findings are limited only by the issues being addressed.

1.3 Therapeutic environments

While there are healing environments that have nothing to do with evidence-based design, many healing environments are the result of an evidence-based design that has demonstrated measurable improvements in the physical and/or psychological states of patients and/or staff, physicians, and visitors. If it meets these standards, a healing environment is therefore a complementary treatment modality that makes a therapeutic contribution to the course of care (van den Berg, 2005). The role played by the environment is certainly not as therapeutically effective as the role of surgery, pharmacology, medical interventions, or perhaps even the caring touch of an empathetic nurse. The therapeutic role of the physical environment is, however, absolutely real and must therefore be considered as contributing to the course of care and the patient outcome.

If the physical environment can contribute to improved clinical outcomes, then surely there is a moral obligation to provide critical care environments that are supportive of the teams of healthcare professionals who work with patients and their families. Designers have a responsibility to provide environments conducive to the safety, health, therapeutic interventions, and recovery of critical care patients. Above all, the environment, like every other aspect of healthcare, should "do no harm."

Design really matters

Maurene A. Harvey, RN, MPH, FCCM

In the first half of my 43 years in critical care nursing, I became increasingly incensed at how poorly intensive care units were designed. Having been in over 100 U.S. units and dozens in other countries, I was frequently dismayed by how poorly they met the needs of patients, families and/or caregivers, and how frequently the same general design templates were repeated even though they were inefficient, ineffective or starkly non-healing.

Many design teams tried to be more creative and open-minded, but it is difficult to see new possibilities when each team member's experience was often limited to a few units. Hampered by each individual's narrow perspective, teams lacked imagination and ability to develop unique or creative design solutions. They were often focused on solving problems in the existing unit using old engrained frameworks. New ground-breaking ideas that would allow the best possible patient and family care, as well as attract and retain expert staff, were required and lacking. They were doomed to repeat the same mistakes. The result was often just an improved version of the same outdated, flawed, dysfunctional design.

In the last two decades, my frustration has been decreasing. Building a new critical care unit is a high stakes investment. There is motivation to create a unit of the best possible design to meet patient, family and staff needs while recognizing fiscal constraints. Successful teams are those that are putting aside their assumptions, thinking creatively, and actively seeking and embracing what evidence is available.

Evidence-based design is a new concept. The success of future teams depends on continuing to build a robust and evolving body of research on the impact of design on a variety of outcomes. Each new building project presents an opportunity to evaluate the impact of design elements on outcomes pre- and post occupancy, and add to our understanding of key design features. The information presented in this book will be of value to both critical care design and research teams.

Maurene A. Harvey is a nurse and past President of the Society of Critical Care Medicine.

1.4 Interpretation of research findings

The challenge for the designer is to discover what research is relevant to his or her design issue, and to use critical thinking to draw careful conclusions about the implications of the research as they apply to the design. Research studies generally focus on a narrowly defined topic in order to eliminate confounding variables. Such specificity means no study is likely to precisely match the situation faced by the designer. Each design is in some way unique, and the designer must make a thoughtful interpretation of the research findings as they apply to the unique design decision under consideration.

Critical thinking is required to make thoughtful interpretations of research findings that are suited to specific design issues. The interpretation might need to extrapolate narrow findings to the larger context of the project. The interpretation also might need to combine multiple findings to serve a single design decision for a project. And the interpretation may often require sorting out conflicting findings to make an important design decision in the face of ambiguity.

One of the benefits of an evidence-based practice model is that when decisions cannot be based on the findings from research, an experiment can be conducted to help find an answer. It is possible to think of a facility design as an experiment. The designer may hypothesize the intended result of a design and measure the outcome to see if the hypothesis is supported. This will in turn lead to a better understanding of design and the outcomes that can be associated with it. Reporting these results to the field will offer others the benefit of additional and potentially relevant findings.

1.5 Applied research by design and clinical practitioners

Having made the important case for the use of evidence-based design, it is now equally important to make the case for ongoing contributions to the growing knowledge about critical care facilities. It is the responsibility of the architects, designers, and users of these critical care facilities to examine the results of their design efforts and to publicly share the results (Hamilton, 2003, 2004a).

Jarvis (1999) has pointed out that more and more research is occurring in the workplace. He describes the dual role of "practitioner-researchers." Both medical professionals and design professionals in practice can play these dual roles in an effort to track the results of design decisions associated with critical care projects. Jarvis contends that the pace of change and the tendency toward reflective practice are leading to growth in the number of practitioner-researchers.

Chapter 9 will continue the discussion about applied research by practitioners. Much of what is done in the way of applied practitioner research in the field is not described as research. Design practitioners do not always understand how much they can contribute in the way of field-based research. Many practitioners who perform simple or less complex types of research in the field do not consider themselves to be researchers (Jarvis, 1999). They may not feel their work is relevant to others or that it's sufficiently "scientific" to be credible. Architects rarely have training in traditional research methods (Shepley, 1997).

Environmental research is not the research of test tubes, beakers, and microscopes. It is more likely to be based on social science methods that include field observations, participant observation, instrument measurements of environmental factors, interviews, surveys, videotaping, and ethnographic techniques (Babbie, 2002; Bailey, 1978). As part of this type of environmental research, design interventions may be matched to medical records of the occupants of an altered space. Or a design might be measured by observations of staff productivity, or by a simple calculation of staff travel distances before and after a design change. The study may include measurements of sound, light levels, or temperatures.

Science is the study of principles, laws, rules, or structures that can be observed in a tangible existing reality, while design is the act of imagining something which does not yet exist. Once implemented and constructed, a design becomes "an object for study by any of the arts and sciences" (Buchanan, 1995, p. 17). The reader should not be tempted to hold emerging research related to the multi-factorial physical environment and its influence on human behavior to the standards of the randomized and controlled clinical trials of medicine. While the evidence for design purposes will certainly grow, it will never be as robust as the massive pool of rigorous medical evidence. Similarly, the design evidence will not fit into the same hierarchy of evidence quality that is currently accepted in medicine. This does not suggest environmental findings should be ignored or discarded. As the process of research-informed design matures, a consensus will surely develop around a hierarchy of quality for environmental findings.

Environments for quality care and a healthy work experience

Connie A. Jastremski, RN, MS, MBA, ANP, FCCM

Today's hospitalized patients are sicker than ever before. As a chief nursing officer I am focused on providing the highest quality care to these patients, especially those in the critical care units. In addition, I am also concerned about the staff's ability to provide that quality care.

Creating a healthcare environment that supports high quality patient care and a healthy work environment for staff is critical. With evidence-based design as a conscientious, explicit use of evidence from research and practice, a design can be created to embrace the concepts of quality, workflow, patient care, family care and support, and staff satisfaction.

Much research has been done over the years to focus an organization's attention on the workplace. Efforts to create quiet zones for patients to improve healing have been incorporated into many designs. Capitalizing on the work of Florence Nightingale concerning light and healing, ICUs are required to have windows to allow natural light and some ICUs have even added skylights above the beds. In addition to improving the physical look of the units, the more pleasant environment does promote healing.

Bringing families closer to the patient is another concept that increases patient comfort and decreases stress for the patient and family. Dr. Cathie Guzzetta, a 2005 SCCM keynoter, has done a great deal of research on the effects of family presence on stress reduction and healing (Guzzetta et al., 2004). ICU rooms can have a space for a bed and family can be welcome to stay in the room. Nearby kitchens are available for family use, to allow the family to leave the room and stay close to the unit. The addition of family as part of the care team at times challenges the staff, but it is so important to the patient care.

Work areas near to the patient and away from a central desk allow for closer observation of the patient and promote higher interaction with the family. Caregivers must have time to think and refresh the spirit, away from the hectic workplace. Creating healing work environments for staff includes respite areas to escape the stress of the care environment. This has become central in most new or remodelled plans.

The critical care team needs to be engaged in any design efforts on their units. The authors are providing what is needed to bring forward the best environmental designs for critical care, through their research, their critical care connections, and a comprehensive review of relevant evidence. This book will be seen as a true guide for the physicians, nurses, respiratory therapists, pharmacists, and other team members who become involved in creating the environment that helps heal.

Reference

Guzzetta, C.E., Meyers, T.A., Eichhorn, D.J., et al., 2004, January/February/March. Family presence during invasive procedures and resuscitation: the experience of family members, nurses, and physicians. Top. Emerg. Med. 26 (1), 61–73.

Connie A. Jastremski is the Chief Nursing Officer and Vice-President, Patient Care Services, at Bassett Healthcare in Cooperstown, New York.

One of the aims of this book is to offer both design and clinical practitioners some simple and practical ways to enter into the world of environmental research, and to encourage an active participation that helps advance the state of knowledge about the relationship between facility design and critical care. A further hope is that those who turn to this book will find effective ways to design and build their own high performance critical care units. We hope they will be inclined to openly share their findings and the lessons learned.

Facility design for critical care 2

The concept of critical care is to provide a place in which the most qualified staff can use the appropriate supplies and equipment to make intensive interventions in the course of care for patients at high risk. There is much leeway in such a description.

A hospital in Tatarstan, one of the former Soviet republics, in the late 1990s had a second position located inside the operating room because the only staff qualified to care for a recovering patient would be in the operating room. The ICU was a single room which contained the only heart monitor in the building. A small rural hospital in Utah has an oversized room that can serve as a birthing room, but becomes the ICU whenever the "ICU cart" is placed there to replace the birthing cart. At the other extreme, large teaching hospitals such as Richmond's Medical College of Virginia or the Stanford University Medical Center can have seven or more intensive care units devoted to different narrow clinical specialties.

2.1 A brief history of design for critical care

Early models

It is plausible that the earliest equivalent of a critical care treatment might have been the care associated with post-surgical recovery and complications. The history of contemporary critical care must surely date from the introduction of scientific medicine in the 1800s. Treatment for trauma and shock benefited from lessons in military medicine. Knowledge gained in the Crimea in the 1850s was taken to the United States' Civil War of the 1860s, and refined in the Franco-Prussian War of the 1870s. Florence Nightingale advocated keeping the most acute patients in front of the nurse's desk in the ward and Louisa May Alcott reported on her use of different rooms for patients of differing acuity (Fairman & Lynaugh, 1998).

The availability of anesthetics dating from the 1840s, Lister's development of aseptic techniques, scientific studies of anatomy, Roentgen's discovery of X-rays, experimentation with new surgical techniques, and the important observations of Florence Nightingale made possible many advances in the art of surgery and treatment of those who survived it. By the turn of the century, surgery had become more widely used as survival became more predictable and anesthesia made it more bearable. As surgery became more frequent and new techniques evolved, it became important for it to be performed in a hospital where equipment was available and the recovery process could be monitored by trained nurses. Previously, anyone of stature and with financial resources would have been treated at home, including surgical procedures. This shift away from care in the home for those who could afford it led to better hospitals (Guzzanti, 2006).

World War I brought the horrors of battlefield wounds, mass casualties, the development of triage concepts, and the army field hospital. Johns Hopkins in Baltimore has published reports that it had an early intensive care unit dating from the 1920s (Varon & Fromm, 2002). In 1923, Dr. Dandy created a three-bed space for post operative neurosurgical patients at Johns Hopkins (Harvey, 1974). Dr. Kirschner designed and built a 30-bed combined recovery room and intensive care ward at the University of Tuebingen's surgical hospital (Hilberman, 1975). The concept of a "recovery room" in which post surgical patients could be closely observed gained acceptance in the period between the wars.

Post World War II development: 1940s through the 1960s

The World War II period brought battlefield lessons in treatment for trauma, methods for rapid intervention, and the introduction of new drugs in the form of penicillin and sulfa (Cowdery, 1994). The triage concept was further developed and the field hospital became more sophisticated. In at least one account, renowned heart surgeon Michael E. DeBakey, MD is credited with development of the modern recovery room while working in the office of the U.S. Army Surgeon General (Mitka, 2005). Since qualified staff were at a premium in the battle zone, DeBakey is said to have introduced the grouping of recovering patients to improve care and observation.

The domestic shortage of nurses during World War II had accelerated the opening of recovery rooms in the United States (Charbon, 1949). The Oschner Clinic's Dr. Alton Oschner advocated for specially trained recovery room nurses based on his experience in New Orleans (Oschner, 1950). In the post war period of the late 1940s through the mid-1960s much construction of hospitals occurred in the United States as a result of the Hill-Burton funding program (Lave & Lave, 1974). The typical designs for small town hospitals had recovery rooms connected to the surgery suites, but most did not include a critical care unit. Larger, urban hospitals were, however, developing surgical intensive care beds as the precursors to full blown critical care units (Diaz, 2000). Advances in surgery, higher levels of post operative acuity, and the evolution of the recovery room led directly to development of the surgical ICU concept.

Mechanical ventilation was improved and developed for use in the 1950s in response to the poliomyelitis epidemic. Ventilator devices were made practical in Denmark, and then England, and respiratory units which became prototypes for the respiratory ICU opened in Denmark, Sweden, England, Canada, and the United States (Hilberman, 1975).

Advances in cardiac resuscitation in the 1950s, and the introduction of defibrillation in 1956, contributed to the concept of specialized coronary care. In 1962 the first coronary care units appeared in Toronto, Kansas City, and Philadelphia (Hilberman, 1975). Development of cardiac surgery interventions produced the need for a post operative unit that had both a coronary aspect and a surgical aspect suited to cardiovascular patients.

A period of technical upgrades and increasing sophistication of hospital design occurred during the 1960s. In addition to renovations to upgrade surgery and radiology departments, many U.S. hospitals became air-conditioned. This period saw the broad introduction of ICUs in most North American hospitals (Fairman & Lynaugh, 1998). The first intensive care units were general units without specialty designations, and the majority of their patients were still trauma and surgical cases. The surgical ICU, respiratory units, coronary units, and cardiovascular surgical units were the first to evolve. The teaching hospitals began to develop specialized units and to use them in the training of young physicians.

Post medicare development: 1970s through the 1990s

The next period of intensive care development includes the wide acceptance of critical care specialization. As bright, young physicians moved to community hospitals, they brought the idea of units similar to those in which they had trained. Intensive care units began to be split into the medical-surgical ICU and the cardiac unit, as occurred at Peninsula General Hospital in Salisbury, Maryland in the mid-1970s. Some began to operate surgical and medical ICUs separately, along with coronary units for heart attack victims (Tai & Ng, 2001). Large teaching hospitals and academic medical centers introduced cardiovascular ICUs, trauma ICUs, burn units, neuro and neurosurgery units, nephrology and dialysis centers, neonatal intensive care nurseries, and numerous other highly specialized units (Hilberman, 1975).

Many international physicians who trained in the United States, Canada, and the United Kingdom took the concept of intensive care units back to their own countries. The ICU model spread widely around the world, although significant variations in coverage, unit organization, technology, and resources continue to exist today (Vincent, Thijs & Cerny, 1997; Yoshiya & Baik, 1997; Dobb, 1998).

The decade of the 1980s seemed to focus in the United States on development of sophisticated equipment, such as physiologic monitors, new variations of life support systems, and the continuous advancement of imaging technologies (Hendee, 2002). This period saw the widespread introduction of computerized tomography and the beginnings of magnetic resonance.

The decade of the 1990s saw the promotion of critical care as a specialty unto itself, with intensivists beginning to develop best practice models and clinical pathways (Rainey, 2000). The Society of Critical Care Medicine began a campaign to promote the use of intensivists.

2000 and beyond

At the turn of the Millennium, the focus of critical care in the United States seemed to be on outcome improvement and safety. The Institute for Healthcare Improvement (IHI), in response to the challenge of the Institute of Medicine reports (Kohn et al., 2000; IOM, 2001), assembled working collaboratives of hospitals to study the ICU and patient flow (Haraden & Resar, 2004). These efforts produced recommendations for improved critical care performance. The Leapfrog Group, a coalition of large businesses frustrated by the rising cost and low quality in healthcare, proposed a series of initiatives designed to make major improvements (Birkmeyer et al., 2000; Lovern, 2002; Morrissey, 2003). One of the Leapfrog requirements was to have a specially trained intensivist for every intensive care unit.

2.2 Contemporary trends in critical care

Some trends in the use and delivery of critical care appear to have a potential impact on design. New design concepts may develop out of the issues these trends are raising.

Demographic imperative

The population cohort about to enter the age of higher levels of healthcare utilization is enormous. The leading edge of the so-called Baby Boom generation in the United States is just turning

60 and prepared to become voracious users of healthcare services, including critical care (Lumsdon, 1993). This new cohort of the elderly is likely to live somewhat longer than their predecessors, potentially increasing the period in which they will consume a disproportionate percentage of healthcare resources. Increased demand for healthcare, including critical care, is predictable.

Changes in mortality and morbidity

The patients who survive a critical care experience today, in many cases would not have survived in the past. Medical advances have made it possible to treat conditions that would have been fatal (Schwartz, 2000). These advances mean that more and sicker elderly patients will be able to be treated in the future. More and sicker patients will mean more beds and units, and this will mean designs for higher acuities.

Shortage of skilled healthcare workers

There is a significant shortage of trained critical care nurses, pharmacists, respiratory technicians, and specialty-trained intensivists in the United States (Pittman, 2006). Conditions are equally dire in most other countries.

The persistent shortage of trained professionals in healthcare will have an impact on facility design as the need for efficiency and labor savings increases. Designs to help the staff be more efficient, and to reduce the effort required to deliver care, will be preferred.

Intensivist-led teams

There is a trend toward care delivery in the form of interdisciplinary teams led by a specialty-trained intensivist (Rainey, 2000). The intensivist, or some other dedicated physician, is expected to devote all of their time and practice to the critical care service. In the past, the physician directing the care of the patient may have been one of several attending physicians who care for critical patients along with their other obligations.

The full-time physician presence on the unit, and this change in the delivery model, has implications for the design of units. Consideration for office and on-call space increases, and the likelihood of more rapid intervention may reduce the typical patient's length of stay. These physician intensivists are more likely to demand access to point-of-care testing and satellite services for their units.

All is not rosy, however. At the present time, there are not sufficient numbers of intensivists to serve every hospital that has a critical care unit. Some organizations in which the attending physicians resent the potential loss of control over their patients have resisted the change to an intensivist model.

Virtual ICU

The concept of remote electronic monitoring to provide 24-hour support of physician intensivists and specialty certified critical care nurses is spreading from a few entrepreneurial experiments to broad adoption within major healthcare systems (Field & Grigsby, 2002; Leong, Sirio, & Rotondi, 2005). The physical design implications of this innovative model have not yet been fully explored. The early versions employ a camera in the room, sufficiently powerful to show facial color and detail, along with a control center from which multiple rooms, units, or hospital locations can be monitored. The highly trained staff in the control room can monitor many more patients electronically than they would be able to cover by live rounding. The control center staff is able to advise the staff at the bedside in real time. Early adopters, such as the Sentara system in Virginia, have had excellent results and the concept of the e-ICU has spread to other systems, such as the Memorial Hermann Healthcare System in the Houston area, and the Intermountain Health Care system based in Utah.

Leveraging critical care resources via optimal design

Erkan Hassan, Pharm. D., FCCM

The current critical care landscape depicts a care delivery model of limited resources to meet the needs of an ever growing population of patients with increasing illness severity. This current scenario is expected to continue for the foreseeable future. As various methods of healthcare overhaul are discussed and debated, an often overlooked approach is to consider the redistribution of limited resources via creative design and technology. Redesign of the care of the critically ill patient has recently been reported in the form of an extra layer of care via a physically remote location with clinicians and staff. The electronic ICU or e-ICU is a proven, innovative design which uses technology to leverage limited critical care clinicians. Recent results indicate a statistically significant reduction in mortality by 30–50%, decreased length of stay as well as decreased morbidity. Although the e-ICU consists of hardware and software, the megabytes and pixels are not what make this concept work. Rather, the technology is the tool used in the redesign in the care delivery model.

Distance from the patient care site is not a consideration. Currently, remote sites range from being physically on campus to being in a different state and even continent. The future may have to account for services provided during part of the day at one remote facility and at another facility (potentially in another time zone or country) at other times of the day. Also consider remote services provided by nursing, medical, pharmacy, case management, etc., each provided at different facilities.

The initial consideration in designing the remote physical environment is the selection of a site with an adequate amount of space. Currently, e-ICUs monitor and manage up to approximately 500 patients. Therefore, site selection should account for the current and future number of workstations necessary to support the desired staffing model. Keep in mind that a critically ill patient is not defined by a geographic location, therefore future expansion of beds is not necessarily limited to ICU beds. The emergency department, pediatrics, Ob-Gyn patients, stroke patients, step down, operating room and medical/surgical floors may all provide locations to expand remote services.

Based on the volume of patients to be monitored by the e-ICU, the approach to patient management has to shift from one at a time specific patient management to population-based individual selected patient management. Therefore, the tools used in the e-ICU may be vastly different than at the bedside. Population-based patient management requires knowledge and application of best practices to a large number of patients. This is best accomplished with various decision support tools. Although these tools will vary, their primary purpose is to evaluate and prioritize patients requiring attention.

The technology components making remote monitoring and management possible are critical in the design consideration process. A high quality audio-video system (camera, video, speaker system) achieves several goals:

a. Two-way video capability.
b. Remote providers may see and/or interact with patient, family, bedside clinicians, medical equipment.

c. Either the remote or bedside team should be able to initiate contact.
d. Privacy indicators to the remote team for times when entering the patient's room is not desired.
e. Technological systems should be able to accommodate remote care providers to observe breathing patterns, read mechanical device settings (i.e., infusion pumps, mechanical ventilators, etc.) and be expandable for additional equipment such as electronic remote stethoscopes, etc.

Such remote networks involve both local and wide area networks. These networks are necessary to ensure seamless and secure transmission of clinical data, and require adequate bandwidth, data encryption and strict security measures as well as redundancy. Since the program consists of two-way video into each patient's room, the designer needs to be cognizant of the view of the remote facility from the patient's perspective. An uncluttered, clean, organized view is optimal. In addition, keeping any patient identifier information from view via the patient's room around and behind the remote clinician is important.

Within the clinical setting, a complete separate system connected to the remote center should also be considered. This private location can be used for times when the remote and bedside teams need to discuss clinical issues without the presence of the patient. In addition, this additional site can be used for private rounds as well as family conferences.

One of the primary concerns with the design of the onsite bedside facility is interoperability. Currently, two, three or more different systems/components are used at the bedside in the care of ICU patients. These various devices are not able to easily communicate with each other. Adding additional tasks, such as multiple sign-ins, double documentation, etc., to already busy bedside clinicians is not an acceptable solution. The interoperability of these various devices/applications is paramount now and in the future as technology grows.

The remote team must have access to all relevant patient data, laboratory results, medications, progress notes and bedside flowsheet documentation in order to provide a complete, current clinical status of every patient. With this information, the remote team can help ensure the consistent and timely attainment of the therapeutic plan established by the bedside clinicians by monitoring the patient's progress, titrating therapies when necessary and identifying emerging problems. In order to attain these goals, communication to and from all members of the care team must be easily facilitated. In addition, the actual division of responsibilities between onsite and remote team members must be established. Issues to consider include:

a. Do personnel and/or equipment require some type of permanent tracking (i.e., radiofrequency device monitoring) so resources can be allocated as appropriate in the most efficient manner?
b. Effective communication between all necessary members of the multi-professional critical care team and the remote site.
c. Optimal location of onsite workstations (i.e., each patient room vs. a smaller number of access/workstations throughout the ICU).
d. As more health systems move toward the concept of universal beds and rapid response teams to floor patients, how will these teams interact with the remote team (mobile vs. fixed units)?

As health systems need to leverage limited resources, the use of remote site clinicians will continue to experiment with novel approaches to optimally evolve clinicians and technology to improve financial and clinical outcomes.

Erkan Hassan is the Director of Pharmacotherapy for the VISICU telemedicine corporation.

Decentralized nursing

The ability to use electronic documentation has encouraged the decentralization of nursing and caregiver functions closer to the bedside, usually associated with one or two patient beds rather than at a central "nurses' station". This change in practice suggests a change in the design of the central station, and the need to design multiple effective satellite positions in appropriate locations.

One reoccurring design is for a charting station to be located on the corridor wall outside a pair of rooms. An ideal version of this configuration has the person at the position looking at the head and face of the patient on the opposite wall. In some versions the beds are back-to-back on a common wall in front of the charting position, offering a view to the side of the patient's head.

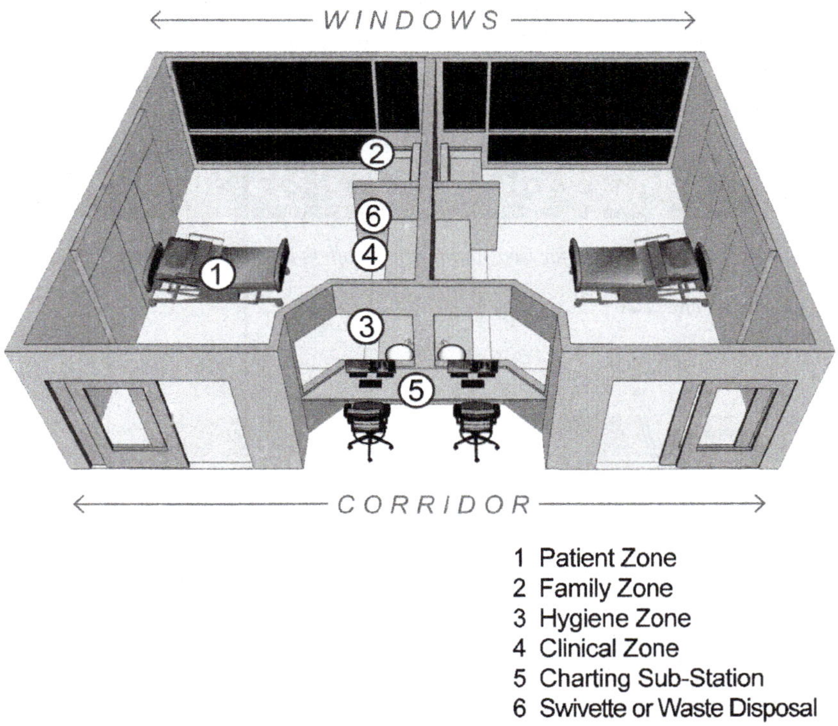

Figure 2.1: *Patient bed perpendicular to corridor*
Architect: WHR Architects
Drawing: Elizabeth Viets

As the trend to decentralize caregiving continues, designers are faced with questions about the location of medications, supplies, and equipment. If medication remains centralized, for example, much of the benefit of decentralization and reduced travel distance can be lost. Other relevant issues include the important need for socialization and mentorship of inexperienced staff that tend to feel isolated in decentralized positions. What seems to be needed is a model which simultaneously moves the caregiver and required supplies closer to the bedside, and offers the centralized social and professional support of a common interdisciplinary team.

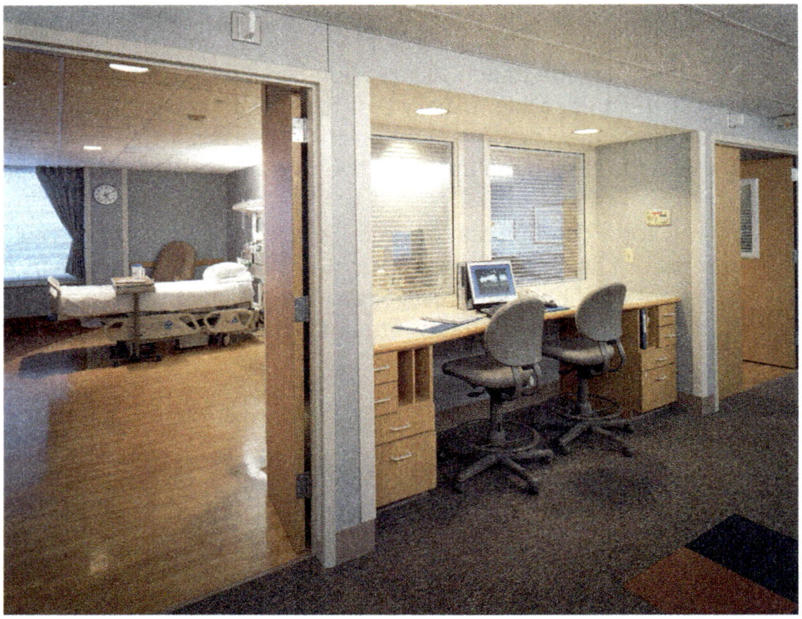

Figure 2.2: *A decentralized position sized for two staff members offers a side view of the patient's head; note the storage drawers and integral blinds*
Location: Methodist Omaha Hospital
Architect: HDR
Photo credit: Tom Kessler

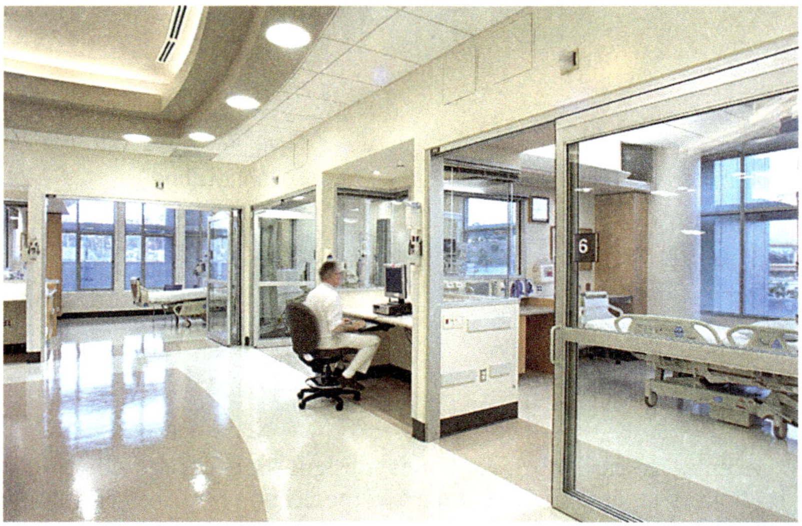

Figure 2.3: *Decentralized positions provide direct observation of two rooms; note privacy can be achieved with the blinds located inside the patient's room*
Location: Grossmont
Architect: Design Partnership
Photo credit: Dennis Sullivan

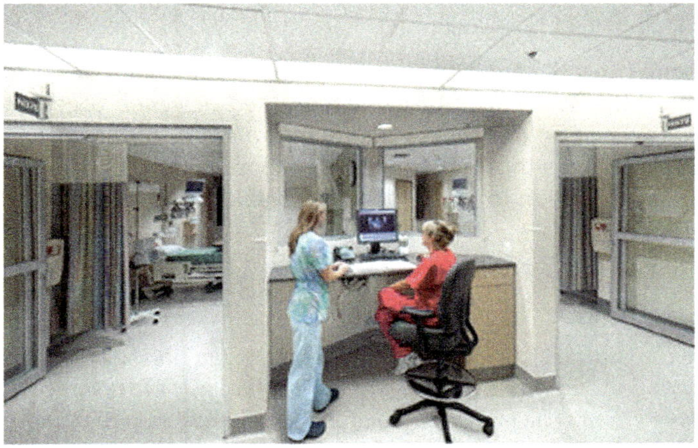

Figure 2.4: *Note the stand-up height of this decentralized position and the stool height seating*
Location: Boswell Memorial Hospital ICU, nurses station
Architect: Orcutt/Winslow
Photo Credit: Al Payne

Proliferation of electronic media

Critical care units were among the first to embrace the use of computerized physiologic monitors, computerized medical records, electronic reporting of lab results, reading of digital diagnostic images, decision support software, and access to the Internet for inquiry. The use of automated, digital, and computerized systems in the ICU will only increase.

Physicians who work in the critical care arena are generally computer savvy, but many of today's healthcare workers were originally trained without computers. We are witnessing the transition from "people of the book" to "people of the screen" as the next generation of healthcare workers is totally at home in the world of computers.

Ultimately, when the transition to electronic record keeping is complete, a problem arises whenever the system is down and the staff must revert to the now unfamiliar model of manual record entry. This is when the productivity increases resulting from computerization become obvious. Doing the same work manually is not possible in the same span of time.

Miniaturization of equipment

The continuing direction of size reduction in medical devices is making it possible to bring more technology onto the critical care unit, and into the patient room. This trend is permitting more portable equipment to be brought to the bedside, and fuelling advances in point-of-care testing. Further advances are expected in the integrated technologies that will be used with beds and monitoring devices.

Evidence-based medicine

The early 1990s marked a period in which the concept of evidence-based medicine was described. Sackett and his colleagues (1996) have defined evidence-based medicine as "the conscientious, explicit and judicious use of current best evidence in making decisions about the care of individual patients." The evolution of this trend has resulted in studies based in critical care and produced clinical pathways.

Evidence-based design

A parallel development in healthcare architecture has been the analogous evolution of evidence-based design. Hamilton has said that "*An evidence-based designer, together with an informed client, makes decisions based on the best available information from research and project evaluations*" (2003, p.20). It appears that some are finding positive results (Cassidy, 2003). This book is intended to make a contribution to the evidence available in the healthcare design literature.

An evidence-based approach to design for critical care

Peter J. Pronovost, M. D., Ph.D.

In the intensive care unit (ICU), form drives function. If the closest sink is halfway down the unit from the patient's bed and a central-line insertion is needed, the distance traveled adds time to prepare for this insertion. The probability that a clinician will skip washing their hands increases exponentially if the line insertion is needed in an emergency. Timeliness and sterile care are both recommended practices, and the mechanisms to achieve both in this case are closely linked.

I have learned through clinical and research experiences over the last decade that architecture (e.g., placement of sinks and oxygen) influences system performance, and ultimately clinical outcomes. My colleagues and I routinely train healthcare professionals from various disciplines about the science of safety. The learning objectives of this training are to: a) understand that safety is dependent on the system in which we work, b) understand the basic principles of a safe system design (standardize work, create independent checklists for key processes, and learn from mistakes) and recognize that these principles apply to technical and team work, and c) understand that teams make wise decisions when there is diverse and independent input.

Interdisciplinary daily patient rounds and a daily goals checklist are examples of redesigning systems to be safer. The goals checklist is completed during rounds to clarify the plan of care for each patient and to discuss any safety concerns that a nurse or other staff member may have for the day. Interdisciplinary rounds bring together the collective wisdom of staff from different clinical disciplines, levels of training, and even cultural backgrounds to discuss the best care plan for the patient. Both of these examples were initially implemented as quality improvement interventions. They have created more reliable and safer systems of care, and improved communication, collaboration, safety culture and quality in hundreds of ICUs.

Using science to redesign broken systems is one method to improve the architecture of critical care. Another way would be to develop a blueprint of the ideal ICU design that facilitates quality performance and safe care, such as installing sinks outside every patient room to increase hand-washing compliance. However, there remain many unanswered questions about the ideal ICU design, and it may be that architecture is relative to the local unit and healthcare professionals. Some guiding principles to follow are best described by the Institute of Medicine's Crossing the Quality Chasm *report (2001), which states that care should be safe, effective, efficient, patient-centered, timely, and equitable. In the end, the wisdom of those working on the front lines will be invaluable when redesigning the physical space and processes of care in a clinical area.*

This book provides state-of-the-art evidence and a research agenda for the safe design of critical care. It offers up-to-date science coupled with practical solutions, and will be a guidebook for those building or designing ICUs.

Peter J. Pronovost, M.D., Ph.D. is a practicing anesthesiologist and critical care physician at Johns Hopkins, and is on the faculty of the Institute for Healthcare Improvement.

Patient and family-centered care

Since the 1980s healthcare has been influenced by a growing realization that physician-centric hospitals might offer more attention to the needs of patients and their families. Consumer organizations like the Planetree organization have influenced major change in the philosophy of care, policies, procedures, space, and furnishings of hospitals (Orr, 1992; Frampton, Gilpin, & Charmel, 2003). It seems likely that critical care units will be influenced in this direction as well.

Family presence in a crisis

There has been a trend in emergency departments and intensive care units to allow the family to be present during a resuscitation attempt or other aggressive clinical intervention. Studies have shown that families respond with greater understanding of the staff's attempts to care for their loved one, and are less likely to sue the organization or individuals involved (Snoby, 2005; Spittler, 2006).

The space required to safely and comfortably accommodate family members has not always been included in critical care designs. Most units still ask families to leave during a code situation, and there is rarely room for anyone other than the code team in rooms that were never designed to accommodate the family, much less the proliferation of equipment.

A design that respected the role of family members during a crisis would have space allocated to family use that would not intrude on the activity of a code team working around the patient. At a meeting of the Institute for Family-Centered Care a nurse told the following story about a pediatric ICU which had a fairly generous visitation policy but asked family members to leave during a crisis or a code blue intervention. A young girl was in a precarious state and members of the family had been in nearly constant attendance. When the arrest occurred, by chance the grandmother was the only family member in the room, the parents having taken a short break to go home to shower and change clothes. As was the custom, the code team asked her to leave, but she stayed. As the team desperately worked on the child, she sat out of the way and quietly sang *Amazing Grace*. The child did not survive. The grandmother thanked the team for their heroic effort, apologized for not following instructions, and said, "I just thought that when someone was dying, they should know they were loved". The next day, when the story made the rounds of the rest of the unit staff, the policy was changed to allow families to remain in the room in a crisis.

Other ideas

Designers and their healthcare professional clients should be alert for other potential trends that will influence the delivery of critical care, and thus should be accounted for in the facility design. Productive ideas can be inspired by observations from other fields or industries.

2.3 North American case studies

There is benefit to the study of facilities that can serve as examples, in whole or in part, positive or negative. When planning new facilities, tours of other comparable facilities offer the opportunity to observe new design ideas in a real setting and the chance to talk with staff members who work there every day. An often overlooked benefit of such tours is the opportunity to find things that should not be repeated.

It should be easy to say that there is no single "perfect" design for a critical care unit. There are far too many unique situations for any one design to be universally suited to any condition. At the same time, the force of continuous change means that designs once well suited to their purpose may no longer perform at optimum levels. Most architects will say they have yet to accomplish their best work, and any critical care staff member could suggest improvements to the best of designs.

The following case studies are offered in the hope that readers may see several different ways to arrive at design success.

Medical ICU, The Methodist Hospital, Houston, Texas (Architect: WHR)

The Medical ICU at The Methodist Hospital features all private rooms in renovated space. The patient rooms feature a prototype of a dual power column life support system in which power columns with very narrow profiles are placed on either side of the patient's head. The rooms are spartan with an upholstered bench at the window for families. The corridors utilize vinyl floor covering in attractive patterns.

Decentralized documentation stations occur outside pairs of patient rooms, and there are substations for nursing for clusters of six rooms. What is unexpected is that the central station on the unit has no observation of the patient rooms, and serves for greeting and unit clerical functions. Caregiving is truly decentralized.

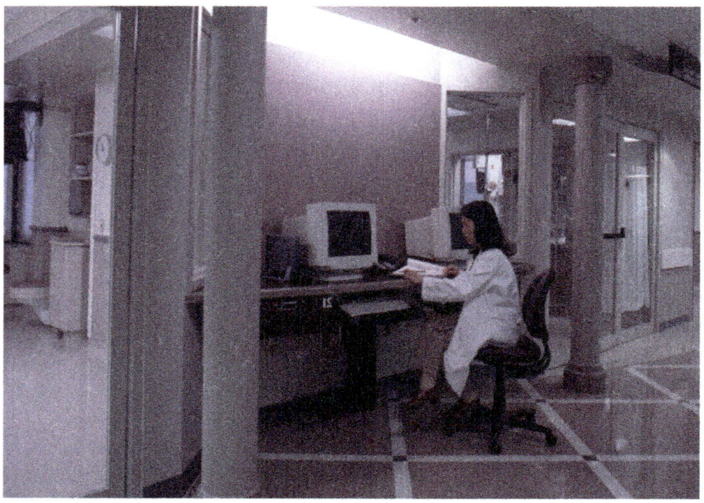

Figure 2.5: *The staff workspace occurs in the corridor between pairs of rooms*
Location: Methodist MICU
Architect: WHR Architects
Photo credit: Debra Burge

Planetree ICU, Griffin Hospital, Derby, Connecticut (Architect: SLAM Collaborative)

This design features the extraordinary use of a full external perimeter corridor for family and visitor access. Patients get "borrowed light" through a glass block to the exterior corridor and in turn from windows on the exterior wall of the corridor. The carpeted internal corridor is dedicated to staff use and is very quiet. Staff support, utility, and supply functions are located on another central "off-stage" corridor providing an uncluttered appearance.

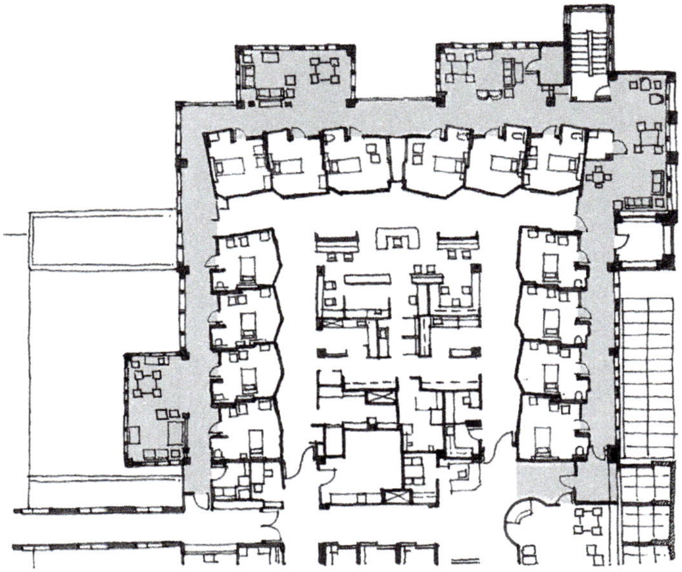

Figure 2.6: *Planetree Derby floor plan, Griffin Hospital, Derby, CT*
Architect: SLAM Cooperative
Illustration: Diana Anderson

The private patient rooms feature a full floor to ceiling glass wall facing the staff corridor. There is a headwall life support system and a moderately sized room. The design is simple and features the accents of light colored wood. There are accordion doors for the patient toilets which provide wide and accessible openings for assisted patient access.

The central station for staff observes the rooms in a horseshoe configuration. Task lighting at the central workstation is effective. The glass walls at the patient rooms are angled slightly to reduce glare and provide some visual relief along the corridor.

Meiklejohn Critical Care Pavilion, Saddleback Medical Center, Laguna Hills, CA (Architect: TAYLOR)

Consideration for dignity and the human spirit were key factors for the designers. The modernization and expansion project features natural daylighting and an open operational arena. Use of clerestory/skylights over the main caregiver workstation spills natural daylight into the open arena and patient rooms, benefiting patients, patient families, and, equally important, the caregivers. Decentralized nursing workstations are positioned with direct views into pairs of patient rooms to optimize clinical observation. An exterior patio provides the caregiver an opportunity to

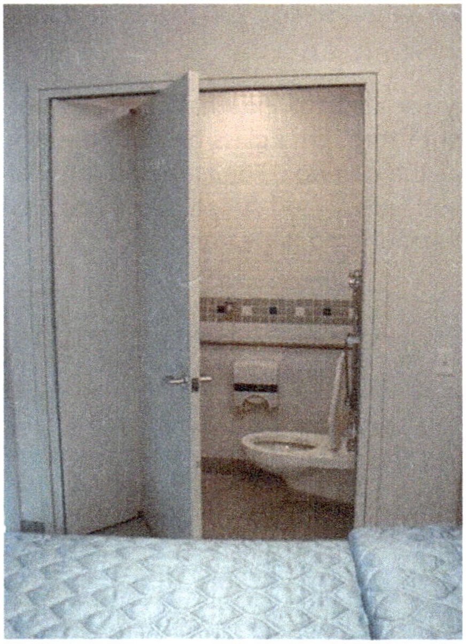

Figure 2.7: *Folding toilet door creates wide opening*
Location: Griffin Hospital, Derby, CT
Photo: Kirk Hamilton

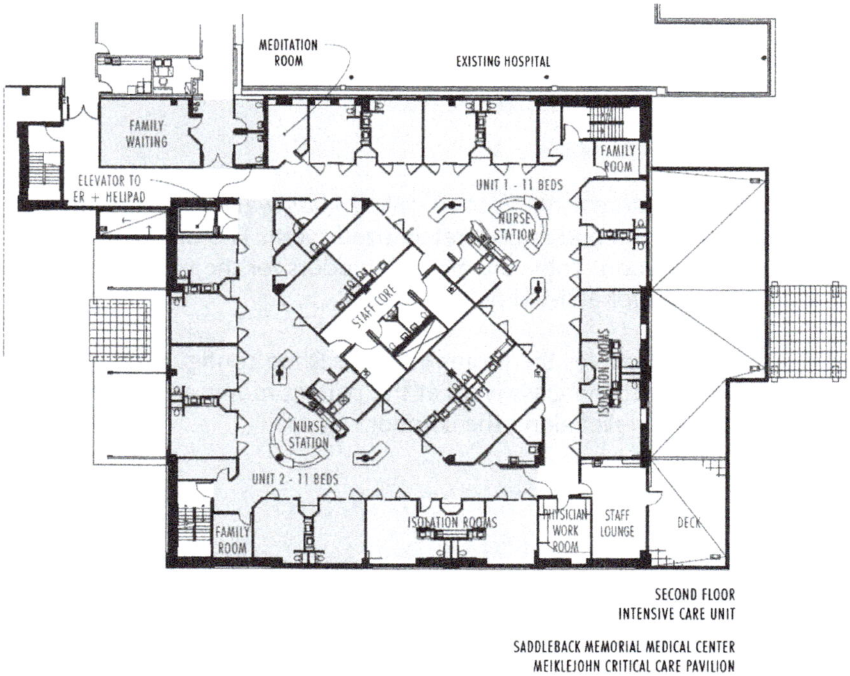

Figure 2.8: *Second floor, intensive care unit, Laguna Hills, CA*
Location: Meiklejohn Critical Care Pavilion, Saddleback Memorial Medical Center
Architect: TAYLOR and Questar Construction

regenerate while off stage and outdoors. This feature has become significant for recruiting and retention. The design gives family members comfortable access and accommodations within the patient room, all of which are private. The rooms feature headwall life support systems.

Saperstein Critical Care Tower, Cedars-Sinai Medical Center, Los Angeles, CA (Architect: Langdon Wilson)

The new Saperstein Critical Care Tower features a group of intensive care and stepdown units arranged on similarly designed floors. The unit is composed entirely of private rooms designed with the concept of standardization as a means of reducing error and confusion. The patient room is in every case precisely identical, a "same handed" orientation rather than the more common back-to-back designs to reduce plumbing cost. In fact, the head of the bed is positioned towards the exterior wall, so observation from the corridor and staff positions is ideal, but there is glare from the window behind the patient.

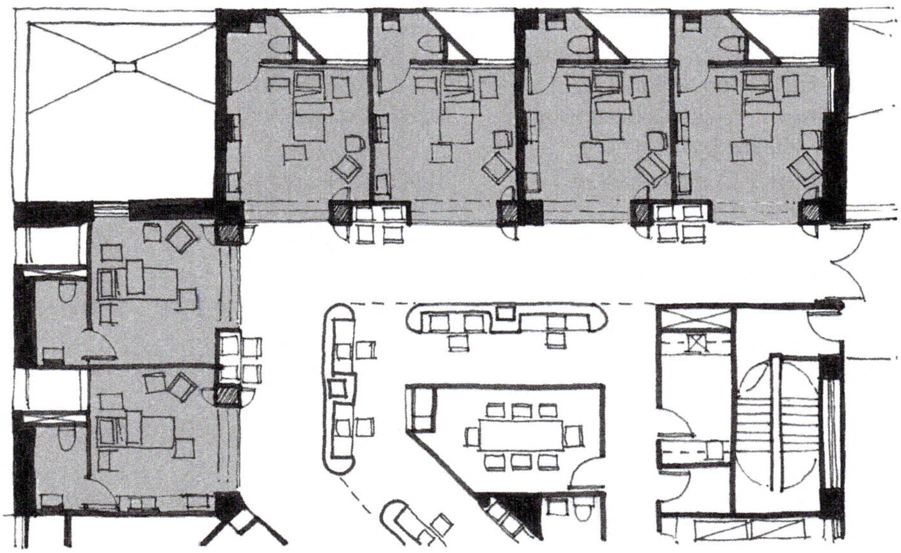

Figure 2.9: *Same-handed rooms are identical*
Location: Saperstein Tower, Cedars-Sinai, Los Angeles, CA
Illustration: Diana Anderson

Lessons learned from 16 years of SCCM design awards

Charles D. Cadenhead, FAIA, FACHA

Diana C. Anderson, M.D., LEED® AP

Robert G. Uhlenhake, AIA, ACHA, LEED® AP

In 1992, the Society of Critical Care Medicine (SCCM), with the American Association of Critical Care Nurses (AACN) and the American Institute of Architects/Academy of Architecture for Health (AIA/AAH), held the first SCCM ICU Design Competition. In February 2009, at the SCCM Annual Congress, this unique design competition presented awards to the medical director and architect of the 16th design winning ICUs. Each of the sponsoring organizations, composed of physicians, nurses and architects, is represented in judging competition entries, leading to selections judged from multi-professional perspectives. Over the history of the design competition, an impressive array of ICUs have been identified, all with varying attributes. The richness of information and best-practice examples that these winning designs offer encouraged us to look at the similarities and differences between them.

Our hope in sharing this growing body of knowledge is that the quality of critical care facilities will continue to improve, leading to improved patient outcomes and better places for people to work. This analysis presents 13 of the best-practice adult ICUs designed between 1992 and 2009. Each of these units is a winning entry from the SCCM Design Competition and together they constitute some of the best examples for critical care design within the United States and Canada. Although a number of Neonatal (NICU) and Pediatric (PICU) units have won the SCCM design award over the years, only the 13 adult facilities are included in this analysis.

The following table lists the units referenced.

	Year	*SCCM Citation Winners*	*Type of Critical Care Unit*	*Beds*	*Construction Type*
1	1992	The Swedish Medical Center Englewood, Colorado	CCU/Multidisciplinary	32	New Construction
2	1993	East Jefferson General Hospital Metairie, Louisiana	Medical/Surgical	20	New Construction
3	1996	Legacy Good Samaritan Portland, Oregon	Multidisciplinary	28	Remodel Addition
4	1997	Southeast Missouri Hospital Cape Girardeau, Missouri	Cardiothoracic Surgery	12	New Construction
5	1998	Loyola University Medical Center Maywood, Illinois	Burn/Trauma	21	Renovation
6	2000	Clarian Health Group Methodist Hospital Indianapolis, Indiana	CCU/Cardiovascular Medical	56	New Construction
7	2001	St. Joseph's Health Center Kansas City, Missouri	Med/Surg/ Cardiovascular	16	New Construction
8	2003	Harris Methodist Fort Worth Hospital Fort Worth, Texas	Multidisciplinary	20	New Construction
9	2003	McGill University Health Center Montreal, Quebec, Canada	Surg/Med/ Cardiovascular/Trauma	26	Renovation
10	2005	The Queen's Medical Center Honolulu, Hawaii	Cardiac & Thoracic	40	Renovation
11	2006	Sharp Grossmont Hospital La Mesa, California	Adult Medical/Surgical	24	New Construction
12	2008	Emory University Hospital Atlanta, Georgia	Neurology/ Neurosurgical	20	New Construction
13	2009	Memorial Sloan-Kettering Cancer Center New York, New York	Adult Medical/Surgical	20	Renovation

Lessons learned: eight critical care design trends identified

(1) *The family zone*

Several of the winning designs have completely re-evaluated the patient room to incorporate designated family space, thereby including families as an integral part of the healing process and central to the entire unit's functioning. Perhaps the most distinctive unit in this category is the

2008 winner, Emory University Hospital's Neurosciences ICU. This unit is unique in its allocation of 115 square feet of space for a family zone within the patient room, separated by a glass block partition complete with a closable door allowing natural light to penetrate through the family room into the patient zone. This "adjacent studio apartment" acts as a private place for respite just steps away from the patient room. The patient room size, including this family space, is over 350 square feet. Interestingly, 18% of the unit's departmental gross square footage (DGSF) is dedicated to family space in this ICU, including each family zone within the patient rooms, waiting areas, lounge and amenities such as a kitchen, showers, and laundry facilities. Similarly, the 2000 winning design, the cardiac unit at Clarian Health System's Methodist Hospital in Indiana, incorporates a similar family zone as an alcove within the patient room plan, located towards the exterior wall with no physical divider. In conjunction with the design trend of considering family needs, the field of clinical medicine has been moving towards a greater understanding of the importance of patient autonomy and family involvement in the care process.

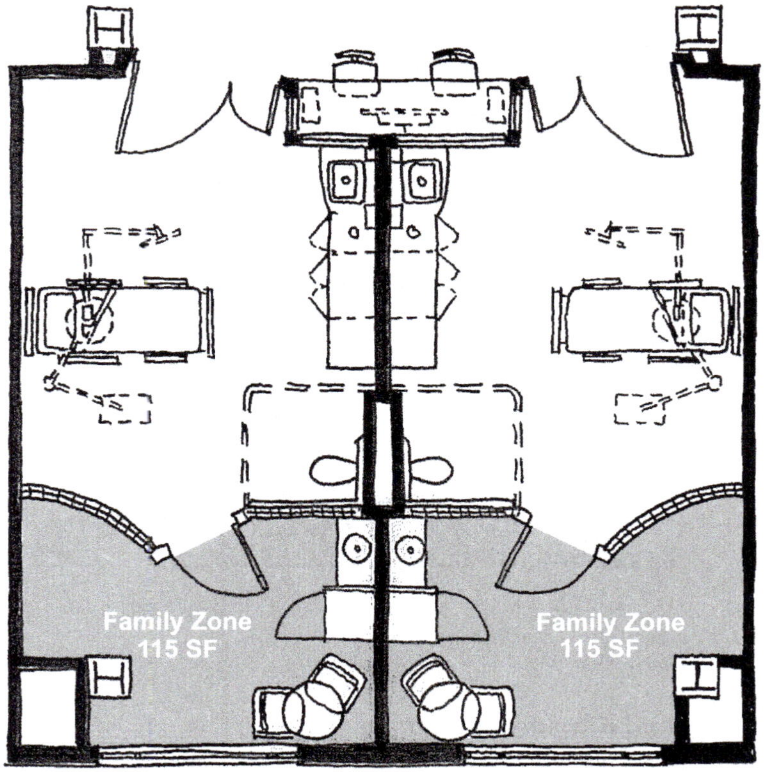

Exemplary Case: Emory University Hospital, Neurosciences ICU, Atlanta, Georgia, 2009 winner. Each patient room incorporates a family zone separated by a glass block partition
Illustration Credit: Diana Anderson

(2) *Design for interdisciplinary teams*

Interestingly, all ICUs surveyed for this study had some form of decentralized charting space with none employing exclusively centralized nursing positions for patient care support. The 1992 design for the Swedish Medical Center ICU allocates space for four central stations, each serving an eight-bed pod, but at the same time incorporating computer charting terminals inside each patient room. Both the 2001 St. Joseph's Health Center and the 2005 Queen's Medical Center winners are unique to the group in that they eliminate the central nursing station altogether to become a completely decentralized unit, each stating in their narratives the main reason for this design shift being noise control. Although nursing support areas do not appear to have grown in overall area over the last two decades, the notion of decentralization is seen throughout by way of charting stations within patient rooms or within corridors looking into single or pairs of patient rooms. Proximity of caregivers to the patient for reasons of patient safety and decreased walking distance, in addition to high nurse/patient ratios have likely contributed to the shift of documentation to closer to the bedside. It remains to be seen whether pure decentralization will be utilized in future designs or whether a hybrid model will continue, perhaps indicating the value of communication and socialization between caregivers.

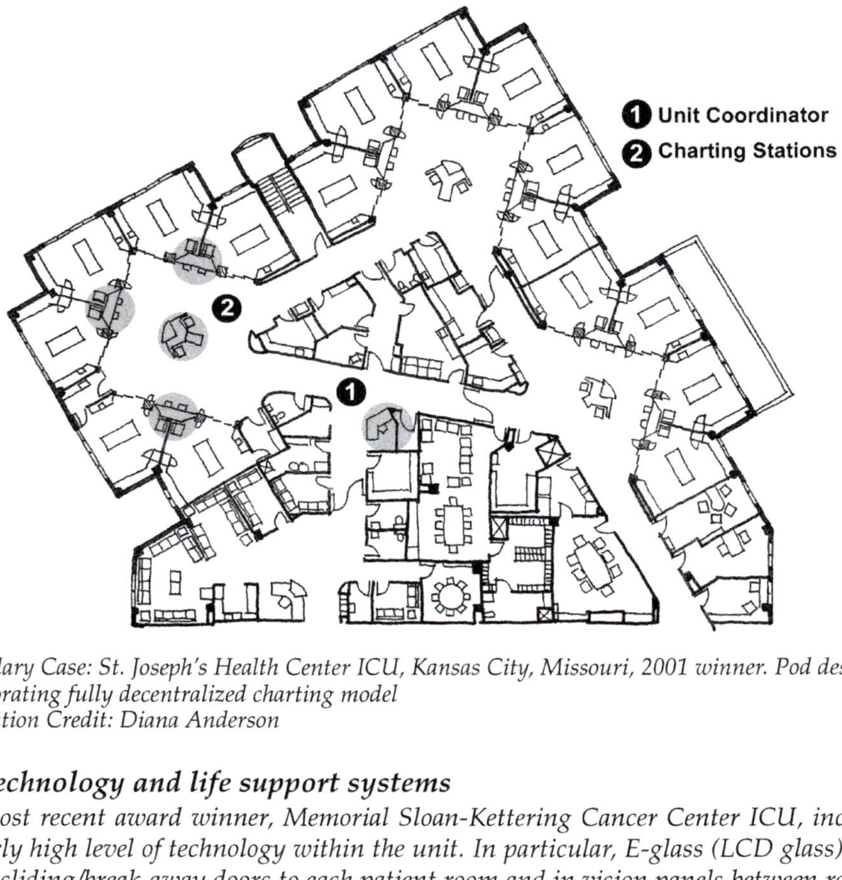

Exemplary Case: St. Joseph's Health Center ICU, Kansas City, Missouri, 2001 winner. Pod design incorporating fully decentralized charting model
Illustration Credit: Diana Anderson

(3) *Technology and life support systems*

The most recent award winner, Memorial Sloan-Kettering Cancer Center ICU, includes a particularly high level of technology within the unit. In particular, E-glass (LCD glass) is employed for all sliding/break-away doors to each patient room and in vision panels between rooms, changing from transparent to opaque at the flick of a switch, allowing for instant privacy. Other high-tech devices include web cameras enabling staff to observe patients from other locations, and specifically from a conference center adjacent to the unit equipped with multimedia technologies and multiple high definition projection screens, enhancing review of patient data and teaching though simultaneous display of historical and real-time images, including the patient, lab reports, hospital Electronic Medical Record (EMR) and bedside monitors and ventilators. Each patient room is equipped with a laboratory label printer that facilitates immediate and proper labeling of specimens while the unit is outfitted with wireless systems integrated into web-based applications enhancing patient care and safety. Evolution in monitoring technology, now allowing centralized monitoring of any patient anywhere, as seen at Memorial Sloan-Kettering Cancer Center, allows great flexibility in design. With healthcare moving towards the EMR, in addition to diagnostic and treatment modalities becoming more reliant on technological advances, it is likely this trend will continue with the incorporation of high-tech devices into the design of the physical environment.

Life support systems: headwalls versus power columns

The first winning design entry in 1992, the Swedish Medical Center, employed a fixed power column in their patient room design. The most recent winning design, Memorial Sloan-Kettering Cancer Center's ICU has provided twin ceiling booms in each patient room, allowing the bed to rotate in any direction, particularly toward the outside windows if the patient is medically stable, to be able to be turned to appreciate outside views. The choice for the twin booms in this project was also based on their goal of unimpeded access to the patient. For similar reasons, a single boom, double arm system is seen in the Legacy Good Samaritan Hospital's ICU allowing for flexibility in patient bed orientation, potentially providing patient views of the unit's large exterior plaza and roofscape located directly outside the patient rooms. The Emory University Hospital ICU also utilized ceiling booms for their flexibility by allowing access to the patient's head for airway and brain monitoring procedures and emergencies, particularly important in this neurological critical care setting.

Although about half of the projects (five) used fixed headwalls in their patient room designs, ceiling-mounted booms were installed in the majority (eight), and have appeared to replace headwalls and fixed columns in more recent years. In addition, the dual arm booms have added enormous flexibility by freeing the bed from the wall, efficiently integrating technology to deliver critical monitoring, telemetry, gases and IV pumps, and access to radiologic imaging. Current research demonstrates that booms have an advantage over headwalls in the case of high-acuity ICU patients, and when procedures are performed inside patient rooms. However, booms may not provide a proportionate level of advantage when compared with the additional cost involved in their procurement in the case of lower-acuity ICU patients, as well as when procedures are not typically conducted in the patient room (Pati et al., 2008).

(4) *The patient room*

The current sample of intensive care environments dates back almost two decades. At that time, the trends of private patient rooms and decentralized nursing stations appeared to be rapidly becoming the norm. This is further supported by the fact that no double occupancy rooms were noted in any of the adult units surveyed. Several of the more recent pediatric and neonatal ICU winning designs still appear to employ shared patient rooms in the event of siblings. Regarding patient room size, it appears that rooms have not been increasing in area. Patient room areas, including toilet facilities, range from 189 square feet in the 2003 McGill University Health Center renovation project to 353 square feet in the Emory University Hospital's unit which incorporates a substantial family zone in each patient room of about 115 square feet.

Toilet solutions

Concerning waste disposal systems and toilet rooms, often included in patient room square footage, all of the ICU patient rooms in the sample include either a modulav within the same room, or a toilet room directly accessible from the patient bed. Of the 13 projects, both Queen's Medical Center and Clarian Health Group's Methodist Hospital were found to have private enclosed toilet

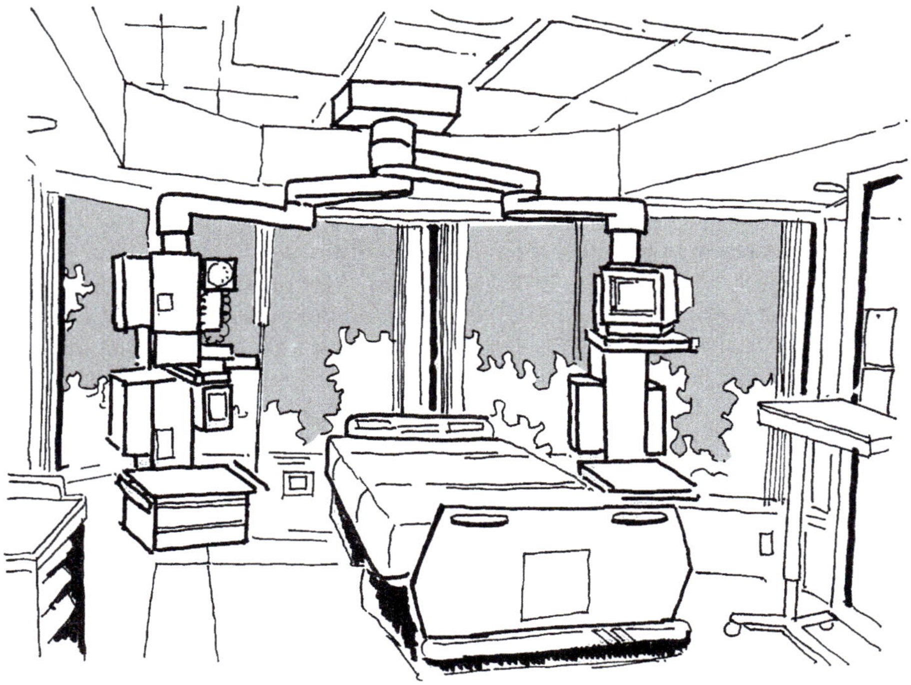

Exemplary Case: Legacy Good Samaritan Multidisciplinary ICU, Portland, Oregon, 1996 winner. Ceiling boom with twin arms allowing for flexibility in bed orientation and access to the patient
Illustration Credit: Diana Anderson

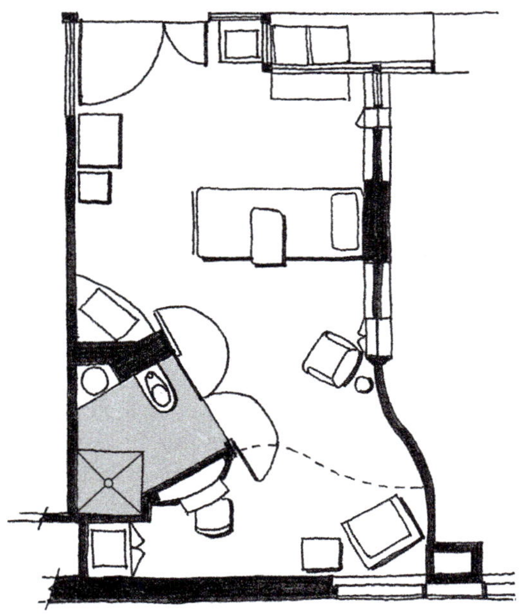

Exemplary Case: Clarian Health Group's Methodist Hospital Cardiac ICU,. Indianapolis, Indiana, 2000 winner. Single patient room with private toilet facility

rooms adjoining the patient room, while three others (Swedish Medical Center, Legacy Good Samaritan, and Loyola University Medical Center) have a combination of private and shared toilet rooms, with the remaining employing waste disposal systems adjacent to the bed space. No award winning facility built or renovated after 1998 has shared toilet rooms. The trend appears to be toward a dedicated toilet for each patient room, although there does not seem to be a preference for either modulav or an enclosed room for a toilet facility. The use of enclosed toilet rooms increases overall size and expense of unit construction, while not necessarily contributing to improved safety of the patient who needs routine assistance. Critically ill patients most often use bedpans or portable commodes, which are flushed at the toilet facility. Prevalence of modulavs in most of the recent projects may indicate juror regard for the enclosed room as a family convenience not necessary for patient care.

(5) *Proximity to diagnostic and treatment support*

An interesting trend noted across all units is the proximity to diagnostic and treatment support spaces. In attempting to further classify this tendency, it appears that elements of these diagnostic and treatment services are located either within the actual ICU, close to the unit on the same level, or connected vertically to a location directly above or below the unit by elevator. An example of vertical connection is the 1996 winner, Legacy Good Samaritan ICU, which has designated elevators for patient transport to angiography, surgery, radiology and emergency. The 1992 Swedish Medical Center ICU is located next to the cardiac catheterization suite and was placed strategically within the hospital to allow lateral access to the emergency room, operating room, recovery room, radiology, and laboratory. At the 2009 Memorial Sloan-Kettering Cancer Center, a hemodialysis suite is incorporated within the ICU providing round-the-clock access to renal technicians while at the same time providing two dialysis rooms with ICU surge capacity. The respiratory therapy suite is also located on the floor, serving both the ICU and the overall hospital. In addition, an MRI is situated down the hall from the unit. An integral part of Emory University Hospital's Neurosciences ICU design was the location of a CT scanner within the unit itself, located for convenient access to other services within the hospital without entering the ICU. This allows critically ill patients to conveniently undergo scanning as they are admitted to the ICU and throughout their stay, without the need for transport to the radiology department. Satellite pharmacies are also seen located near or in at least three of the winning units, with the Legacy Good Samaritan ICU having a centrally located satellite pharmacy and laboratory within the unit itself.

This trend of proximity to diagnostic and treatment facilities appears in numerous units in different forms, likely dependent on existing hospital spaces and services. Interestingly, although this decision of placing the diagnostic facilities within the ICU itself can sometimes mean fewer patient rooms for the purposes of space allocation, proximity to services has been chosen over patient rooms in several instances, indicating the importance of these spaces in the view of care providers. The possibility of including these supporting facilities may be a function of the ICU bed number, in part leading to larger units than would have been normally seen before.

(6) *Administrative and support spaces*

Space allocation for administrative areas within units appears to be on an upward trend, most notably in academic medical centers where teaching is an integral part of daily ICU activities. All units surveyed contain some amount of offices on the unit, at the very least one or two for the nurse manager and unit coordinator while others include a series of offices, conference and seminar rooms. This tendency is illustrated by the two most recent winning entries where a significant amount of unit area is given toward administrative and teaching functions.

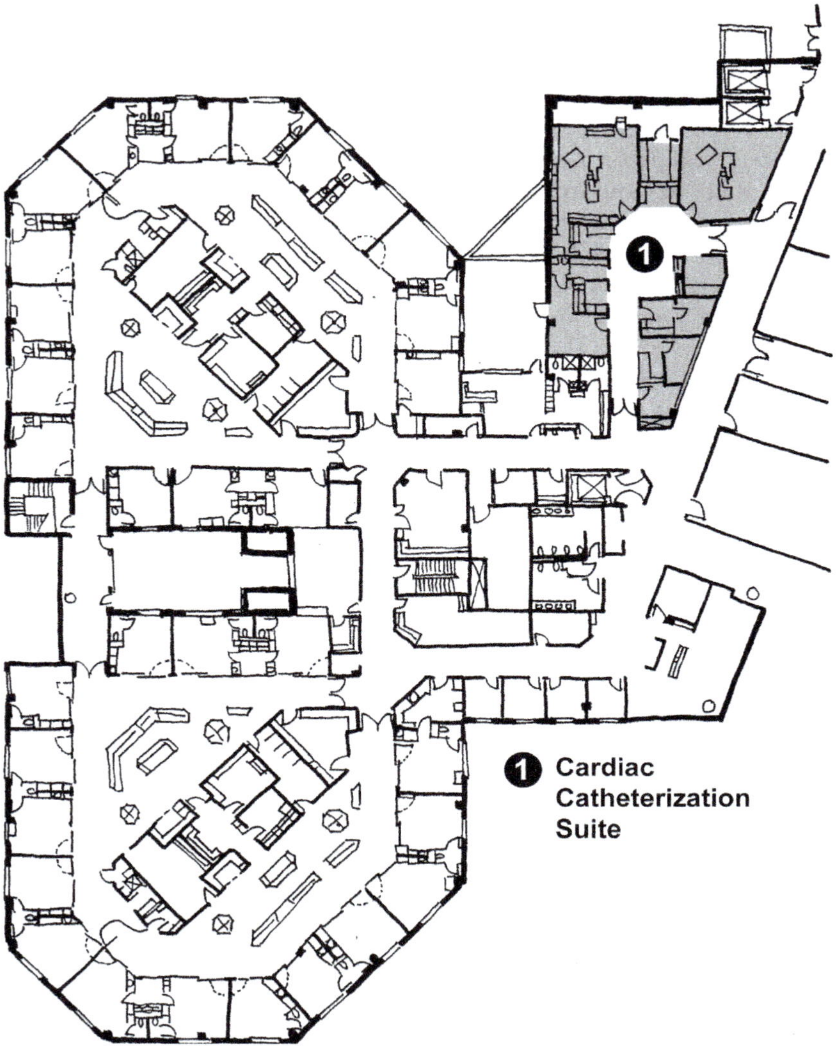

Exemplary Case: Swedish Medical Center ICU, Englewood, Colorado, 1992 winner. Proximity of ICU to cardiac catheterization suite
Illustration Credit: Diana Anderson

In the case of Emory University Hospital, 9% of the departmental gross square footage is dedicated space for this programmatic function, while at Memorial Sloan-Kettering Cancer Center's ICU, this percentage has increased to 14%. Furthermore, there appears to be a preference for staff meeting and education spaces located on the unit itself if this is at all feasible. The team at Emory University Hospital felt that locating these meeting spaces within the ICU was crucial to the success of their unit's functioning, preferring these spaces over additional patient rooms. At Memorial Sloan-Kettering Cancer Center a research lab was relocated to the administrative suite to be located adjacent to the bed unit. Conference rooms incorporating advanced technology to allow for remote patient care planning through the use of cameras or robots are being seen in recent years. It is likely we will observe a continuing trend of administrative and education space incorporated into the designs of critical care environments, especially teaching facilities, given the importance placed on proximity and flexibility of these spaces with patient care areas.

Regarding staff support spaces, there appears to be an increased emphasis on stress-relieving spaces for staff incorporating a connection to nature, where clinicians can go for respite during work hours. Memorial Sloan-Kettering Cancer Center's in-unit ICU staff lounge was designed to reduce staff stress through its surrounding large windows with river and city views. The Queen's Medical Center in Honolulu, Hawaii, located a central staff lounge for views to the ocean and maintained three lanais, or outdoor patios, for both staff and family access and benefit. Staff lounge spaces with lockers and staff toilets are provided within all units, with five (Queen's Medical Center, Sharp Grossmont Hospital, Swedish Medical Center, McGill University Health Center and Legacy Good Samaritan Hospital) providing an exterior courtyard or terrace for staff access. On-call suites with sleep rooms and shower facilities located on the unit itself are seen in the majority (eight) of the ICUs surveyed, with several locating the overnight facilities just outside the unit for easy access.

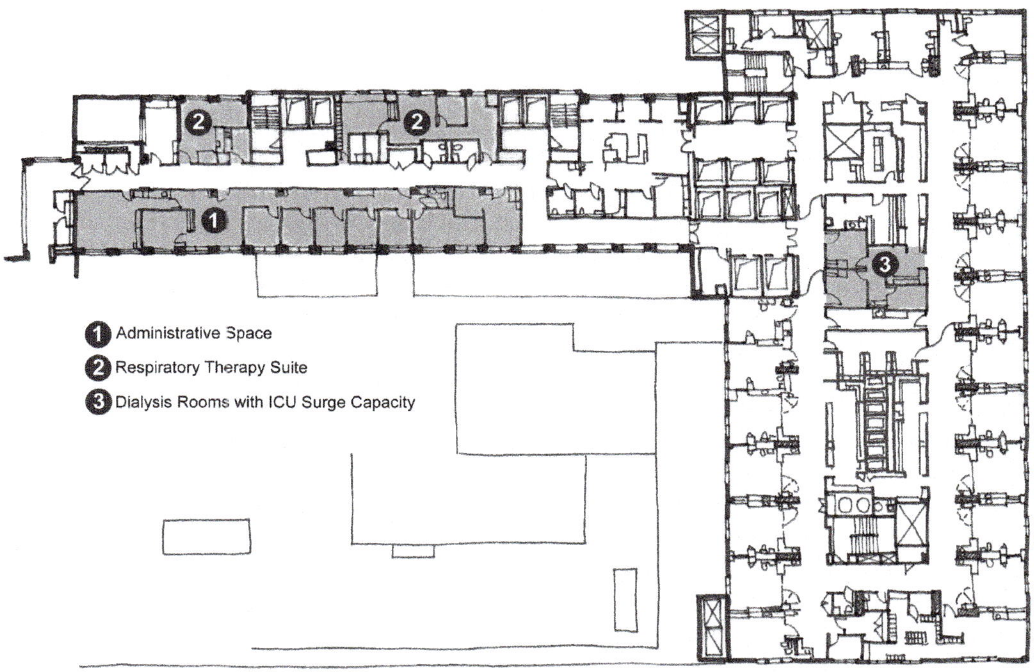

Exemplary Case: Memorial Sloan Kettering ICU, New York, New York, 2009 winner. Administrative and support spaces located within the unit
Illustration Credit: Diana Anderson

(7) *Unit geometry and circulation*

Geometry

In general terms, no single ICU geometry has been found to be superior over another, and a general consensus appears to be that patient room size, unit scale and comprehensive program more effectively impact healing. An overview of the bed numbers in each of the winning entries shows that most have over 20 private beds, with the exception of a few outliers, indicating the need for additional perimeter to gain exterior exposure for each room. This no doubt becomes a design challenge related to window access for both patient rooms and staff spaces, along with proximity to medications, supplies and equipment and visibility into patient rooms by staff. Over half the units (seven) were in new construction, with the minority of the projects (four) constructed strictly as renovations, seen mostly in recent years, and several (two) were a mix of renovation and expansions.

The Swedish Medical Center's ICU was best suited to an octagonal configuration in order to incorporate their pod concept and design. Interestingly, the majority of units utilized the pod concept of decentralization with varying bed numbers ranging from 4–20 beds per pod. The pod arrangement appears to be the most frequently employed concept amongst winning designs, likely for ease of patient monitoring and decreased walking distances by staff. Three of the units demonstrate more of a linear configuration, including Memorial Sloan-Kettering Cancer Center, Harris Methodist Fort Worth Hospital, and Southeast Missouri Hospital. East Jefferson General Hospital and Memorial Sloan-Kettering present racetrack configurations. With the improvements of communication technologies and distributed documentation stations, neither building age nor configuration of available space seems to compromise patient safety and efficiency, in the view of the committees who select the winning designs.

Circulation

The designation of space for circulation appears to have moved towards an on-stage/off-stage model in more recent years. The 1992 Swedish Medical Center's ICU demonstrates one method of passage throughout the whole unit for staff, patients and families, likely determined by the octagonal nature of the unit geometry. In contrast, the 1996 Legacy Good Samaritan Hospital demonstrates the other extreme with a separate public corridor to allow visitors to arrive at the unit, a designated service corridor, and a patient and staff corridor for transport and daily care activities within the critical care unit. The 2001 winner, St. Joseph Health Center, provides a separate corridor connected to the main hospital for transport of patients to and from ancillary departments, which not only allows transport to the main part of the hospital building but also provides a direct connection between ICU and surgery. It must be noted that incorporating multiple circulation routes adds to the overall departmental area of an ICU, thus increasing the departmental grossing factor and costs associated with the design and construction of units. However, cost and space allowing, this notion of separate paths of movement and circulation will likely continue to be a tendency seen in future critical care designs.

Geometry and circulation clearly contribute heavily to unit size, and to multiplier factors of net square footage (NSF) to departmental square footage (DGSF). Square footage takeoffs of the units surveyed indicate the following:

Unit Departmental Square Feet Per Bed (DGSF/Bed):

- *New Construction—average = 933 DGSF/Bed*
- *Renovation Construction—average = 809 DGSF/Bed*
- *New and Renovation Construction (Mixed)—average = 902 DGSF/Bed*

It should be noted that a number of the units, including the last two winners, are approximately 1100 DGSF/Bed. These are both comprehensive programs, located in academic centers.

Net to Departmental Square Feet Factors (N:DGSF):

- *New Construction—average N:DGSF factor = 1.57*
- *Renovation Construction—average N:DGSF factor = 1.68*
- *New and Renovation Construction (Mixed)—average N:DGSF = 1.62*

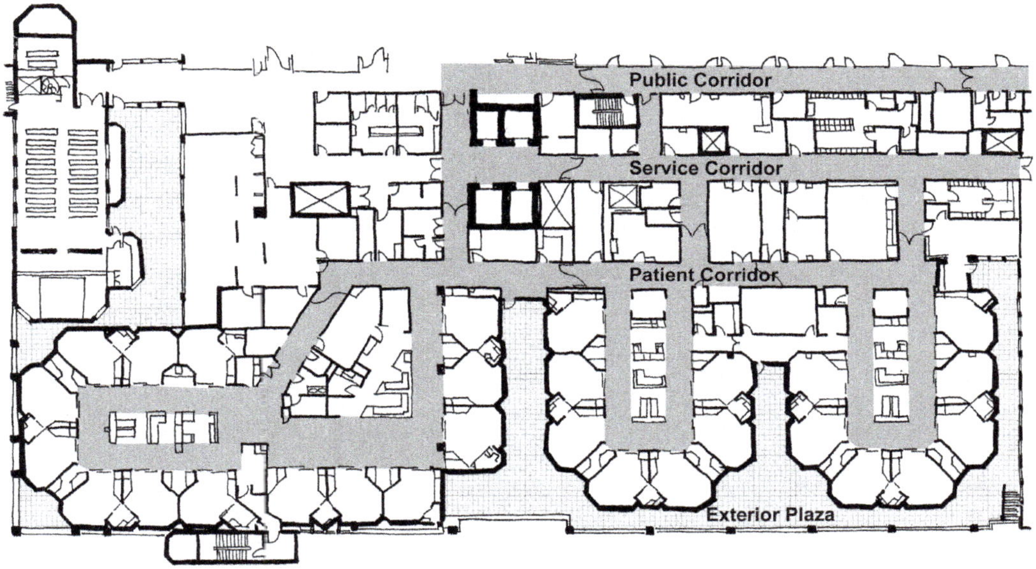

Exemplary Case: Legacy Good Samaritan Multidisciplinary ICU, Portland, Oregon, 1996 winner. Unique geometry allowing increased unit perimeter and plaza access: on-stage/off-stage circulation
Illustration Credit: Diana Anderson

It should be noted that within the renovation and mixed categories, net:departmental factors ranged as high as 1.8, reflecting the inherent inefficiencies of renovation designs.

(8) *Access to nature*

With a number of studies showing the benefits of access to nature and its healing properties (Ulrich, 1984, 1999), it is becoming more common to see the incorporation of natural elements into the intensive care environment. Legacy Good Samaritan Hospital is perhaps the most extreme example of this incorporation of natural elements by the provision of an extensive external plaza surrounding the unit for use by all users, including staff, patients and families. This unit design is all the more impressive in that it was a vertical rooftop expansion. The design intent was to provide patients who may be clinically stable, access to the outdoors directly from their rooms onto the outdoor plaza. The East Jefferson General Hospital provides two large courtyards on either side of the corridor into the unit so that natural light and views surround those entering the space. The McGill University Health Center ICU renovation and the Swedish Medical Center both provide an outdoor terrace for staff just off their lounge space.

Several units analyzed appear to have incorporated light courts into the designs, allowing for an increase in exterior perimeter and patient room numbers. Swedish Medical Center and Emory University Hospital are examples where several patient rooms have exterior views through windows looking out onto courtyards. The 2006 winner, Sharp Grossmont Hospital, has a 1500 square foot exterior courtyard in the center of the critical care unit. The courtyard also contains a skylight feature which allows for daylight access to the emergency department located directly below this space. The majority of units (seven) incorporate some form of outdoor spaces into the unit design. In some of the urban renovation projects, there is little possibility of space to allow for exterior access, such as New York City's Memorial Sloan-Kettering Cancer Center's ICU

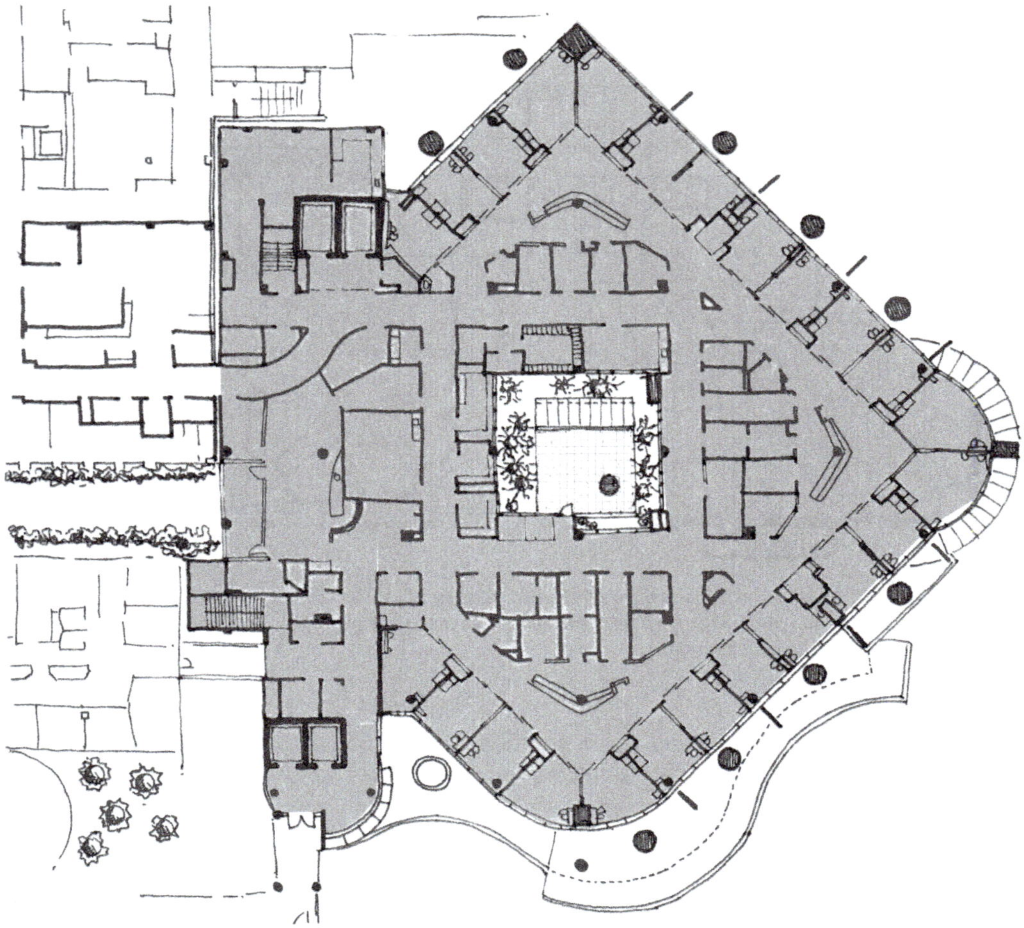

Exemplary Case: Sharp Grossmont Hospital ICU, La Mesa, California, 2006 winner. Centrally located exterior courtyard: 1500 square feet
Illustration Credit: Diana Anderson

renovation. However, the theme of nature through artwork and color sequences is frequently mentioned in the unit narratives as being important in the interior design of most spaces. In addition, a number of family and visitor waiting rooms provide fish tanks for their calming and entertaining effects.

Future design challenges and continuing trends

Larger units

As life expectancy continues to increase along with a rise in aging populations, these demographic changes have the potential to place a greater demand on medical services, particularly in the specialty of intensive care (Wunsch et al., 2008). An analysis of U.S. critical care showed that between 1985 and 2000, the total number of inpatient hospital beds decreased by 26.4%. In contrast, critical care beds increased by 26.2%, illustrating the growing importance for these units within our hospitals (Halpern et al., 2004). Thus, the importance of ICUs in our current healthcare system is enormous. From these statistics, one may postulate that more and larger units will be needed in coming years to accommodate these changing healthcare needs.

Technology and remote care

As technology advances for remote care planning, we may continue to see ICUs incorporating these new technological developments and designed to accommodate these advanced forms of high-tech conference and education spaces with patient viewing capabilities, handheld charting devices and improved electronic records.

Unit adjacencies

Increased diagnostic and treatment support located within ICUs was a trend noted in the survey of winning unit designs. It is likely that this trend will continue with more satellite services and hospital-wide facilities, such as dialysis and respiratory therapy spaces located within units, decreasing the need for patient transports to other areas of the hospital.

Decentralized support

Although most units surveyed employed a decentralized support model, most retained a type of central nursing or workstation. We may begin to see more units which present a complete absence of the central nursing station while providing decentralized charting outside individual or pairs of patient rooms. However, it is also a possibility that certain units and their work cultures may value the need and benefits of socialization and communication, thus retaining the need for some type of centralized space. Staffing shortages may also affect the ability of units to decentralize. The future trend for patient care support remains to be seen.

Nature for staff

With the advent of evidence-based design research, the importance of daylight and nature is more and more recognized. This trend has been seen mainly in the context of the patient room and family spaces. However, access to exterior spaces and nature elements for clinical staff members will likely become more evident in future ICU designs.

Designated circulation

The on-stage and off-stage model of circulation will likely continue in the future of ICU designs. Medical planners and designers are becoming more conscious of the built environment's capability to aid in preventing infection, minimizing patient transport distances, and augmenting the family's experience when entering the hospital and intensive care environment.

Charles D. Cadenhead, FAIA, FACHA, is a Senior Principal at WHR Architects; Diana C. Anderson, M.D., LEED® AP is the 2008–09 Tradewell Fellow at WHR Architects; and Robert G. Uhlenhake, AIA, ACHA, LEED® AP is a Senior Consultant with WHR Advisors.

References

Halpern, N.A., Pastores, S.M., Greenstein, R.J., (2004). Critical care medicine in the United States 1985–2000: an analysis of bed numbers, use, and costs. Crit. Care Med. 32 (6), 1254–1259.

Pati, D., Evans, J., Waggener, L., Harvey, T., 2008. An exploratory examination of medical gas booms versus traditional headwalls in intensive care unit design. Crit. Care Nurs. Quart. 31 (4), 340–356.

Ulrich, R.S., 1984. View through a window may influence recovery from surgery. Science 224, 42–421.

Ulrich, R.S., 1999. Effects of gardens on health outcomes: theory and research. In: Cooper Marcus, C., Barnes, M. (Eds.) Healing Gardens. Wiley, New York, pp. 27–86.
Wunsch, H., Angus, D.C., Harrison, D.A., et al., 2008. Variation in critical care services across North America and Western Europe. Crit. Care Med. 36 (10), 2787–2793.

The following examples are projects which won the SCCM/AIA/AACN Design Award (see the related sidebar above by Cadenhead, Anderson, and Uhlenhake).

Neuro ICU, Emory University Hospital, Atlanta, Georgia (Architect: HKS)

Owen Samuels, M.D., the unit director of the Neuro Intensive Care Unit at Emory University Hospital, was involved in a renovation project. He was not fully satisfied with the design and invited comments from Craig Zimring, Ph.D., an environmental psychologist of Georgia Tech's College of Architecture who focuses his research on healthcare settings. The design was examined and determined to fall short of some evidence-based principles. The proposed unit seemed to lack features to accommodate families and the workspaces for staff did not seem to offer improved efficiency.

Samuels and Zimring convened a group of graduate students to rapidly search for relevant evidence. A "charrette" workshop was held with the architect, the unit staff, and the university, to consider alternatives to the original design. The unit was redesigned to incorporate more design concepts based on evidence from the literature, resulting in redesigned patient rooms, redesigned nursing positions, and the introduction of a small garden space.

Kern Unit, Legacy Good Samaritan, Portland, Oregon (Architect: Tom Sagerser)

The Kern Unit at Good Samaritan in Portland is an extraordinary example of the use of windows and a garden for an ICU. Floor to ceiling glass dramatically affects the appearance of these rooms, each of which looks onto a private garden built on the roof deck. Protocols include 10 minutes per day in the garden for patients who are able to do so whenever the weather permits. The ICU and its garden are on the second floor of the hospital, looking into the branches of the trees on the sidewalk below.

The 28-bed Kern Unit is composed entirely of private rooms divided into three pods. It features dual overhead pendant-mounted life support systems that allow continuous access to the patient's head, and multiple bed orientations. The room is also capable of supporting minor procedures such as line insertions and pacemaker implants when the portable C-arm is brought in.

The staff work at decentralized stations for caregiver documentation, which occur between every two rooms. There is also a central workstation for the team which is bathed in natural light from large skylights.

Supplies are not in rooms with doors. Convenient and centrally accessible alcoves contain clean supplies kept on large carts. They are easily reached by staff within relatively short walking distance on the carpeted corridors.

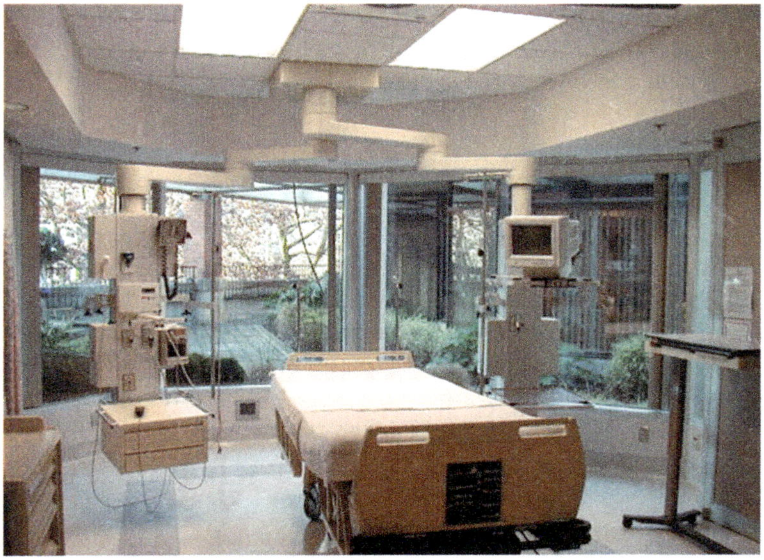

Figure 2.10: *View of patient room, with outside access*
Photo: Kirk Hamilton

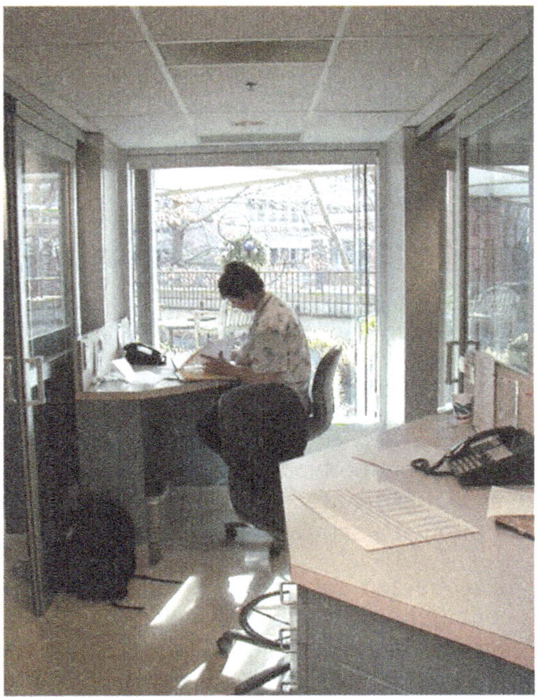

Figure 2.11: *Decentralized positions with a view reduce staff stress*
Location: Legacy Good Samaritan, Portland, OR
Photo: Kirk Hamilton

The unit has provided generous and attractive family waiting space adjacent to the pods. The family lounge has views into a courtyard adjacent to the hospital's chapel. The unit features a pleasant staff lounge with windows and a separate kitchen area.

Cardiac Comprehensive Care Unit, Clarian Methodist, Indianapolis, IN (Architect: BSA LifeStructures)

The cardiac unit was a widely published design for renovation that created an acuity-adaptable room combined with an operational model that combines management of the cardiac critical care unit and the associated stepdown unit (Hendrich, 2003; Hendrich et al., 2003; Hendrich et al., 2004). It features large, oversized private rooms made possible by the renovation configuration. The nearly 400 square foot room accommodates family presence, including a private nook behind the toilet. The headwall-based life support system is capable of flexing between critical and stepdown care levels. Sliding panels conceal unused elements of the system.

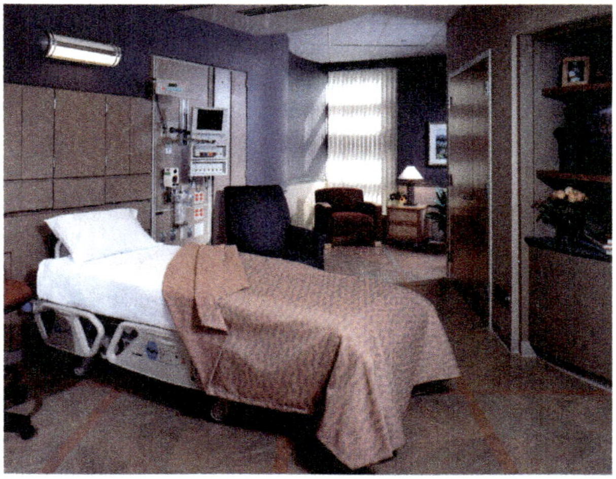

Figure 2.12: *Providing sufficient space for family activities will positively impact a family's experience in the ICU*
Location: Methodist Hospital, Indianapolis, IN
Architect: BSA LifeStructures and Maregatti Interiors
Photo credit: Dan Francis, Mardan Photography

The patient toilet features double doors and the advanced bed design, which folds up into a chair-like configuration, allows for better support of patient toileting, contributing to reduced falls and staff injuries. It seems that many falls occur when the staff member is peeled away from the patient as they maneuver through a narrow doorway.

The attractive unit utilizes decentralized documentation stations just outside the patient room, and the carpeted hallways contribute to the sense of quiet. The project has produced outcome measurements, such as reduced medication errors, reduced falls, increased staff efficiency, and improved patient and family satisfaction (Malkin, 2003; Hendrich et al., 2004).

The unit no longer functions in its original capacity as an acuity-adaptable cardiac setting. The introduction of four new heart hospitals in the Indianapolis market has left Clarian Methodist with the sickest cardiac patients and there is no longer a stepdown feature to the unit.

2.4 A regional example

The regional distribution of critical care capability is an access issue. Critical care facilities range from small generalized ICU units in community hospitals to multiple highly specialized units located in tertiary or quaternary care institutions. Some argue that with the increasing pressure of growing need, and the prospect of shortages of qualified healthcare professionals, that critical care should be more formally organized into regional networks (Kouri, 2002; Moodie, 2003).

Regionalization of critical care

In the face of potential shortages of trained personnel and the uneven distribution of critical care services, some experts have suggested a policy of regionalization to offer a full spectrum of specialized care, as well as to provide each patient with the highest level of experienced personnel, even if such a system requires an increase in the transport of critically ill patients. The independent physician model that prevails in the United States contributes to the lack of acceptance of this model.

The concept of regionalization can be seen in the state of Maryland, where the helicopter transport system, which is dispatched by the state police, conveys patients to a single trauma hospital to provide all critical care for trauma victims anywhere in the state (Franklin & Doelp, 1980). The Maryland Institute for Emergency Medical Services Systems (MIEMSS) in Baltimore is a hospital composed entirely of critical care and stepdown beds. The MIEMSS is open to any trauma patient in the state, so that everyone may receive the highest level of specialized expertise at a single location that is able to sustain a critical mass of staff, equipment, and specialty physicians. Quaternary care can be found at Johns Hopkins. The regional model is intended to ensure that every citizen of Maryland receives the same high quality trauma care. Regionalized networks might be designed to have highly centralized facilities like MIEMSS in Baltimore. Other less intensive care occurs in community hospitals around the state.

In 1994, the American College of Critical Care Medicine challenged the field to consider regionalization. After reviewing 146 articles related to the topic, a task force reported that there was broad agreement that regionalization would be "in the best interest of outcome and has the potential to reduce the cost of healthcare delivery" (Thompson et al., 1994, p. 1308). They, however, concluded that it was premature to recommend it until a system can be designed and built on the basis of defensible scientific and economic data. Little has been done, perhaps because of resistance from communities afraid of losing critical care service and lack of active support from physicians and intensivists who may not be inclined to relocate.

In most of the United States each hospital makes its own entrepreneurial determination of the need for critical care beds and plans accordingly. In many states the decision must be approved through a Certificate of Need process (Campbell & Fournier, 1993). Even when there is a public forum intended to restrain irresponsible growth, the actions are separately initiated by each individual institution or system. National initiatives with centralized planning and approval models are not common. Regardless of top-down or bottom-up planning and implementation models, a case can be made to rationalize the distribution of critical care services in order to provide the most effective support for the population being served.

The example of critical care service distribution in the greater Houston, Texas area might be instructive. There are more than 80 hospitals represented in the Greater Houston-Galveston

Area Hospital Council. The Council has representatives of free-standing community hospitals, regional systems with multiple hospital sites, components of national proprietary systems, public and government sponsored facilities, academic medical centers (most located in the Texas Medical Center), and a variety of specialty hospitals. Each type has some form of critical care capability.

Table 2.1 summarizes the distribution of critical care beds in the region.

Table 2.1 *Adult Hospital & Critical Care Beds for Harris County, Texas*

Facility Name	*Total Beds*	*ICU Beds*
Bayshore Medical Center	369	26
Ben Taub General Hospital	598	80
CHRISTUS St. Catherine Hospital	102	22
CHRISTUS St. John Hospital	178	14
Clear Lake Regional Medical Center	537	51
Cypress Fairbanks Medical Center	181	22
Doctors Hospital—Tidwell	101	16
Doctors Hospital—Parkway	152	8
East Houston Regional Medical Center	131	16
Houston Community Hospital, Inc. *dba* Renaissance Hospital	39	10
Houston Northwest Medical Center	430	48
Kingwood Medical Center	200	32
Lyndon B. Johnson General Hospital	328	24
Memorial Hermann Hospital	1082	228
Memorial Hermann Katy Hospital	127	12
Memorial Hermann Memorial City Medical Center	644	44
Memorial Hermann Northeast Hospital	255	24
Memorial Hermann Northwest Hospital	238	30
Memorial Hermann Southeast Hospital	274	32
Memorial Hermann Southwest Hospital	629	61
Methodist West Pavilion	251	16
Methodist Willowbrook Hospital	119	12
North Cypress Medical Center	91	20
Park Plaza Hospital	444	26
Patients Medical Center	61	4
Plaza Specialty Hospital	65	8
Riverside General Hospital	98	0
San Jacinto Methodist Hospital—Garth Road	190	24
San Jacinto Methodist Hospital—James Bowie Dr.	187	11
Spring Branch Medical Center	299	48
St. Joseph Medical Center	792	36
St. Luke's Episcopal Hospital	912	109
The Methodist Hospital	1101	148
The Woman's Hospital of Texas	275	4
Tomball Regional Hospital	358	28
University General Hospital	72	6
West Houston Medical Center	222	19
TOTALS	**12 132**	**1319**

Data compiled by Avery Imara Kennedy, RN, MSN, APRN-BC

According to publicly available data, the hospitals in the Houston area (Harris County) have 1319 adult critical care beds within their total of 12132 acute adult inpatient beds. Only one acute care hospital in the area does not have a critical care unit: Riverside General Hospital. The smallest critical care units at The Women's Hospital of Texas and Patient's Medical Center have four beds each. The largest number of critical care beds occurs at Memorial Hermann Hospital where there are 228 adult critical care beds. These 1319 adult critical care beds serve an adult population of 2763093, or one critical bed per 2095 citizens (http://quickfacts.census.gov/qfd/states/48/48201.html).

The 1319 adult critical care beds represent 10.9% of the total adult inpatient beds in the greater Houston area. This is close to the national percentage for critical care. The 12132 adult inpatient beds are provided at the rate of 4.39 beds per 1000 population, which is greater than the national average of three beds per 1000 (http://statehealthfacts.org/profileind.jsp?ind=384&cat=8&rgn=45). Houston draws many patients from outside the traditional boundaries of an urban catchment area.

Trauma patients arriving by ambulance will most often find themselves at the county's Ben Taub General Hospital, and patients arriving by Life Flight helicopter will arrive at the helistop on the roof of Memorial Hermann Hospital. The tertiary and quaternary units are in the Texas Medical Center where cardiac cases most often go to the St. Luke's/Texas Heart Institute or The Methodist Hospital, where both coronary care units (CCU) and cardiovascular intensive care units (CVICU) are found. Cancer patients are found at the University of Texas M.D. Anderson Cancer Center where chemotherapy, radiation therapy, cancer surgery, and bone marrow transplant patients can be treated. Transplant units are found at M.D. Anderson, Memorial Hermann, Methodist, and St. Luke's. Trauma and head injury patients are likely to end up in the ICU at The Institute for Rehabilitation and Research (TIRR) after their initial stabilization at another institution's trauma unit.

The Texas Medical Center (TMC) is unique in many ways (Elliott, 2004). There were more than 35 institutions and 6000 beds in the TMC in 2000. It is the world's largest concentration of medical facilities on a single site, and draws patients from well beyond the greater Houston area (Burleson & Burleson, 1987). Patients from all over the world flock to receive cardiac, cancer, and rehabilitation treatment at the TMC in Houston. At the same time, there are many community hospitals located around the city. Many prospective patients find the Texas Medical Center to be too complex and imposing. Parking is terrible, wayfinding is complicated, and the time and energy expended to go there is great. These people prefer to go to community facilities if they do not perceive a need for extraordinary clinical expertise. The majority of these community facilities, as is the case in many other U.S. cities, are located in areas that serve a middle class population whose members are likely to be insured. There are neighborhoods where the poor are disproportionately underserved.

2.5 International comparisons

The authors both teach in a graduate architecture program that specializes in design and research associated with healthcare environments. Interestingly, for the last several years more than half of the students earning a Master of Architecture with a Certificate in Health Systems & Design at Texas A&M University have been international students. There is a strong desire on their part to understand contemporary healthcare design practice in North America and to be exposed to cutting edge research on health environments.

The United Kingdom has long worked with open wards, often exactly as Florence Nightingale would have recommended. More recently the various standardized designs of the National Health Service (NHS), such as the Nuffield designs for six-bed wards of 1955 and the Best Buy hospitals of the 1960s (James & Tatton-Brown, 1986) or the Harness and Nucleus models of the 1970s (Cox & Groves, 1990), were to be replaced by hospitals built by the Private Finance Initiative (PFI), which has since been superseded by the Public Private Partnerships (PPP) program. Several large hospitals have been constructed under these auspices with mixed reviews. All of these projects feature modern critical care environments, but do not feature many private rooms. The NHS engaged Roger Ulrich, Ph.D., for the larger part of two years to consult on issues related to environmental factors associated with infections, which have become a serious problem (Ulrich & Wilson, 2006). Subsequent projects are providing significantly higher percentages of private rooms, as is the case in Ontario and Ireland where Ulrich has also been influential.

St. Mary's Hospital ICU: a current example from the UK

Phil Astley

Nancy Silva

Peter McGinity

Background

The intensive care unit at St. Mary's Hospital, Imperial College Healthcare Trust in London has a total of 16 beds for adults who require the highest level of nursing and medical intensive care. The unit is subdivided into two four-bed intensive care bays, and eight single rooms of which six rooms are engineered isolation rooms with negative pressure, one of which with either positive or negative pressure. All bed spaces have been designed to meet the latest Department of Health space standards as documented in Facilities for Critical Care Health Building Notes (HBN-57). *Patients are admitted to the unit through one of two routes: internally, for example following surgery, or by transfer to St. Mary's Hospital from another hospital.*

Briefing notes

Each bed space is designed to allow:

- *Access and visibility on four sides for staff and families.*
- *Bed space innovative design—"double handed" as medical gases, electrical sockets, data points are arranged on pendants on either side of bed to give maximum flexibility of use.*
- *Space at bed side allows equipment size to change depending on need.*
- *Every bed space has access to a hand wash basin.*
- *Every bed space or room has natural light.*
- *Access management system innovative design—audio/visual access management system developed to allow nurses to manage the access of visitors to the unit from each bed space via an audio/visual system that controls the door entry system. System can be used to instruct visitors to particular bays via a "follow-me" lighting system which also unlocks access control doors as necessary.*
- *Video conference system developed to enable video conferencing at every bed linked to MDT room, seminar room, main nurse stations and several other offices. System allows for consultation, training and supervision, and also allows for nurses to communicate with each other between beds on the unit without leaving the patient.*

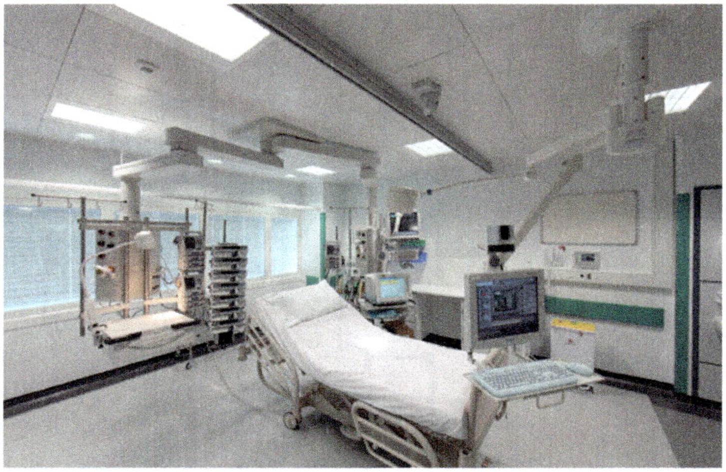

Technology for critical care bed at St. Mary's Hospital, London

- *Clinical information system innovative design—an extensive clinical information system has been implemented on the unit to link in with the video conferencing system such that clinicians can view both the patient directly and all information relating to that patient. A third pendant has been installed at the foot of each bed for the clinical information system, which doubles with the video conferencing system.*
- *Independent environmental control—each bed space has control over their immediate environment via a touch screen panel, which allows for control of lights, blinds, intelligent glass, TV, and heating +/− 3 degrees.*

From observation, two activities illustrate required performance of the unit space.

Activity one: Perform procedures on patient

1. *Staff gather necessary equipment*
2. *Wash hands, go to the patient*
3. *Notify CIS (clinical information system) of intended procedure*
4. *Check identity, perform procedures, wash hands*
5. *Log in details of procedure on CIS*

Activity analysis:

- *Infection control—considered for each procedure and equipment used*
- *Frequency and necessity of procedure*
- *Work flow, location of equipment*
- *Workload measure—how many staff involved in one procedure*
- *Equipment size and working space—ergonomics*
- *Duration—time taken for one procedure*
- *Lighting—artificial lighting level can be varied for time of day, patient comfort and care needed*
- *Natural daylight to bed spaces.*

Activity two: Data input

1. *Staff confirm patient and staff identity on CIS*
2. *Input data on the computer*

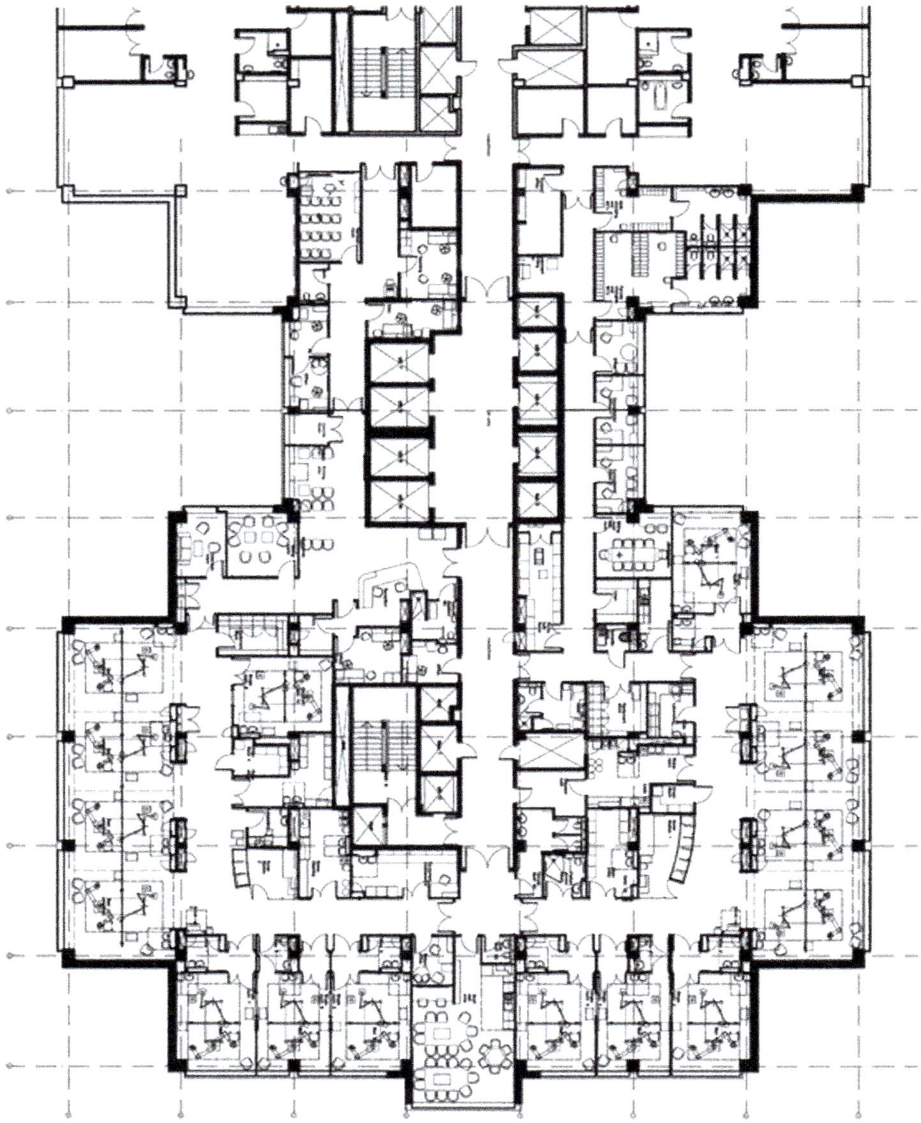

3. *Staff save data by password confirmation (audit trail)*
4. *Automated entry of data from any medical device connected to the patient*
5. *Staff log out on completion of data entry.*

Activity analysis:

- *Equipment needed—computer, CIS, patient testing*
- *Pendant at foot of bed to house clinical grade monitor and keyboard*
- *Privacy—on patient data.*

Summary: briefing and design implications

Staff and patient perspective

- *Bed spaces work clinically but space for staff and family can be compromised by equipment size and quantity*
- *Noise can be an issue because of hard, easy to clean surfaces and operational activity in open plan space, mitigated in part by provision of single rooms and smaller bed bays.*

Design guidance recommendation

Findings

The space at this ICU is fully utilized; furniture arrangement must support staff efficiency. Therefore:

- The user *needs to address the operational policy/procedures clearly and predict future activity and services.*
- *The furniture/equipment location needs to reflect the staff working flows (better working environment).*
- Designers *need to check published design standards and requirements (ergonomic, dimensional, grids) and the design strategies, and evaluate whether they support those work flows.*

Phil Astley is a Senior Lecturer and Architect at the Medical Architecture Research Unit (MARU) at London South Bank University. Nancy Silva is Associate Director for Capital Developments at St. Mary's Hospital. Peter McGinity is Associate Director of Redevelopments at St. Mary's Hospital.

Critical care has only been formally recognized as a specialty in the UK since 1999 (Intensive Care Society, 2003). In 1962 the Department of Health's "Progressive Patient Care" document recommended that 2–5% of a hospital's acute care beds should be devoted to intensive care. By 1998, the median size of ICUs in the UK was just under six beds, the size of the typical open ward from 1955 through the 1970s (Intensive Care Society, 2003). Phil Astley, a senior lecturer and architect at the Medical Architecture Research Unit (MARU) at London South Bank University, indicates that the current group of hospital projects in the UK all feature larger critical care units with higher percentages of private rooms, decentralized charting positions, numerous hand hygiene stations, and attention paid to infection control.

Northern European critical care in the Netherlands, Germany, and Scandinavia seems to have much in common. Architects and physicians in these countries have a history of open ward designs with many windows and natural light. The finishes are often white ceramic tiles and the units are kept spotless. More recent designs feature sophisticated monitoring, robust life support systems, and some are introducing color on the walls, as in the Netherlands at the Academic

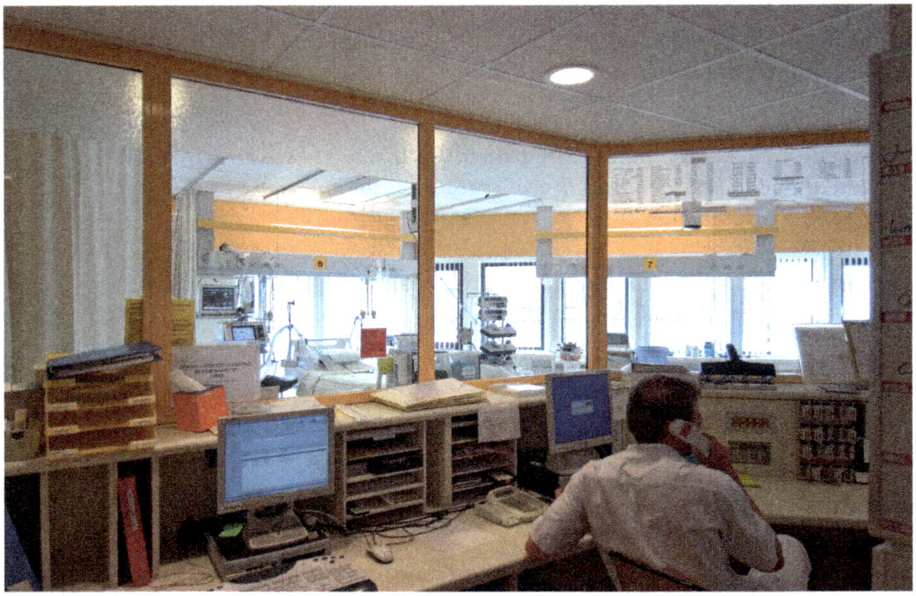

Figure 2.13: *ICU nursing station*
Location: Groningen Academic Medical Center, The Netherlands
Photo: By permission of GAMC

Medical Center in Groningen, or the Erasmus Medical Center in Rotterdam. The Bouwcollege of the Netherlands Board for Healthcare Institutions is responsible for reviews of health facility planning, and it is actively pursuing research into evidence-based design. They have begun to hold an annual forum for Dutch health environment researchers.

In Germany, intensive care units at the Ulm University Clinical Center feature 22 beds in double rooms and three in private isolation rooms (Nickl-Weller & Nickl, 2007). The Würzburg University Clinical Center also features nearly all patient rooms with two beds. The Vivantes Clinical Center Friedrichshain in Berlin, however, has a 15-bed unit adjacent to surgery which has only eight of its beds in double rooms (Nickl-Weller & Nickl, 2007) and the Vivantes-Klinikum Spandau in Berlin has a 14-bed unit with only six beds in double rooms (Meuser & Shirmer, 2006). There would seem to be a trend toward a higher proportion of private rooms and isolation rooms.

There are notable new hospitals in Norway, including the Rijkshospital in Oslo and the University Hospital in Trondheim. Sweden has a new facility for the Karolinska University Hospital in Stockholm, and there is apparently planning for a new University Hospital in MalmÄ. In Denmark, the Gentofte Hospital plans a new addition for surgical operating theatres and an intensive care unit. The Åarhus New University Hospital is planned like a town and will have four small wards totaling 16 beds for isolation of infectious patients, such as SARS or Ebola victims. Finnish architects Paatela & Paatela have designed the 1996 First Affiliated Teaching Hospital at Beijing Medical University, as well as projects in Iraq, Turkmenistan, and Russia.

Intensive care units in Norway and Scandinavia

Knut Bergsland

The need for intensive care in Norway and the rest of Scandinavia is growing steadily. It will continue to do so, due to the rapid growth of the over-70 population, the main user group in ICUs. NEMS scores (Nine Equivalents of Nursing Manpower use Score), the scoring system for ICU resource use, have already been going up for years. Length of stay (LOS) in ICUs is supposed to rise, as is the complexity and severity of patients' problems. Combined with hospital reform that demands that all hospital trusts should be in economic balance, this will put great pressure on hospitals at all levels.

Most hospitals trusts are at the moment facing severe economic problems and thus not living up to the reform demands, which will affect critical care design. On one hand, new projects have to reduce planned ICU space—often by 20–30%—when they apply for government approval. Operational and life cycle costs are to be kept at minimum levels. The coming elderly boom (2015 and onwards) will not make the situation any easier. On the other hand, higher demands for patient privacy and integrity, patient safety, better patient environments, space for families, efficient work environments, infection control, and other quality and space driving forces make planning ICUs a great challenge to Norwegian hospital planners.

The ideal size for ICU level 3 is traditionally considered to be 8–12 beds. In the new university hospitals with a need for more beds, 8-bed units are grouped together, sharing support functions such as utility rooms, storage rooms, rooms for relatives and meeting rooms to ensure that maximum space can be devoted to the area round the patient's bed. Step-down units (intermediate units or HDUs) may also be planned so as to share staff with ICUs, and thus need to be located close to these units. In an 8-bed unit, there would typically be a small workspace for each two patient rooms, with a workstation in the middle. This physical organization is supposed to minimize nurses' travel distances, maintaining present day staffing levels into the future.

ICUs are increasingly being planned with single room accommodation, replacing the typical, conventional open bay or ward solution with a centrally located nursing station within a horseshoe configuration. The two newest completed Norwegian hospitals, however, both have a few double rooms. Single rooms will typically have an area of 25 square meters, although some rooms have up to 30 square meters for isolation purposes or for accommodating future needs. Daylight to as many spaces as possible and good soundproofing is considered essential in ICUs, regardless of size. Relatives do not have designated sleeping spaces within the ICU but will, in most cases, spend the night at the patient hotel, which is a part of the hospital.

There are no set rules or standards for the dimensioning of hospital areas, or any structured evidence base for planners to consult. Basically planners learn from project to project, building evidence at an office level. Whole units in the latest university hospital projects are at present using 40 net square meters per intensive care bed as a standard, including support spaces, but excluding offices. Planned bed usage or occupancy is usually 75%. In the upcoming Århus hospital project in Denmark, however, the standard is raised to 60 net square meters per bed in the primary planning phase, for future proofing purposes. It is anticipated that these standards may be reduced, as the Danish government wants better space economy in all projects receiving government funding.

Norwegian ICUs are being planned within a system that at present focuses on economy. Planning for effective use of space and personnel seem to be the main themes at this stage. Whether the solutions have the necessary flexibility in use during the coming years remains to be seen.

Knut Bergsland is an architect and senior adviser of Norway's SINTEF Health Research.

In France, recent critical care designs by NMS-Architecture include a 20-bed surgical critical care unit at the Centre Hospitalier Universitaire de Rennes and a 24-bed medical critical care unit at the Centre Hospitalier Universitaire d'Angers. The French have built a number of new facilities, including the Centre Hospitalier de la Région d'Annecy (CHRA)—a 608-bed hospital which opened in 2007. The more famous Hôpital Européen Georges Pompidou, a 758-bed flagship facility on the west side of Paris, opened in 2001 with a scandal of deaths from Legionnaires Disease (Weber, 2001). French hospitals have had problems with hospital-acquired infections (HAI) including resistant strains of MRSA.

Safety and well-being in Intensive Care Units. Research-driven design for an integrated system: the Italian challenge

Prof. Arch. Romano Del Nord

Dealing with research and practice, I constantly face new challenges to keep at the forefront of international innovation.

The contemporary national debate declares a condition of double standards: on one hand, scientific research is deeply committed to the understanding and improvement of safety and psychologically-driven design principles; on the other hand, architects practicing in this specific field are not yet adequately aware of the interaction and implication between the environment and the care process. This condition becomes more critical when applied to the state of the intensive care units.

In Italy we count on 300 intensive care units for a grand total of 2000 beds. The aim of our Italian national healthcare policy is to implement organization models able to provide different levels of ICU care inside every hospital. The contemporary trend toward open space intensive care (eight-bed) wards is caused by a general lack of specialized staff. A limited number of highly trained nurses, able to provide intensive care treatment and monitoring for people who are in a critically ill or unstable condition, clashes with the principles of humanization that we promote today.

Humanization is at the core of innovation: a new approach that must become an integral part of the design process from its very earliest stage. There are, however, a wide range of critical factors that need to be evaluated and, most of all, integrated to launch innovative strategies for ICU design of the future.

The aims and commitment of scientific research can be summed up in two mainstream fields: the first concerns highlighting the main critical factors shaping ICU design; the second, in balancing the conflicting aspects of each individual factor, without each one missing their full potential benefits for patients (an example is the positive contribution of family care and involvement that may be the cause of infection).

Hospital borne infections involve approximately 100 000 cases being diagnosed per annum, with 5000 deaths. When the increased stay in hospital is 2.5 times the expected hospital stay, the impact on the system is significant.

The presence of the family is scientifically recognized as an integral part of caregiving. Family involvement, even in extremely critical conditions, may help chances of health recovery. As family incorporation becomes more and more desirable, ICUs must develop an appropriate space to accommodate parents and relatives. On the other hand, the in-room family presence may be the cause of an infection. Infection control, especially within acute healthcare environments, is a serious issue that requires a holistic and multidiscipline approach.

The correct and appropriate design related to the clarity of controls, display, and indicators affects patient safety and reduces the risk of injury for patients and staff. It is important to improve the culture of safety and integrate all related strategies in the design of ICU settings.

The room layout and its ease of maintenance contribute to facilitate caregiving. A successful morphology is the starting point for a more advanced environmental quality affecting patients, families, and staff well-being.

Thermal comfort, indoor air quality (IAQ) performance, natural light, color, location, sound, and view of the exterior are considered to be elements that improve well-being even in patients with acute conditions. Although each factor may well deserve a separate analysis, on the whole evidence-based research has proved that many biological processes and behavioral patterns are influenced by environmental conditions. The psycho-sensorial environment is therefore as important as the physical one; in fact the two cannot be separated. Furthermore, the environment for healing is considered an integral component of the care delivery process.

Patient-centered care refers to a healthcare policy that establishes a relationship among medical staff, patients, and their family to ensure that a patient's physical and emotional needs are respected and equally cared for. Reducing stress is therefore a key factor and the evidence is impressive.

The successful ICU of the future will be based on the importance of the interaction between innovation in healthcare technologies, safety, patient, and family focused design.

The concept of the healing environment for which psychology, art, and landscape are vital components is now part of mainstream thinking in hospital design. Although its benefits have been internationally shown to support evidence-based design theory, in Italy it still tends to be an add-on rather than being integrated into the design concept from its early stages.

We must therefore change our design process towards a much more integrated system.

Romano Del Nord is a Professor of Architecture at the University of Florence.

Turkey is a fairly modern country with aspirations to join the European Union. Most critical care available in Turkey is currently in urban hospitals, especially in Istanbul and Ankara. Some international organizations have built private hospitals in Turkey to offer a supposedly higher level of medicine, along the lines of European or North American models. This includes a commitment to critical care. Care in Turkey is complicated by the Muslim requirement to separate male and female patients.

On the other hand, large areas of countries like Turkey remain medically underserved. Dr. Michael DeBakey was invited by Turkey's then President, Turgut Ozal, to design and construct a hospital in his home town of Malatya, in eastern Anatolia. The Inonu University Medical Center was built with 880 beds, including multiple critical care units, to serve a population of some 2 million citizens.

Another of Dr. DeBakey's international contributions was a hospital redesign for the oil industry in Almetyevsk, Tatarstan—one of the former Soviet republics. Free healthcare is provided in the former Soviet Union by the military, and by large industries formerly run by the state. The design team observed an existing situation in which the only ICU bed was in a single room without windows. It was staffed by a single young nurse and contained the only bed in the house with a physiologic monitor. It can be presumed that this example was fairly typical of most of the former Soviet Union.

Russia today continues to have sophisticated critical care capability limited to the major urban hospitals. Dr. Renat Akchurin, recognized as the heart surgeon who cared for Boris Yeltsin, has pioneered a high-tech surgery institute in Moscow which included very sophisticated critical care capability for recovering surgical patients.

China is making great strides in hospital construction, as it has made strides in manufacturing, power production, and urban development. In 2003, Hamilton visited a major hospital in Shen Yang which was an example of a hospital built in the era of Mao and since expanded. It featured small amounts of space for departments, open ward designs, and largely manual record keeping. The ICU was a multi-bed space with glass walls used as dividers and an obvious high usage of gowning, masks and infection control technique. By Western standards, there were only moderate levels of monitoring and equipment available.

Today, with modernization examples like the 2008 Beijing Olympics, we see a completely different picture. Chinese design institutes, which are similar to design firms, are designing many new hospitals. Designs by U.S. firms teamed with Chinese design institutes are also being constructed. An example is the Shenzhen Third People's Hospital designed by TRO Jung & Brannen and the Shenzhen General Institute of Architects Design and Research. The project is designed to meet especially high standards for isolation of infectious patients while respecting traditional Chinese cultural models.

Taiwan has had advanced medical facilities for a longer period. The most respected physicians in Taiwan have usually had an international education, and have been responsible for bringing Western-style designs to the island. The Kao Hsiung Veteran's General Hospital in Kao Hsiung is an example of an 830-bed hospital with multiple critical care units that feature advanced technology and equipment.

There have been prominently publicized hospital projects in Korea that have been designed by North American architects. The Samsung Hospital in Seoul was designed by NBBJ. This large urban hospital contains sophisticated critical care units modeled after western examples. The contemporary and advanced Cha Women's Hospital was designed by KMD.

Contemporary Intensive Care in Japan

Yasushi Nagasawa, Dr. Eng. Dip.HFP, JIA

It is well known that among the developed countries Japan has a far longer length of stay in hospitals; it was approximately 30 days in the 1990s. This astonishing situation stemmed from the lack of financial incentives to reduce the length of stay, that is to say, hospital fees were paid by insurance bodies at the end of every month on the basis of the total number of inpatients in hospitals, not on the basis of the number of patients discharged from hospitals. However the payment system was recently amended. A clear distinction was made between "acute" hospitals and "non-acute" hospitals. In the case of the former, acute hospital fees are paid on the basis of fee for service, but after a certain period of days the fee scale related to the diagnosis is cut down , similar to the DRG system. In the latter non-acute case, hospital fees are paid on the basis of a lump sum fee for a month. Even though the non-acute hospitals treat patients using sophisticated medical technology, the amount of money paid is to be the same as pre-indicated. As a result, the length of stay in acute hospitals has become shorter and shorter. Now the national average length of stay is about 18 days.

Under the circumstances mentioned above, the provision of ICUs in Japanese hospitals becomes financially significant. For example, at NTT Kanto Hospital, which with 550 general beds is recognized as one of the typical acute hospitals in Tokyo, the average length of stay is 10.5 days. Eight ICU beds treat 710 patients per year. The length of stay in ICU beds was 4.1 days in 2007. This figure is very similar to that in U.S. hospitals. The characteristics of the ICU patients are serious medical and surgical cases from the emergency department and those who experienced neurological, gastronomic, and respiratory surgery, along with specialized stoke care in the SCU (Stoke Care Unit). The number of surgeries in this hospital in 2007 was 5700, which were carried out in 10 operating theaters. The number of medical staff for the ICU beds is three to five. The number of nursing staff, who work in three shifts a day, is 30 in total. This number seems very low compared with the U.S.

Like most of the other hospitals in Japan, 80% of the ICU beds are provided in the form of open wards, and there are several private rooms for infectious and/or terminal stage patients. Medical equipment for each ICU bed is sophisticated, similar to most Western hospitals. However, in terms of floor area per bed, the typical Japanese ICU seems to be too tight to accommodate ideal treatment for critical care patients.

One of the current problems in acute hospitals in Japan is the profile of patients. There are many patients aged over 80 in acute beds, which is due to the fact that Japan has the world's highest life expectancy. Critical care in Japan can be described, in short, as concentrated medical treatment and nursing care carried out for a large number of aged patients.

Yasushi Nagasawa is Vice-President of Kogakuin University in Tokyo, Japan.

The authors do not have information on the state of critical care in the South-East Asia locations of "medical tourism." These locations prominently feature in advertising that suggests modern and high-tech hospitals with internationally trained physicians. It can be assumed that they have also adopted Western standards for post-operative critical care. ParkwayHealth of Singapore describes their Hospital of the Future which is expected to open in 2011 to complement their three existing hospitals. The Praram 9 Hospital in Bangkok features a Kidney Transplant Institute, a Cardiovascular Institute, and all of the services of a tertiary care hospital. Bangkok's Bumrungrad International, the first Asian hospital to be accredited by Joint Commission International, is a 554-bed tertiary care hospital which advertises its "American management." The bulk of their campus dates from 1997.

In India, there is a notable shift towards private hospitals to serve the rapidly growing middle class. One example is the Apollo Hospitals Group which has 43 hospitals and more than 7500 beds. Apollo Hospitals Chennai has a major Centre for Cardiology and Cardiothoracic Surgery. In Delhi, the Apollo hospital features a Cancer Institute, Heart Centre, Neurosciences Centre, a Centre for Advanced Pediatrics, and a Surgical Science Centre associated with their Multi Organ Transplantation program. Critical care is at the core of their enterprise.

Cost of labor versus capital

It is interesting to note that in North America and the fully industrialized countries of Europe, the cost of hospital labor is high, and the capital cost of facilities and equipment can rapidly be equaled by the salaries paid to staff in only a few years. By contrast, in countries like the former Soviet Union, China of a few years ago, and most underdeveloped nations, the cost of labor (including physicians) is dramatically lower, and thus by comparison the cost of construction materials and medical equipment is precious. This explains in part why countries with underdeveloped or developing economies do not often build new, modern, high-tech healthcare facilities. It would take decades for the personnel cost to nearly equal such a capital investment in facilities. Critical care facilities and technology, of course, are among the most expensive components of a hospital.

While science and medical knowledge spreads across the world more evenly than ever, there remains wide variation in the quality and functionality of facilities and equipment that accommodate delivery of critical care. The authors hope for a broader sharing of design lessons and for a productive mix of reduced variation around the concept of "best practice," while simultaneously enriching the international exchange with robust dialog around new and interesting concepts.

Part Two: The Physical Setting

Design of the unit

3

An architecture firm working with the staff at Emory Hospital in Atlanta, Georgia, presented a design for a replacement Neuro ICU (see Chapter 2). The unit's medical director, Owen Samuels, M.D., was concerned that the intended design might not address some of his issues. Dr. Samuels approached Craig Zimring, Ph.D. of Georgia Tech's School of Architecture to see if there was any relevant literature on ICU design. Zimring shared examples of publications that could be relevant and was asked to involve his graduate students in an exercise to search the literature and develop design concepts based on research findings. This exercise ultimately led to an interdisciplinary design charrette with the architectural firm and a redesign of the project.

The end result of this process was a revised Neuro ICU design for Emory that took into account the design implications of findings from relevant literature. Dr. Samuels and the architects are pleased with the new design, which better serves the needs of the unit. Patient rooms were redesigned on the basis of evidence, as were nursing positions, lounges, family areas, and a courtyard garden. No additional spaces were created.

Neuroscience ICU tale: Redesigning the unit to enhance family participation and improve outcomes

Owen Samuels, M.D. and Craig Zimring, Ph.D.

Fulfilling a promise to our patients, their families, and hospital staff, Emory University Hospital's new neuroscience critical care unit (2D NCCU) opened its doors in February 2007. Our effort in creating this unit, which combined evidenced-based design and principles of patient family-centered care (PFCC), has resulted in an innovative healing environment. Here we describe the impetus for the new unit, the process of the initial design and then redesign, as well as early results and lessons learned.

Evidence for a better way

The need for a larger critical care unit came from our rapid growth, with neurocritical care admissions rising from 587 patients in 1999 to more than 1400 patients in 2007. We treat patients with severe brain and nervous systems diseases, such as traumatic brain injury, meningitis, brain aneurysms, strokes, and other severe brain and spinal cord diseases. By 2007, we were literally out of beds and turning patients away. We were caring for these patients in three geographically-separated small units (two seven-bed units, and one nine-bed unit), which was inherently inefficient and compromised patient safety and delivery of high quality care.

When we initially proposed a replacement neurocritical care unit, we appealed to the bottom line: if we had more beds and could attract more patients, we would generate more revenue and, most importantly, satisfy our mission as the hospital of last resort for many of these patients with complex brain injury. The hospital's mission stated that we had to take care of patients with neurological emergencies, because no one else in town could or would.

The hospital agreed to build a new unit, but with predictable restrictions; because Emory University, at that time, was in the early phases of planning a replacement hospital, estimated at over a billion dollars, the administration did not want to spend a lot of money on an new unit, which would be demolished in five years with the new hospital coming online. In fact, the new unit, early on, was described as the "throw away" neuroscience ICU. They agreed only to meet the state and federal requirements so that we could quickly open to meet the immediate ICU bed shortages.

The initial design was for a 24-bed intensive care unit (ICU) with a "track" around it; visitors would enter the patient rooms from the back so as not to disrupt the central area used by the doctors and nurses. The rooms measured 200 square feet, as required by the state of Georgia, with no dedicated space for family members. This design essentially duplicated the current ICUs at

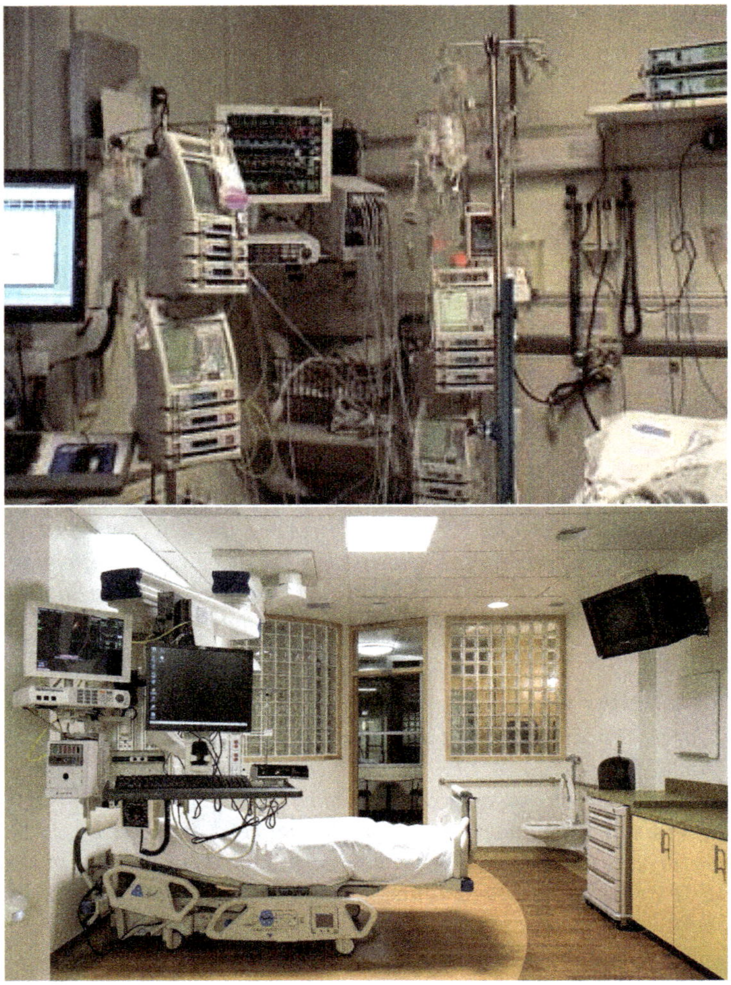

Figure 1 Illustrates crowded initial conditions and completed project

that time. In these units, the typical patient room was so crowded and cluttered with specialized equipment that it was virtually impossible to get to the patient without tripping over cords and knocking out invasive lines from the patient (Figure 1 shows a comparison of the ICU before and after construction). It took some time to respond to an emergency and maintaining sterility in such an environment was near impossible. During patient care rounds, the ICU team's numerous members practically fell over one another in crowded rooms and hallways. Actually seeing the patient in the midst of all this was a challenge. In the central areas, nurses were crowded around desks with charts spread all over tables, increasing the potential for mistakes in documentation, record keeping and medication administration.

Where were the families? They were often banished to dark, dingy, common spaces in the outside hall, well away from patients. Families were restricted to visiting during morning rounds for fear they should misinterpret or be alarmed by something they heard. Discussions between doctor and families took place either in the cluttered patient rooms or in public hallways with no privacy. This is where discussions of a patient's poor prognosis, as well as discussions regarding brain death, organ donation and end of life, occurred. The new proposed space promised little more than some new converter chairs.

As a neurologist and intensive care specialist, I did not have a clear idea of what new ICU design we needed, but I knew the proposed design was not it!

To convince the administration that we should pursue a completely new concept, we focused on key people: the Chief Nursing Officer for neurosciences and the Chief Executive Officer of Emory Healthcare. We told them that our current ICUs were terrible for families and the space was inherently dangerous. The potential for avoidable medical mistakes was enormous and largely unrecognized. Staff burnout was also an issue: we reminded them of the tremendous nursing turnover, especially with our aging nursing population. We also told them that we believed there was a better way.

Doctors and nurses make clinical decisions, such as choosing a drug to treat infection, on evidence from the literature. Shouldn't such evidence also inform how we design hospitals and ICUs? We rapidly learned that convincing scientific evidence exists that the physical environment affects patient outcome and staff effectiveness (Ulrich et al., 2004). The literature shows that we can empower families and staff, and reduce costs.

We proposed a new design founded on an evidenced-based approach for patient and family-centered care supported by a healing environment. We were confident that an improved design could reduce staff stress and enhance performance. As an academic institution, we wanted to measure such factors and continue to study this by building a living laboratory of a new type of ICU. We also needed every high-tech treatment tool available, while remaining flexible enough that we could continue to change in the future. Most importantly, we wanted to keep patients and their families the center of our focus.

Emphasis on family involvement

We sometimes fool ourselves into thinking that technology alone improves outcome, when, in fact, many other factors may be even more beneficial. When we designed the ICU, we had several goals or "design drivers" (Table 1) in mind, with accompanying measurable outcome variables to be tracked.

A primary driver for the new ICU was support of families. We proposed completely eliminating all the signs restricting family visitation. We were tempted to replace the sign "PHYSICIAN ROUNDS IN PROGRESS" with "PHYSICIAN ROUNDS IN PROGRESS, FAMILY PRESENCE ENCOURAGED."

Design Drivers	*Design Response*	*Outcome Measures*
Support families	Family zone in patient room Kids' room Lockers and showers Family quiet room	Greater satisfaction on Press-Ganey and Emory ICU surveys Fewer complaints and litigation
Support more procedures at the bedside	Medical gas booms	Fewer patient transfer complications and lower costs
	Larger patient zone Improved ergonomics	Fewer errors Shorter stays More time spent by ICU staff in the ICU area
Reduce infection	Numerous rubs and handwashing stations	Improved handwashing compliance Lower MRSA and nosocomial infection rates
Reduce medical errors and increase patient safety	Improved ceiling tiles Carpet where appropriate Charting niches Zoned caregiver area	Fewer medical and medication errors Less litigation Reduced self-extubation Decreased falls and injuries related to patients leaving beds

ICU = intensive care unit: MRSA = methicillin-resistant Staphylococcus aureus

We planned for a family zone located within the patient's room, as the "family studio", a children's area located immediately outside the ICU, family lockers and showers, clothing washers and dryers, and a quiet room for families and close friends. Outcome measures collected included patient and family satisfaction scores, hospital-acquired infections, nursing retention rates, ICU length of stay, organ donation success, and number of litigation filings.

Other important drivers were: to support more procedures at the bedside; turning the patient ICU room into a mini-operating room, thereby reducing patient transfers; reduction of medical errors; and increase of patient safety. Each goal had measureable outcomes to be tracked.

A dynamic design process

To help determine factors such as patient room size and configuration, as well as the design of family spaces, we analyzed best practices of the prior 10 years' winners of the ICU Design Citation Award, which is given jointly by the Society of Critical Care Medicine, the American Association of Critical Care Nurses, and the American Institute of Architects. We partnered with the division of healthcare design at Georgia Institute of Technology's College of Architecture, led by an environmental psychologist specializing in the utilization of architectural design as a healing tool. Several charrette sessions were held, which included key stakeholders from Emory, the architects (HKS) and Georgia Tech.

We then created a mock-up of the proposed ICU, including a nurses' station, patient rooms, wall-to-ceiling booms, and family areas. We spent a great deal of time role-playing a variety of procedures, including resuscitation, intubation, implantation of a brain monitor, nursing shift-change, and interactions between families and staff. Videographers recorded everything for later analysis. A mock-up of the family studio allowed analysis of functionality and family flow.

As we learned from such experiences, we altered the design of the ICU even as construction was underway. We originally planned to distribute the nurses' stations throughout the unit, but later decided to keep a communal area as well, recognizing that nurses and doctors at times need to be in the same area in order to better support one another.

Family members of patients who had recently been discharged from or were still in the ICU were involved with the unit's design throughout the process.

Proposal becomes reality

The new unit opened February 2007. The rooms range from 345–450 square feet (Figure 2), compared with 120–200 square feet for the old rooms. Each room is a suite, consisting of the patient room and a family area separated by a curved wall with large glass-block windows that let in light, creating a cocoon-like effect (Figure 3). The family studio has a table, chairs, comfortable sleeping arrangements, a flat-screen television, wireless Internet access, music and a white-noise system to blunt surrounding noises.

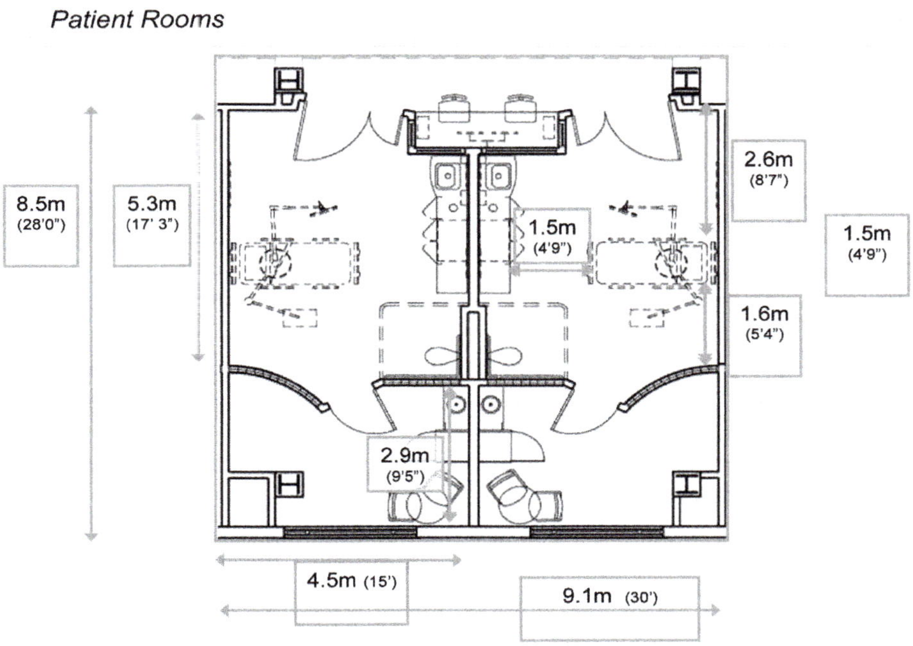

Figure 2

The new unit allows us to do things we could not do before. We can now easily hold a private conversation with a family member when we visit a patient. Family members can leave the room for some respite and still be just a stone's throw away from their loved one.

Patient rooms are significantly larger, and pneumatic booms lift equipment off the floor, minimizing cords, cables and clutter, and allow rapid 360 degree access to the patient's head in emergency situations. The beds and doors are configured so that patients who are awake have a direct line of sight to the nurse's station or a bay window.

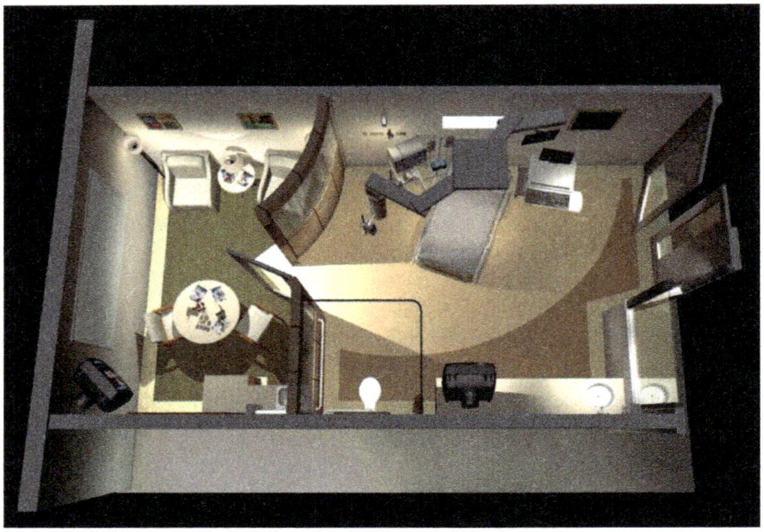

Figure 3

Benefits of family-centered units: a case study

The following case study illustrates some of the advantages of our new family-centered unit. David was a 31-year-old computer programmer, the father of a three-year-old girl, and about to be married. He came in with a ruptured brain aneurysm. He was in the old neurocritical care unit for four or five days, and then was moved to the new unit when it opened.

The family—David's parents and his fiancée—kept a rotating vigil. They always felt they were in the way in the old ICU, whereas they felt welcome in the new facility. The family often stood at David's bedside as the team explained the purpose of the complex monitors and instruments. The mother said, "This was our home for a month, and it got so that the nurses could tell when we needed a hug." (Landro, 2007)

After two weeks, David developed neurogenic pulmonary edema, severe pneumonia, acute respiratory distress syndrome, and heart failure. We induced a coma to protect his brain from high intracranial pressure and placed hypothermia catheters to lower his core temperature in an attempt to better oxygenate him. Just as he was getting better, the aneurysm ruptured again, and we knew that recovery was hopeless.

The family was by his bedside 24 hours a day and knew that the medical team was as well. They witnessed the whole situation and understood when we ran out of options. As David's parents and fiancée gathered at the bedside, I told them that David had progressed to brain death. Shortly after that, the team that arranged organ donation came to speak with David's parents, and they elected to donate. They were grateful for the time they had with him and for the way they were treated. David's father said, "No one ever misled us or told us anything but the truth. . . and most importantly, we were there for everything." (Mantone, 2007)

We did everything we could for David, and nothing could change his ultimate outcome. But I think that the way someone dies is incredibly important. The circumstances of how he was treated probably helped allow the family to donate David's organs and better come to terms with his death. They later generously donated their time to help the neurocritical care unit develop the family-centered approach we wanted by participating in many discussions about their experiences.

Family-centered units pose challenges

Units that are designed for both patients and their families raise enormous issues that arise in the ICU daily. How does one care for patients and their families simultaneously? Some of the many challenges have included:

- *Team rounding. Many doctors and nurses were apprehensive about inviting families to rounds. Training doctors and nurses with families present is a real paradigm shift and raises many controversial issues.*
- *Nursing handoffs. Imagine a nurse operating six or seven intravenous pumps and trying to figure out medications while having a family member—or three or four members— continuously present.*
- *Urgent or frightening treatment. How do you deal with resuscitation? What if the family is right by the bedside: do you ask them to leave? What kind of support do they need?*

We do not have all the answers to such problems. We are currently studying them and trying to figure out best practices.

Successes and future directions

Emory's neurosciences critical care unit won the 2008 ICU Design Citation Award from the Society of Critical Care Medicine, the American Association of Critical Care Nurses, and the American Institute of Architects Academy on Architecture for Health.

We are now beginning to look at outcomes resulting from the unit redesign, and they all are going in the right direction. ICU patient satisfaction and staff satisfaction have increased, according to self-assessments. Most recent Press-Ganey Family Satisfaction scores have been greater than 85% overall satisfaction. Other variables of benchmarks of quality care include significant decrease in pneumonia rates and central venous line bloodstream infections, increased compliance with critical care pathways, increased nursing retention, and a trend towards decreased medical legal litigation.

Although the concept of care centered around the patient and their family seems as acceptable as motherhood and apple pie, there is enormous resistance to it, even from the most dedicated health-care workers. The process was long and laborious: we spent about a year and a half preparing for it with a family-centered team and involved all sorts of charters and directors along the way. Starting the changes is the real challenge.

Fact sheet: Emory Neuroscience Critical Care Unit

- *The Emory Neuroscience Critical Care Unit provides tertiary care for acutely ill patients with complex neurologic and neurosurgical conditions such as hemorrhagic and ischemic stroke, brain aneurysms and traumatic brain injury*
- *1500 patients admitted each year*
- *Average stay: 14.5 days, with 10% staying 30 days or more*
- *15–25% ICU mortality rate*
- *Focus on patient-and-family-centered care*
- *27 beds, 20 in the 2D-ICU that opened Feb 1, 2007; 7 located in an older unit*
- *2D-ICU (newly constructed)*
  - *Departmental gross square feet: 22 097*
  - *20 patient suites, 390–410 sq. ft which includes a dedicated 130 sq. ft private family studio area*
  - *Family studio (130 sq. ft) within the patient room that includes two chairs that convert to beds, table, sink, white board, Wi-Fi, TV, wardrobe for family personal items*
  - *Family studio provides family members privacy and allows staff to talk to family privately.*

References

Ulrich, R., Quan, X., Zimring, C., et al., (2004). *The role of the physical environment in the hospital of the 21st century: a once-in-a-lifetime opportunity*. Research report from the Center for Health Design; September. <http://www.healthdesign.org/research/reports/physical_environ.php/>. (accessed 30.10.2008).

Landro, L., (2007) 12 July. ICUs' new message: welcome, families. *Wall St. J. p.* <http://online.wsj.com/article/SB118419577614963880.html/>. (accessed 30.10.2008).

Mantone, J., (2007) 12 July. Building family-friendly ICUs. *Wall St. J. p.* <http://blogs.wsj.com/health/2007/07/12/building-familyfriendly-icus/>. (accessed 30.10.2008).

Dr. Owen Samuels is the director of the Neuroscience Critical Care and Stroke unit at The Emery Clinic in Atlanta, Georgia. Craig Zimring, Ph.D., is a faculty member in the College of Architecture at the Georgia Institute of Technology.

The places in which critical care occurs can be defined as the space that constitutes the physical setting for the activity. The setting is a collection of distinct spaces dedicated to various intended purposes; each space exhibits varying degrees of distinct characteristics, such as size, amount of enclosure, privacy, lighting, comfort, functionality, and so forth. A skilled designer may create observable differences between spaces that share common characteristics but for which the ambiance somehow varies.

Many different types of spaces may be found within a typical critical care unit. Most will appear in any such unit; a number of them are repetitive in form, while a few are individual and singular. Together these spaces can be arranged in a variety of configurations. Some spaces are enclosed within a room, while others may be adjacent to a room or combined with other spaces without the separation of walls. A common way of identifying a space is to describe the function that occurs within it.

3.1 Quantifying the need for space

Designers have long wrestled with the questions of how to size each space and how to most effectively configure the combination of spaces. In the United States, the listing of spaces to be planned is usually called the program of space requirements or the space program. In most of the rest of the world it is called the project brief. A good program or brief will list each space to be planned and will define each on the basis of size, function, and the equipment and furnishings it is expected to contain (Peña & Parshall, 2001).

Architects who specialize in the design of healthcare facilities will often be qualified to develop a program of space requirements for a critical care unit. In many cases, the client or the architect may elect to engage a consultant who specializes even further in the creation of the carefully quantified space programs required for a properly functioning critical care unit (Durham & Hayward, 1996).

Interview-based programming

One way to develop a listing of required spaces is to use the interview method. The architect or consultant asks the client and the users of the current space to give their opinion as to what a new critical care unit would entail, including the number of beds, major equipment items, a list of rooms, and the amount of space required for each of these elements. This information can be obtained by comparing the proposed unit with an existing unit to be replaced, or with a unit that shares some characteristics with the intended unit. The primary benefit of such a method is the ability to acquire explicit knowledge from those directly involved in doing the work. A drawback is that such knowledge may not be based on the full range of possibilities, and that there may be unfounded assumptions built into the opinions of those being interviewed.

Volume or demand-based programming

A demand model is an evidence-based tool used to quantify space requirements. The architect or consultant examines historical and projected demographic data to identify the current and projected incidence of demand for critical care services, along with the market share for such services among the population served. This method of quantifying future demand for services leads to a data-driven decision about the number of critical care beds needed to serve the population. The demand data is often important when the number of beds has become the subject of arguments based on strongly held beliefs, or when regulatory requirements mandate a justification for the major program elements. Once the number of critical care beds has been determined, the architect and/or consultant can use a variety of guidelines, regulations, formulas and experience-based "rules of thumb" to identify the other spaces required to support the beds.

The "Right Sized" critical care unit

Terry Ritchey, RN, MBA

Determining the right number of beds for an efficient and functional critical care unit that is also adaptable to change over time is a bit like Goldilocks' search for just the right space. There are many factors to be considered during planning and programming to create the unit that is operationally neither "too big" nor "too small" but one that is "just right." We find that a decision-making grid that takes into account the organization's key performance measures is useful in finding the suitable answer to this complex problem.

Critical Care Unit Bed Size Decision Grid

Consider management, ancillary and support staff, students and skill mix to determine maximum number of staff on unit as well as percent occupancy.

Unit Bed Size (beds)	Noise Impact **(Patient Quality and Safety)**	Peer/ Support, Teamwork Back-up **(Patient Safety and Staff Satisfaction)**	Staffing, Efficiency and Productivity **(Financial)**	Available Peer Support and Line of Site **(Staff Satisfaction)**	Walking Distance **(Staff Satisfaction)**
4–8					
8–12					
12–16					
16–20					
20–24					

Rating Scale	**Very Good**	**Good**	**Average**	**Fair**	**Poor**
	●	◕	◑	◔	○

Finding the sweet spot in determining the number of beds for a critical care unit is a mix of strategy, theory, the hospital's service line structure, model of patient care, as well as site and cost constraints. The solution is unique to each facility and project. However, using a framework to balance and assess the impact of unit size on 1) patient safety 2) financial performance 3) patient satisfaction and 4) staff efficiency and satisfaction aids in the decision-making process.

Units that are too large may lead to excessive walking distances for caregivers, noise and distractions which could contribute to errors and impact both staff and patient safety and satisfaction. In addition, it may be more difficult to achieve patient visibility and line of sight for colleagues in larger units which are configured with corridor twists, turns and isolated pods due to their size.

Units that are sized too small may be challenged with achieving productivity targets, have limited flexibility to accommodate census surges, and provide poor peer back-up and support which can affect both safety and satisfaction measures.

In planning the size of a unit, it's important to consider the caregiver's visibility of the patient, peers, space for multidisciplinary team collaboration, as well as the visibility of overall activity of the unit. The standardization of patient room and unit design can also influence quality and safety outcomes.

Staff satisfaction in critical care units is often reflected by how efficient the unit is to work in, relative to the distance between patients, team members and the manager. With the average size of critical care patient rooms larger than in the past, it is important to balance the size of the unit with support space to reduce unnecessary walking and improve staff satisfaction.

Cost considerations take into account productivity targets as well as the number of support spaces, such as medication rooms and supply areas which support clusters of patient rooms while maximizing staff efficiency. Critical care nurses and physicians thrive in an environment which fosters collaboration, mentoring and back-up support during emergencies. With an average ratio of one nurse for two patients, four to six nurses will likely be on a unit with 8–12 beds at any given time, providing a good mix of staff to complement the physicians and other members of the critical care team, as well as helping to achieve most financial targets.

Larger units may result in a decrease in employee productivity caused by time lost in excess walking to provide patient care, deliver medication and retrieve supplies. Likewise units that are too small have limited flexibility to accommodate census surges and are challenged in providing space for peer back-up and support. Units with minimal staffing could also lead to a sense of isolation for both patient and family.

A "right sized" critical care unit balances caregiver team support, visibility, productivity and support for the patient and family while offering space which is functional and easy to maneuver for the staff. It offers opportunity for growth and expansion, for flexibility in the model of care such as the acuity adaptable or "one transfer" process, and for changes in service line structure over time. Employment of a decision-making grid, which takes into account the organization's key performance drivers, offers the chance for design of a critical care unit that is sized appropriately for your current and future needs.

Terry Ritchey is Vice-President of Clinical Solutions and Research at HKS.

Number of beds

A principal element in the design of any critical care unit is the number of beds to be included. The volume of patients that can be expected is predictable based on an understanding of demographics

within the organization's service area, the incidence of disease and trauma, market share, and past performance statistics. Experts recommend using a statistically-based service-volume projection method to determine the number of beds needed.

The traditional ICU design of the past, as it has evolved from the original recovery room concept, has been based on the ability to see the face of each patient from a single central position. The concept was based on the observer's need to be able to rapidly identify any significant change in the patient's condition and allow for the timely summoning of help. This concept was instituted before the advent of heart monitors and other continuous physiologic reporting. In a traditional configuration, the size of the space allotted to each patient room or bed position has generally limited the number of beds that can be seen from such a central position to somewhere between 8 and 10 beds. Many units have attempted to include larger numbers of beds and have experienced corresponding reductions in bed visibility from a central position (Hamilton, 2000).

This limitation on the number of beds that can be observed from a central station has resulted in a pattern in which many larger ICUs have been divided into clusters, pods, or separate units, each fitting the 8–10-bed size range. Some have proposed that the smallest unit that can be managed efficiently is a unit of six beds (Hamilton, 1999).

Assignment equity

In the United States, the standard critical care ratio for nurses to patients is 1:1 or 1:2. The physical arrangement of patient rooms and bed locations should allow for optimal assignment equity among the nursing staff. Equity means that particular rooms or groups of rooms should not give any nurse an unusually difficult assignment. The design should not result in one room that is so unlike the others that it becomes a dreaded assignment or is always the last bed to be filled. Groupings or clusters of rooms should not result in patterns in which one nurse must always travel significantly greater distances than those assigned to other rooms. When we are touring facilities and ask to see an unoccupied room, there invariably seems to be a less desirable room that is the last bed to be filled.

Size of unit

An issue for planners of critical care units is determining the amount of space that should be allocated to serve the expected need. A convenient measure is the unit area (square feet or square meters) divided by the number of beds. Charles Cadenhead, an architect specializing in design for critical care, has collected data on the physical space devoted to critical care units (2005). He suggests that in the United States a range from 850 to 1100 departmental gross square feet per bed can be expected. His review of winners of the ICU Design Award, which is jointly sponsored by the American Institute of Architects (AIA), Society of Critical Care Medicine (SCCM), and the American Association of Critical Care Nurses (AACN), seems to show a trend toward providing a larger area per bed in newer units (see p. 15). This trend can likely be attributed to the availability of new technologies like power columns and pendant life support systems, as well as the use of larger beds and more equipment to serve higher acuity patients, and provision of space to accommodate families.

3.2 Unit design issues for critical care

The planning team, including design professionals, representatives of the clinical users, members of hospital administration, as well as patients and their families, should consider a number of design issues when planning a critical care unit. These issues should be addressed and resolved before the program of space requirements is completed, as their resolution will influence the number and types of spaces required.

Unit geometry and configuration

Critical care units are designed in many types of configurations. As additions to a hospital complex they can be found in round, square, triangular, rectangular, and irregular shapes. Critical care units have been designed both as original elements of a structure as well as renovated within preexisting configurations. There are three principal elements that influence a unit's configuration:

1. The requirement for all patient rooms to have an exterior window results in a large perimeter.
2. The desire for high levels of observation from a central monitoring location suggests some variation of a concentric shape.
3. Critical care units are generally smaller and more idiosyncratic than other units or departments of a hospital and thus do not always conform well to shapes intended for other units above or below.

The first suggestion from a clinician on how to design a critical care unit is usually a radial or circular design in order to maximize the observation of patients arrayed around a central point (Cawood, 1993). Radial designs work effectively until the number of rooms surrounding such a central point increases the unit's circumference and the center becomes too large and unmanageable. Since the relationship of the circumference of a circle to its area is a fixed ratio, problems can occur when there are not enough rooms to surround the area needed for support functions, or, as happens more often, when the perimeter for a large number of rooms forces an area in the center to be greater than the area needed for support functions.

Optimal ICU design—one architect's view

James W. Harrell, FAIA, FACHA

Intensive care providers in general have a common point of view regarding the design of an ICU. They are concerned about patient safety. To that end they wish to be able to keep an eye on the patients even from outside of the patient room. Invariably, when asked to diagram their ideal layout, they illustrate a radial plan with patients around the perimeter and the caregivers in the center. The position of the bed around this perimeter is dependent upon the type and condition of the patient. Very sick patients are aligned with feet facing the center—this allows maximal visualization of the patient. Other patients, i.e., cardiology cases, can enjoy and benefit from looking out of the exterior window, so these patients are more or less perpendicular to caregiver line-of-sight. To further accommodate patient safety, it is crucial that care providers can get to all sides of the bed, including the head.

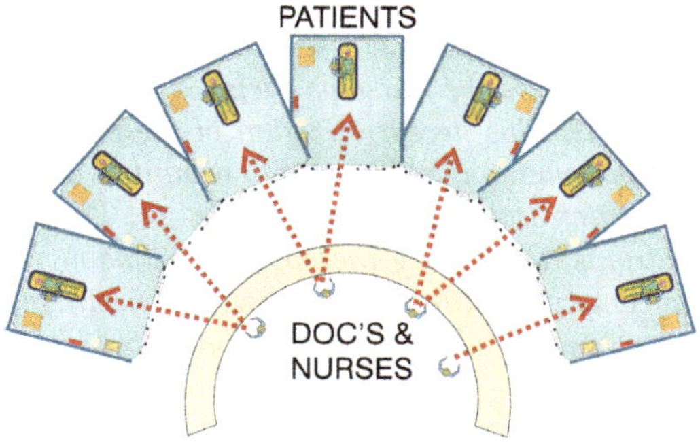

Figure 1

Evidence shows that family-centered care supports patient safety; therefore provision for family members at the patient bedside and for their comfort in the room is a key factor in space allocation. Patient and family privacy is a cardinal aspect of ICU design; consequently each patient should be in a single-bed room.

Fundamental considerations for ICU room design are:

- *Circulation all around the bed*
- *Unencumbered access to medical gas, electric and data outlets*
- *Hand hygiene stations*
- *Accommodation for electronic data entry*
- *Accommodation for fluids disposal*
- *Large exterior window area*
- *Space and accommodation for families to stay through the night*
- *Accommodation for patient toileting*
- *Space for soiled linen hampers and trash containers*
- *Door system that provides transparency and at least six feet of clear width.*

Easy and quick access to supplies is imperative to an efficient ICU. The consummate arrangement for efficiency would have all things the nurse needs in or at the patient room. However, the cost in space and inventory to attain that level is onerous. Therefore, the optimal ICU design has a three tier supply system. Tier I items are in each room—emesis basins, blood draw tubes, tape, tissues, wipes, etc. Tier II items—procedural trays, IV solutions, dressing, etc. are decentralized and replicated so that they are within just a few steps from any given patient room. Tier III items—those of infrequent use and the restock for Tier I and Tier II are located in a room(s) at the periphery of the unit.

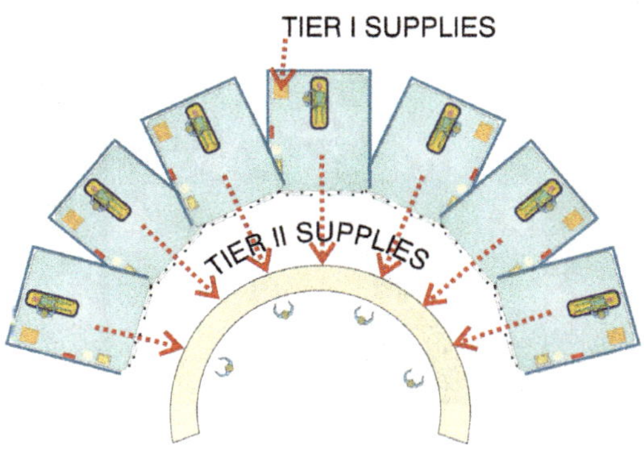

Figure 2

Data and communication networks together with mobile computers promote record keeping at and near the patient bedside. A caregiver (nurse) station in an alcove immediately outside of a bedroom or pair of bedrooms allows the nurse/physician a place for detailed charting while keeping a close eye on the patient. This decentralization of the charting tasks does not preclude a centralized area in which the many other tasks and encounters in the daily routine of ICU care ensue. This central area—Interdisciplinary Team Center (ITC)—is the locus where physicians, nurses, pharmacists, dietitians, respiratory therapists, case managers, and more, confer, mentor, and socialize. Unfettered computer access for charting, diagnostic results, and research should be included. Medicine preparation and nourishment stations should be located in this central area.

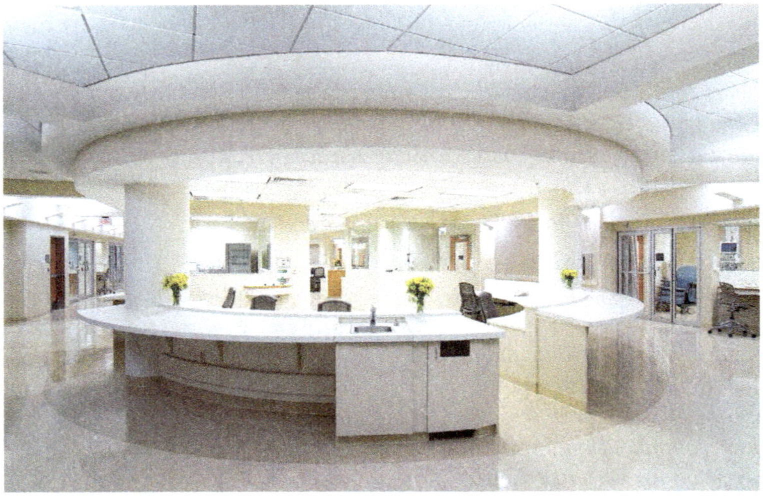

Figure 3

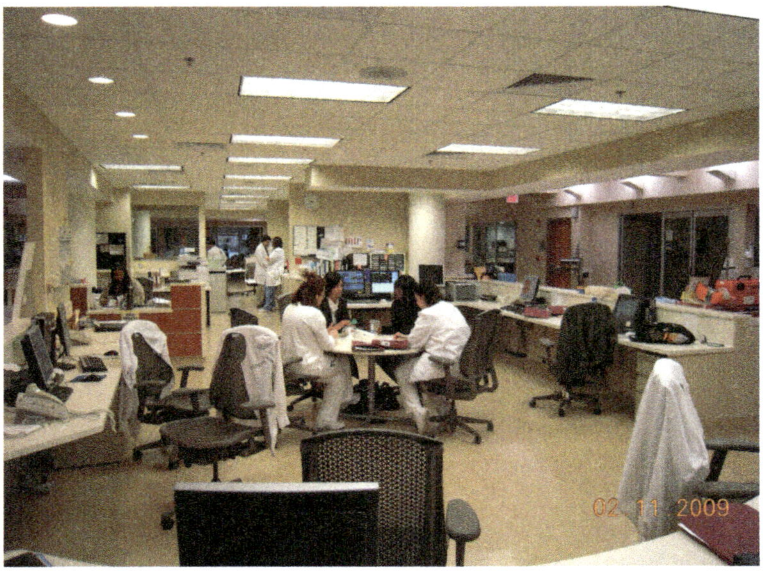

Figure 4

To make the ITC work in terms of patient safety as previously discussed, visualization of the patient rooms from anywhere within ITC should be possible. Therefore no solid walls above countertop height should exist on the sightlines to patient rooms. In the case of rooms that require acoustic isolation—medicine preparation, rooms with noisy equipment like ice-makers—transparent glass can be used.

As patient visualization and observation is the primary axiom for the architectural layout of the ICU, this aspect can be enhanced by elevating the floor of the ITC. Two risers, 14", is enough to allow staff seated at counters or desks across the corridor, opposite the patient rooms, to better see the patient lying in bed.

In the critical care environment, especially in teaching institutions, there is much activity in the corridors. Carts of all sizes and types, beds, and sundry equipment are found—in motion or parked—nearly constantly. Staff rounding with 6–10 people and computer carts can create a significant "clot" in the corridor. The code minimum corridor width of eight feet easily becomes congested with this bustle; therefore the optimal ICU has corridors 10 feet wide.

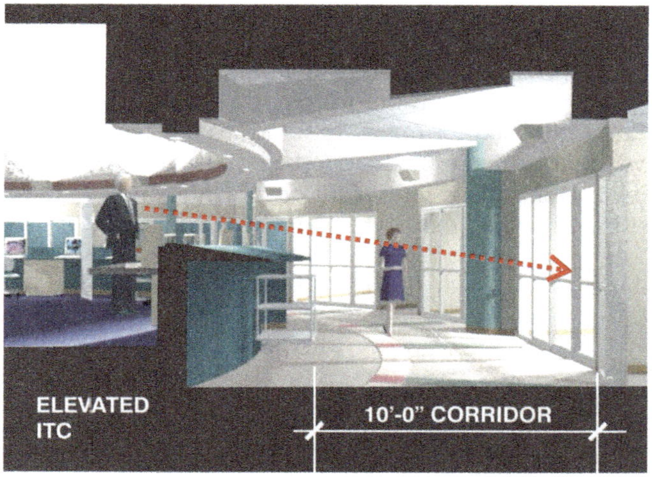

Figure 5

In addition to sufficient space and accommodation within the patient bed room, families need access to tend to basic needs. A common area for families to gather and gain respite from the patient's bedside is a fundamental requirement. Adjunct to this should be toilet and shower facilities. Food and beverage services should also be available at all times. These family amenities should be proximate to the ICU patient care areas.

James Harrell is design leader of Healthcare Group at GBBN Architects, Inc.

There is no single geometry that has proven to be superior to another (Hamilton, 1999). Efficient and effective critical care units that report good outcomes exist in the full range of known configurations. Issues such as observation, travel distance for nurses, location of frequently used supplies, placement of hand hygiene, and design for communication among the staff seem to be more important than geometric shape.

The trend toward decentralized nursing positions near a small number of beds, the wider use of electronic records and computerized hospital information systems, and the evolving technologies associated with remote monitoring in the virtual e-ICU, all suggest a diminishing need for observation and control from a single central position. It remains to be seen how the configuration of future critical care units will evolve under these changing conditions.

Centralized versus decentralized

In the past, critical care units have almost always been designed on the basis of a centralized model. The concept was to enable a high level of observation from a central position, usually described as a nurses' station. This central space was a location for the single paper record, patient monitors, workspace for nurses, medication preparation and dispensing, a unit clerk or secretary, the main telephone and communications center for the unit, and space for physician chart review and dictation. Each patient in a centralized design should be able to be seen from the central position, where physiological data from multiple patients is visible on monitors.

A sign of the need for an alternative to the totally centralized station is the frequency with which nurses establish an ad hoc solution to their charting requirements. At the bedside, nurses commonly use a scrap of paper, a Post-it note, or a uniform sleeve to record important information that must be entered into the chart, so as not to forget the data before they return to the central station. In order to reduce the need for nurses to return to the central station to record information, some nurses have appropriated an extra overbed table to locate the nurse's flow sheet just outside the patient room. Using these temporary documentation sites often becomes the "normal" procedure, as illustrated by the frequency with which such a table is accompanied by a chair.

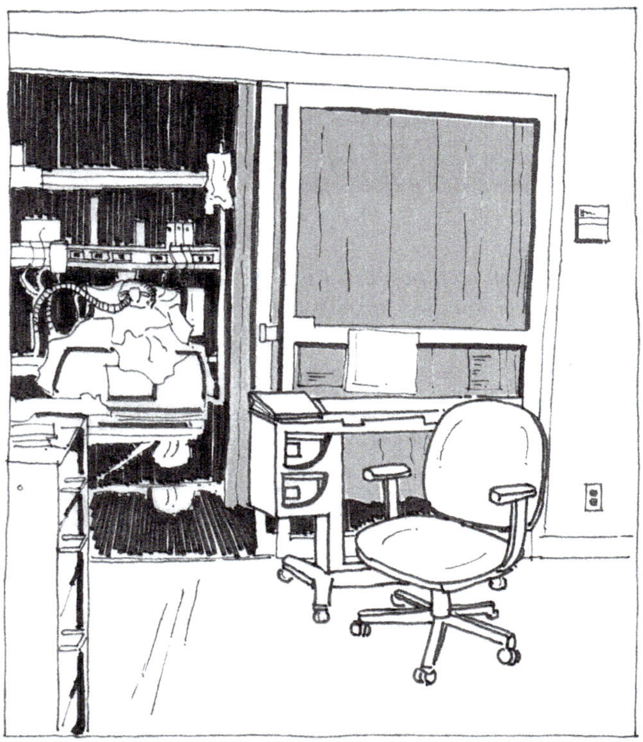

Figure 3.1: *Nurses adopt an overbed table for charting close to the patient when the design hasn't provided a convenient place for it*
Drawing: Diana Anderson

As the patient record has become more digitized, the necessity for a centralized unit design has diminished. An electronic record makes it increasingly possible for important information to be available in more than one location simultaneously. As the record becomes less committed to a single location, and as patient acuity increases, there is a growing trend toward decentralized positions for caregivers closer to the bedside.

These decentralized positions may range from a simple writing surface inside or just outside the patient room, to stations with observation windows into two rooms, to stations that serve clusters of four to six rooms. The intent of such a design is to move caregivers, along with items they use most often, closer to the patient and the bedside. The goal is to reduce the number of steps caregivers must take and to provide documentation capability as close as possible to where the data is gathered. An important element of a decentralized design is considering where hand hygiene stations should be located, which encourages compliance with guidelines, such as those offered by the Centers for Disease Control (CDC, 2002). Should hand hygiene be at a decentralized position outside the patient room doorway, or just inside the door to the patient room? In either location, it should be convenient to normal travel paths and within the caregiver's natural cone of vision.

A variation of decentralized documentation positions occurs with the use of mobile stations. A trend found in some critical care units is the adoption of computers on wheels, sometimes called COWs. These computers are mounted on the same sort of column with wheels that one would find on an IV pole or other rolling hospital equipment. They are supported by a battery that can be recharged when plugged into a wall receptacle. These rolling computers are useful for rounding by nurses, and have been teamed with medication carts or other portable devices. One of the physicians at Emory's new Neuro ICU uses a mobile rounding method which features wireless COWs for both hospital information and for digital images of brain studies. There are rolling stools and writing surfaces for the physicians, nurses, residents, and interdisciplinary team members as they move from patient to patient. Another colleague rounds using the decentralized positions outside the door to pairs of rooms and takes the large team to a conference room for discussions of cases.

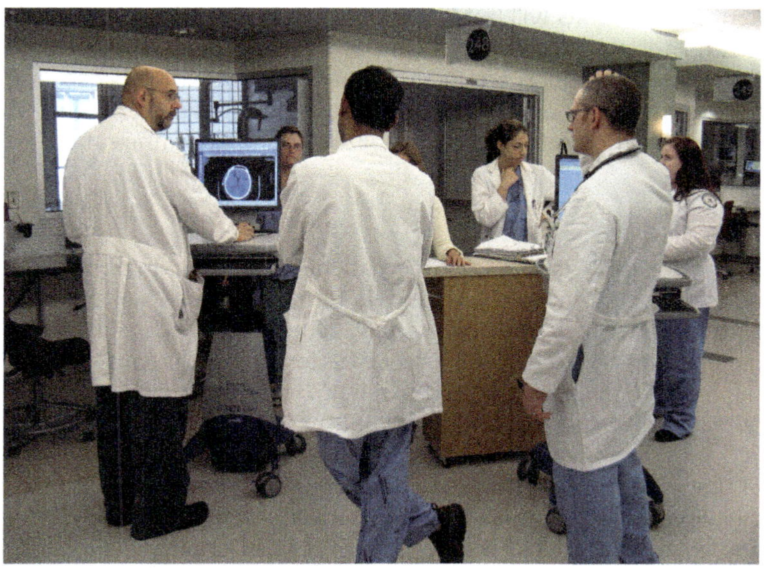

Figure 3.2: *Rounding with wireless computers on wheels Photo: Charles Cadenhead*

A further level of mobility will occur when routine nursing documentation can be performed on a hand-held computing device. The prospect of improved wireless connectivity suggests that nurses should be able to move from room to room, have data from physiologic monitors automatically download to the patient record, and be able to make notes along with simplified charting by exception. The authors have yet to see such a system in use but some nurses are looking forward to its arrival.

There are still relatively few examples of completely decentralized designs in which no observation occurs at a centralized location. There is an example at the Royal Alexandra Hospital in Edmonton, Alberta, Canada, by WSAG Architects. Another example is the medical ICU at The Methodist Hospital in Houston, Texas, designed by WHR Architects. There appear to be a growing number of units that explore this model.

Central stations have continued to be the most common configuration seen in critical care units, although a rapidly increasing number of unit designs feature a combination of centralized and decentralized elements. While decentralized positions move nurses, medications, documentation, and some supplies closer to the bedside, the central station continues to provide a location for staff interaction, socialization, and mentoring, as well as emotional support for individuals involved in highly stressful tasks.

In spite of the advantages offered by moving caregivers and items for their immediate support closer to the patient bedside, there appear to be important reasons to continue to design for some centralized activities on the unit. In addition to staff interaction, socialization, and mentoring, a central location can be home for the core activities of a unit clerk or secretary, along with telephone answering for the unit and monitoring of the nurse-call or intercom functions. A central station can provide space for the many medical professionals who need to work on the unit but who are not housed there, such as pharmacists, therapists, dieticians, social workers, chaplains, record coders, and numerous others.

The users and designers of new critical care units will not likely anguish over the decision to centralize or decentralize workstations for the interdisciplinary team, as neither model seems to provide for all the needs of the team. These individuals are most likely to spend their time deciding what features to include in either or both types of locations. The best practice answer seems to point to a blended model which optimizes the best of both centralization and decentralization.

Specialized versus general units

Some critical care units are organized to serve segments of the patient population, matching the specialized training of physicians and staff. Others are organized to accommodate all types of critical patients. A small community hospital may have only a few general critical care beds in a unit managed by nurses, with patient care directed by a variety of attending physicians. On the other end of the scale, a very large academic medical center might have many distinct critical care units run by interdisciplinary teams led by specially trained intensivists.

The case for designing a general unit is most often made on the basis of economy of resources. Smaller organizations may not have the particular staff to carve out a specialized unit from the overall critical care patient population. A smaller facility may not have enough patients to justify either multiple critical care units or physicians prepared to dedicate themselves to a single specialty.

A specialized unit must be justified on the basis of having a consistent volume of patients within a specialty, enough to support an efficient and effective use of staff and equipment. The unit must also have an interdisciplinary group of clinicians with the unique and complementary skills to work in a dedicated unit; such a unit should exhibit improved outcomes over the care that would be delivered in a general, undifferentiated setting.

In practice, a cardiac unit is usually the first specialized unit to be developed from a general ICU. The next most likely division appears to be between medical and surgical critical care. Thus, the first three specialized units observed might be a medical, surgical, and a cardiac unit. A typical allocation of four units might further subdivide the cardiac care unit, resulting in the following groups: surgical ICU, medical ICU, cardiovascular (surgical) ICU, and a coronary (medical) care unit.

	Surgical Model	*Medical Model*
Cardiac patients	CV ICU	CCU
Non-Cardiac patients	SICU	MICU

Once the four basic units have been developed, further specialties may arise in which patient volumes and dedicated clinician support are present. The medical and surgical differences may continue to be present, as with a neurological ICU (medical) and a neurosurgery ICU (surgical). Other differences may be seen with severity (e.g. trauma ICU versus intermediate care) or population (e.g. pediatric ICU, neonatal ICU). The availability of clinical specialists and the potential volume of patients drive decisions to develop highly specialized units such as a respiratory ICU, a burn unit, or a transplant unit.

Innovative ICUs

Joan Saba, AIA, FACHA and Sarah Markovitz, AIA

Spending time in a hospital can be a sensitive experience for both patients and their families. To make the experience less taxing, the new intensive care unit at Massachusetts General Hospital includes several design features that increase comfort and emphasize compassion.

Whereas the hospital's Neuroscience Department was formerly spread across the medical campus, the new Building for the Third Century merges them into a single location and serves as one of the hospital's premier Centers of Excellence. The consolidation will increase staff efficiency and enable multidisciplinary care teams to provide the best care to ICU patients.

In many hospitals, patients must be taken to different floors for diagnostic imaging. Mass General's Neuro ICU includes its own MRI and PET/CT suite within the department. For continuity of care, a nurse will accompany patients to the suite and remain with them until the test is complete.

Patient rooms within the Neuro ICU utilize state-of-the-art ceiling-mounted booms that, unlike traditional headwalls, give greater flexibility, allow for the better positioning of medical teams around the bed, and provide places to plug in new technology. The ceiling booms also accommodate advanced mobile medical equipment that enables imaging and diagnostic testing in the patient room. Computers were placed bedside to make it possible for nurses to document and access information on the spot.

The combination of precise programmatic planning and rapid advancements in medical technology has made it possible to perform many of the ICU's tests and examinations bedside. By reducing the number of transfers of information and handing off of responsibilities between caregivers, staff efficiency is increased and the risk of further injury to the patient is prevented. Since there are instances when the patient must be moved, ceiling lift tracks in each patient room assist with the safe transferring of patients between beds and stretchers.

All 22 of the ICU's patient rooms are private and include dedicated space for family members so they can remain near the patient. To provide patients with access to natural light and a continuous connection with the outdoors, each room includes full-height glass walls. A lounge within the ICU provides a respite for family members and doubles as a private consult room where they can meet with caregivers to discuss medical decisions.

While the design of Massachusetts General Hospital's intensive care unit successfully utilizes state-of-the-art technology, it does not compromise on maintaining a patient-centered focus. The department's flexible design and efficient layout will provide patients and their families with a comfortable place to focus on their top priority—healing.

Joan Saba, AIA, FACHA, is a partner at NBBJ. Sarah Markovitz, AIA, is a senior associate at NBBJ.

Patient flow and the ICU

The flow of patients into and out of the critical care unit becomes a factor in design. If it is physically or operationally difficult to discharge patients from critical care to environments of lower acuity, such as stepdown beds, acute units, skilled nursing facilities, or rehabilitation settings, then the length of stay will increase for other than clinical reasons. Such increases may constrain admissions to critical care, as having fully occupied beds in a critical care unit reduces a unit's ability to accept new patients from the emergency department, surgery, or other interventional procedures such as catheterization.

The Institute for Healthcare Improvement (IHI) has conducted important research on patient flow through the efforts of a collaborative among hospitals that are interested in the problem (Haraden & Resar, 2004). The first lesson is that critical care units cannot be viewed and planned in isolation. The upstream sources of critical patient admissions must be considered, along with the downstream avenues for their discharge.

Transfers to stepdown and acute beds

In order to maintain a steady flow of patients out of the ICU, some other beds in the organization must be prepared to accept patients who need to be discharged from a critical care unit. A typical practice is to provide another unit, given a variety of designations such as "stepdown," "progressive care," "TCU," "IMU," or "intermediate care," that receives patients who have been discharged from intensive care but who are not ready for an acute unit or for discharge from the hospital. In some cases, such a unit may be within a similar specialty as the intensive care unit, as in the case of a cardiac intensive care unit associated with a dedicated cardiac stepdown unit that features telemetry for cardiac monitoring. Patients discharged from stepdown care are generally moved to an acute medical/surgical unit or are discharged directly home. Some have advocated simplifying this prevailing three-step model to provide only two levels of care (Harvey, 2000).

Standardization and safety

Examination of high-reliability organizations, such as nuclear power plants, and tasks, such as aircraft operations, suggests that safety is enhanced by standardization and the development of redundant or overlapping systems to prevent failures. Some in the field have proposed that single-handed rooms, described below, will produce safer conditions and fewer errors (Reiling, 2005).

The Saperstein Critical Care Tower, designed by Langdon Wilson, at Cedars-Sinai in Los Angeles, California, features single-handed rooms. In these rooms, the head of the bed is placed against the outside wall, providing excellent patient observation from the corridor and decentralized charting positions near the door. The window brings in daylight from behind the patient. Each room is laid out in precisely the same arrangement, in order to reduce any possible confusion in a crisis.

The e-ICU model

A growing number of critical care units are adopting an electronic model for critical care in which there is an electronic connection of both the unit and the patient to a central electronic monitoring location that can be physically separated from the unit. The more robust examples include access to intensivists, specialty-certified critical care nurses, pharmacists, and respiratory therapists. These models offer the ability to remotely monitor patient conditions, providing early intervention and specialty advice to the onsite caregivers (Breslow et al., 2004).

The Sentara Health System in Virginia and the Memorial Hermann Healthcare System in Texas have been early adopters of the e-ICU model. Other systems, such as Intermountain Health Care (IHC), have long used electronic connections to provide remote monitoring, remote reading of digital imaging, and telemedicine consultation. IHC has connections between the central resources in Salt Lake City and multiple critical care units in Utah and Wyoming.

3.3 Design for an uncertain future

Management prizes flexibility because it appears to offer the prospect of fewer and less frequent facility changes that might result in financial savings. Clinicians prize flexibility because their experience tells them that advances in clinical practice will lead to inevitable changes in protocols, equipment, and best practices. Flexibility is desired to allow for a new and superior clinical response, as soon as evidence indicates a change can be justified. Architects are asked to deliver increased flexibility in their designs, but flexibility has a cost. Flexibility is purchased with additional electrical capacity, routing of utilities that anticipate future needs, and structural capacity, just to name a few types of expenditures associated with flexible designs.

Design with generic parameters

One concept for flexibility is the execution of "loose fit" design. This is based on the recognition that a high percentage of spaces can be accommodated within 150 square feet, so nearly all rooms might be constructed at that size, in spite of known initial requirements for many rooms that do not need more than 100 or 120 square feet. In the future, these rooms can easily be converted to new uses, without concern for some which might have been too small for their second or third role. Similarly, a loose fit design is generous in its arrangements for utility distribution and public circulation, allowing for future construction projects to plug into these main systems, and to be configured in fairly standardized blocks of space that might suit multiple types of departmental occupants if required. In the context of a critical care unit, loose fit design might mean planning for oversized rooms of all sorts to accommodate unknown future uses. It might mean wider than normal corridors, and would certainly mean a robust utility distribution system with some level of redundancy.

On the other hand, clinicians also want a space that performs perfectly for its intended purpose, with no waste or excess. They desire ergonomic simplicity, economy of motion and design characteristics that are totally supportive of the equipment and technology. The design for a room that will contain a basic radiographic machine cannot be the same as that for a biplane catheterization lab, and the physicians who work in these spaces will have different demands for items that make their work effective and efficient. Similarly, the requirements for a critical care patient room may be quite different from those for a pediatric acute care room.

In recent years, designs have consisted largely of "tight-fit" or less flexible plans for money-conscious administrative decision-makers who want to deliver the absolute minimum possible area and lowest cost for building materials in an effort to tightly trim the capital costs of projects. Such idiosyncratic custom designs with precise minimum specifications suffer from more rapid obsolescence and are less prone to successful conversion to other uses. A suggestion for a best practice in the future might be to strike a better balance between design aspects that fully support future flexibility and aspects that serve important current requirements.

Another aspect of appropriate design is the search by the clinician users and the design team for technology that is properly supportive of the unit's goals. There are numerous examples of designs that have employed technologies with unneeded features at unnecessary cost.

High technology innovations in ICU design

Neil A. Halpern, M.D.

The intensive care unit (ICU) at Memorial Sloan-Kettering Cancer Center won the 2009 ICU Design Citation Award co-sponsored by the Society of Critical Care Medicine (SCCM), American Institute of Architects Academy of Architecture for Health (AIA) and the American Association of Critical Care Nurses (AACN). Here we explore some of the "high-tech" design innovations that were included in this ICU.

Telemedicine is a code word in the critical care world for advanced remote monitoring of an ICU by an outside vendor. We developed an in-house telemedicine system so our ICU attending physicians could view all patient data from any mobile location, nurses could visualize their "second" patient, and the critical care medicine (CCM) teams could employ comprehensive conferencing that encompasses every element of the ICU patient. Such systems rely upon a robust infrastructure of wired and wireless networking, as well as web-enabled software and servers.

The essential components of an ICU room include the bedside physiological monitor, mechanical ventilator, and infusion pumps. Viewing of these devices usually occurs directly at the bedside excepting for the monitor whose data can also be viewed at a central station. To enable remote viewing of the bedside physiological monitor and mechanical ventilator, we installed web-servers. Adding the web-server to the monitoring system was simple, as the monitors are already on their own network.

Ventilators, however, are usually not part of an existing network. Thus, transmitters (wired and wireless) were placed on each ventilator to connect the ventilators to the hospital network. Once the web-enabled ventilator management server was added to the hospital network, the ventilators could then be visualized on the ventilator website. The ventilator server also performs other tasks, including the broadcast of alarms to assigned providers and storage of ventilator data (settings and alarms).

Our ICU is using the "smart" infusion pumps. While these devices have uni- or bi-directional wireless capabilities and are connected to the hospital network, the pump server is not web-enabled for remote viewing. However, the wireless infusion pump connectivity is used to transmit medication library updates to the pumps and alerts and quality control data from the pumps. Direct visualization of the pumps on the web is not yet an option available from most pump vendors.

After configuring remote monitoring of bedside devices, we addressed direct visualization of the ICU patient by equipping each ICU room with a ceiling-based webcam. These digital video cameras are connected to the hospital network and a web-enabled webcam server. The cameras feature pan, tilt, zoom (PTZ) and audio capabilities. Image recording is continuous and data is stored for 72 hours in the webcam server. The webcams are viewed only through secure access and can be controlled remotely as well.

The myriad of devices and systems at the ICU bedside (bedside computers, physiologic monitors, mechanical ventilators, webcams, infusion pumps, etc.) are time stamped individually, or through a server. The times on each of these, however, may or may not be synchronized. Time dyssynchrony creates challenges to the formatting of cohesive medical records (paper or electronic) and to the performance of quality control reviews of difficult ICU cases. Bedside computers are usually time synchronized to a central Network Time Protocol (NTP) server. In our ICU we have attempted to link bedside devices to the NTP server as well. Wall clocks, however, are commonly battery operated and adjusted by the bedside teams. We addressed this problem by installing wireless clocks linked to a clock web-server synchronized to the NTP server. Similarly, the servers of the ventilator monitoring system, the infusion pumps, and the webcams are all time synchronized to the NTP server. Time synchronization of the physiologic bedside monitors has posed greater challenges for us, but is possible through placement of a gateway server on the monitoring network.

Viewing multiple hospital and ICU systems simultaneously in search of obtaining a comprehensive picture of the patient is particularly vexing. The most efficient solution is to install a "dashboard" system. The dashboard technology simultaneously launches and displays multiple elements of the patient's record (e.g., laboratory values, radiology, EKG, medications list, bedside physiological monitoring, ventilator monitoring and webcam systems) without the user having to access each individual system. However, dashboard software is expensive and difficult to install and maintain. We chose an alternative approach and constructed a multimedia center that permits four PCs, each selected to portray a different system of the same patient, to transmit images through a high definition projector. Thus, in a less sophisticated and costly approach than the dashboard, we are able to view up to four images at once and the projection system permits multiple types of viewing arrangements (from one to four images).

Rapid communication in the ICU, especially in a physically large unit with multiple teams and staff members, may be an issue. Commonly pagers, overhead speakers, and in-room wall-mounted communication systems are used. These traditional systems may be slow and also create unwanted noise in an environment that requires quiet and calm. We installed a VoIP (Voice over Internet Protocol) system that transmits its signals through the hospital's Wi-Fi network. Each staff member wears a bidirectional communicating badge that enables direct and immediate person-to-person or person-to-group communications.

Privacy and cleanliness are also major concerns of ICU patient rooms. Traditionally, curtains or blinds (embedded within double pane glass windows or doors) are usually used to provide privacy. However, curtains are bulky, take up space and are easily stained. Blinds may malfunction and must be individually adjusted by window pane or door to provide privacy. Thus, in our ICU, we used a different approach to privacy and installed electric glass (E-glass) otherwise known as privacy glass. E-glass is composed of two outer layers of glass surrounding an inner layer of liquid crystal film that is electrically energized. Controls for the E-glass were placed within the ICU room so that the bedside staff can control the system. Housekeepers clean the E-glass in a manner similar to all other glass.

In conclusion, we have taken off-the-shelf "high" tech solutions and applied them to our ICU to achieve our goals of in-house telemedicine, time synchronization, sophisticated conferencing, enhanced communications, and patient privacy.

Neil A. Halpern M.D. is the Chief of the Critical Care Medicine Service and Medical Director of Respiratory Therapy at Memorial Sloan-Kettering Cancer Center in New York. He is a Professor of Medicine and Anesthesiology at the Weill Medical College of Cornell University in New York City. The ICU at Memorial Sloan-Kettering Cancer Center was the winner of the 2009 Society of Critical Care Medicine National ICU Design Citation.

Design for flexibility

Webster defines *flexible* as "adjustable to change" or "capable of modification" (Merriam-Webster, 2005). In the case of hospital construction, there are two types of flexibility: adaptable flexibility and convertible flexibility.

Adaptable flexibility is the ability to accommodate changing conditions without any change in the environment itself. The environment is adaptable to the new requirements. This type of flexibility matches Webster's "adjustable to change."

The ability to accommodate a change after a simple and/or inexpensive physical alteration is *convertible flexibility*. The environment is converted to the new purpose without drastic cost, effort, or time. This type of flexibility is illustrative of Webster's "capable of modification."

When change can be accommodated at a lower cost of time, money, or human resources, such change is more palatable in a time of significant financial constraints. A hospital's census and patient mix can be expected to fluctuate frequently and significantly. The world of medicine and science marches relentlessly forward in a constant process of change based on evolving knowledge. Facilities that can quickly adapt to these changes are better positioned, both now and in the future.

Reversible convertibility between acute and critical care

James Diaz, FAIA, FACHA, and Lari Maria Diaz, AIA

Exemplary flexibility to convert all beds, units and floors from acute to critical care (and vice-versa), innovative planning concepts and principles of evidence-based design (EBD) are hallmarks of a proposed new bed tower for Hoag Memorial Hospital in Newport Beach, California.

Building elements

A 96-bed tower designed by Kaplan McLaughlin Diaz (KMD) sits upon a podium of four levels: two with interventional platforms for heart and vascular procedures and general surgery, a ground floor having a lobby, outpatient cardiology services and central processing, and an intermediate level for mechanical equipment to serve the lower floors, education facilities and access to a rooftop garden.

Podium levels feature a central zone (free of elevator shafts and stairs) for maximum planning flexibility, with interchangeable "boxes" or modules of 750 square feet to accommodate large operating rooms, catheterization labs and procedure rooms requiring contiguous control/observation rooms, space for large equipment and ample electrical/IT rooms. Shelled space has been provided for future technologies such as MRI assisted surgical procedures.

Inpatient care floor design

Four identical inpatient care floors of 24 beds are planned for maximum operational flexibility, with three units of eight beds each that may be converted, one at a time, from acute to critical care (or back to acute care), in accordance with California Licensing Statutes that do not allow the intermixing of the two levels of care on an individual bed basis.

In order to ensure a quiet and calm environment within patient care space (EBD), floors are designed to separate visitor circulation from staff, support and service movement, as well as to minimize the travel of visitors within individual units, past occupied patient rooms. Dedicated sub-corridors allow for medications, supplies, equipment, food and trash to be delivered or removed without traversing patient care corridors. They also allow for staff movement to and from lockers, lounges, toilets and satellite pharmacies, as well as to and from report, office, on-call, physician dictation and staff conference rooms away from visitor areas. Ample staff amenities will contribute to improved staff attraction and retention.

Nursing staff decided against decentralized charting at patient room entrances in favor of a continuous nurse station ensuring unobstructed views into several patient bedrooms from any point along the continuum. Portable devices will allow for bedside charting within patient bedrooms.

Unit clerk workstations are provided at visitor entrances to each eight-bed unit. Visitors are greeted as they enter the floor, and space is provided for family consultation and waiting. The staff lounge, elevator lobbies, the ends of principal corridors and private waiting areas for families all have access to views and natural light.

Such unprecedented operational flexibility, reversible convertibility between acute and critical care for every patient bed, eight-bed unit and floor, dedicated staff circulation, decentralized support services, ample staff and visitor amenities, access to views and natural light, as well as the need for three elevator banks (to allow access from two hospital entrances) create a 24-bed floor of 32 000 gross square feet—substantially larger than floors without such features.

Acuity-adaptable inpatient care rooms

Planned within a 30 foot building module, every patient care room meets or exceeds new AIA minimum requirements for critical care and is provided with a full toilet and shower room to meet standards for acute care as well. Larger than code minimum rooms accessible to the handicapped and patient isolation rooms are provided within each eight-bed unit.

Patient Room Standardization (or "same-handedness") was adopted in the belief that patient care will improve over time through reductions of staff errors. Contributing features to such improved care include the ability for physicians to most directly approach the right-hand side of every patient and uniformity in the location of gases, outlets, monitors and dialysis equipment.

Outboard patient toilet rooms at the periphery of the building improve patient observation from the inboard corridor. Also, they are slightly offset to minimize distance and simplify patient transfers from the bed to the toilet room, along the headwall, with a continuous handrail for patient safety.

After careful evaluation using a fully developed mock-up patient room, staff opted not to install ceiling-mounted patient lifts and selected a standard, surface-mounted patient headwall assembly at both sides of the head. Great attention was placed upon creating a family alcove for sitting as well as sleeping, alongside the very large window to the exterior.

Patient bathrooms have integral showers to conserve space and optimize access to the toilet, lavatory and shower seat so as to improve staff assistance and staff safety. Floor-mounted toilets simplify maintenance and better support the weight of obese patients than do wall-hung fixtures.

Additional advantages of "same-handed" rooms include improved acoustics, by eliminating back-to-back gas and electrical outlets within a common wall, and simplified construction without the need to stagger outlets in mirrored rooms. KMD has concluded that the advantages of standardized details, construction assemblies, and repetitive construction accrue substantial economies, offsetting the cost of an additional plumbing stack for each pair of bedrooms.

The resulting patient care floor design meets or exceeds the planning team's goals for:

1. *patient- and family-centered care*
2. *efficient and effective patient care*
3. *operational flexibility through convertibility between acute and critical care*
4. *enhanced staff and patient safety, and*
5. *better staff productivity attraction, retention and well-being.*

James Diaz and Lari Maria Diaz are Planning Directors with KMD ARCHITECTS.

An example of adaptable flexibility in a critical care patient room is a plan for a somewhat larger space to accommodate the equipment needed to perform procedures such as line insertions. No change is required to adapt to a new, temporary, or occasional use. The adaptable flexibility that allows a patient room to temporarily become a procedure room means the room must accommodate technology, such as the imaging capability provided by mobile C-arm fluoroscopy, along with carts for supplies, instruments, and devices specific to the intended procedure. It must also have appropriate filtration and volumes of fresh air as one means of protecting the patient from infection.

An example of convertible flexibility for critical care might be the progressive care units at CHRISTUS St. Michael Health Center in Texarkana, Texas, located one floor above the ICUs. These units follow the same geometry as the ICUs on the floor below and have been designed to convert to an ICU after a relatively simple addition of gas outlets and power from pre-plumbed and wired systems already installed behind the wall in each patient room. This planning permits an inexpensive conversion to a higher acuity intensive care unit at any time in the future.

Shell space for future buildout, and identified growth zones as part of a master plan for expansion, are both examples of convertible flexibility. Planning for additional future capacity in power systems, extra conduits for future wiring, bandwidth that exceeds current requirements in a fiberoptic network, or larger diameter piping that will support future utility needs are other types of flexibility choices.

Design for unique circumstances

Custom design in the patient room can be seen in the burn ICU designed by James Harrell for the University of Cincinnati, which features a concrete step across the headwall. This fixed, or non-flexible, element serves as a raised step for the respiratory therapist to reach over the headboard for access to the patient's head and airway, and it also serves as a bed-positioning device. Such a design is useful because it makes it easier for medical personnel to reach the critical work area. This permanent feature suits the current requirement perfectly but would be very difficult to change.

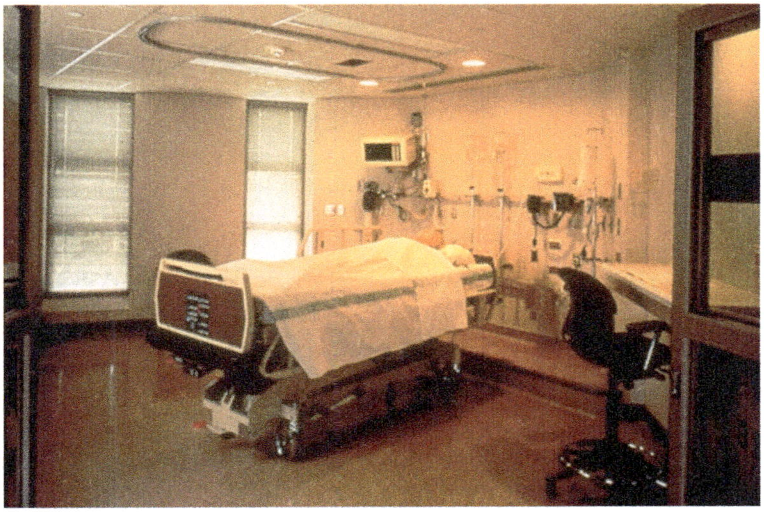

Figure 3.3: *Custom raised step on headwall for access to airway Location: Burn Intensive Care Unit, University of Cincinnati, OH Photo: Kirk Hamilton*

The need for clinicians to have spaces that perform perfectly for their intended purpose, with no waste or excess, has been mentioned. A good design for unique circumstances will be precisely suited to the required equipment and technology. A good custom design will be especially efficient for the work process that occurs in each space. Physicians and staff who work in these spaces will have the exact supportive elements that will allow them to be most effective and efficient in their jobs.

The designers for each critical care project should consciously choose components that suit the unique, adaptable, or convertible requirements of the design. Each of these decisions will have an associated first cost, a likelihood of continued functionality, and a future cost and time associated with any subsequent changes.

Design of patient and family spaces

4

Within the unit, the zone that houses the critical care patient is crucial to delivery of quality care. This is where the patient spends the vast majority of their stay on the unit, and where a significant majority of their care is delivered.

4.1 The patient environment

Design for delivery of care

Patients requiring an intensive level of care are grouped into units where teams of specially trained clinicians can be instantly available and can have access to the appropriate technology. The location where such intense delivery of care takes place is nearly always in the patient's room.

Design for safety

Patient safety is a fundamental goal of all critical care units, and the patient environment is a prime location where harm or adverse events may occur. The design of these environments should, therefore, insofar as possible, contribute directly to reduction of infection, error, and injury.

Similarly, most staff injuries also occur in the patient environment. Nurses experience more workplace injuries than construction workers (Evanoff et al., 2003). The patient environment must also be designed to reduce the chance of injury to the staff involved in delivering patient care (Clarke, Sloane & Aiken, 2002; Retsas & Pinikahana, 2008).

Design for comfort and emotional support

An environment support of the patient and the recovery process will offer the maximum possible comfort, while recognizing that the clinical interventions and treatment plan may involve significant discomfort. At the same time, the emotional distress that accompanies a stay in critical care may be partially alleviated by the support of caring staff and the patient's family and loved ones.

4.2 The patient room

The patient room may be the most important space in the critical care unit. It is the location at which the bulk of care is provided. The design of the patient room is repeated multiple times within each unit.

Number of beds in a room

A long-standing issue associated with patient room design is the question of bed quantities. Critical care began in the tradition of the surgical post anesthesia recovery room, an open bay containing multiple beds. Critical care units most often were based on this open bay model in which multiple patients could be observed simultaneously, allowing caregivers to rapidly support each other as they cared for a group of patients. Over time, some patient populations, notably post infarction coronary care patients, seemed to be better served in a more private environment. The prevailing logic seemed to be that patients who were awake and aware were suited to higher levels of privacy, and the most severe cases, especially those who might be unconscious, were suited to open settings with multiple beds.

Barbara Heulat tells a story about her friend Joe in her book, *Healing Environments* (2003). A routine stress test raised questions which sent Joe to a cardiologist for an angiogram. The procedure resulted in the placement of stents and he was kept overnight at a superb medical facility. Although he received excellent and appropriate treatment for his medical condition, he found himself in a semi-private room with a terminally ill man. Joe and his wife were only separated by a thin curtain from the unconscious man, and as he rasped and gasped for breath, they "found themselves on a deathwatch for a stranger" (Heulat, 2003, p. 4). The wife left after visiting hours and Joe, alone, experienced uncontrollable stress from worries about his roommate, noise on the unit, and his own condition. During the night his roommate passed away, and the stress continued as the grief-stricken family arrived and the body was removed. Joe was administered medication to control his blood pressure and the nurses noted his unexpectedly high readings. Heulat asks pointedly whether Joe, who had received the best clinical care available, had been exposed to a healing environment. She says that although the care was appropriate, healing could not begin until Joe left the hospital.

A trend toward providing private rooms in critical care units has continued to evolve in the United States. Some of this trend can be attributed to clinical preferences for the separation of patients, some to the need to protect patients from nosocomial or hospital-acquired infections, and some to the perception of consumer preference for private environments. Given this trend, the majority of critical care beds in the United States are now housed in private rooms or individual open-fronted cubicles separated by walls or glass. The exceptions continue to include units such as surgical ICUs and trauma units, along with other units in which aggressive care and highly interventional treatment protocols are found.

European countries and most of the rest of the world continue to have many, if not most, critical care beds in open wards of various sizes. The benefits include the ability for a smaller number of specially trained physicians and staff to care for larger numbers of patients. There is an economy of capital cost, as open units require somewhat less space and feature fewer walls, doors, and other physical elements. Opinion in much of the world seems to suggest that the North American model with a high percentage of private rooms was unnecessary, extravagant, and wasteful of valuable resources. Practitioners in most other countries felt that the single room was an example of material excess and an American compulsion for personal privacy.

Research in the last decade has begun to explore the issue of the single patient room. The 2004 study by Chaudhury, Mahmood & Valente for the Coalition for Health Environments Research (CHER) found that the provision of single-bedded rooms has become an issue of safety (Chaudhury et al., 2004, 2006). The 2004 metastudy by Ulrich et al. for the Center for Health Design and the

Robert Wood Johnson Foundation, along with its 2008 update (Ulrich, Zimring, Quan & Joseph, 2004 and 2008), draws the conclusion that the provision of a single-bedded room is no longer a decision for cultural or individual preferences, but is rather an important patient safety issue.

European hospitals have begun to record difficulties with the spread of infection. Outbreaks of resistant strains, such as the methycillin-resistant staphylococcus auraeus (MRSA) virus in the United Kingdom, have begun to provide pointed examples of the case now being made for providing private rooms as a safety issue (Johnson, Pearson & Duckworth, 2005). It is difficult to properly disinfect a multi-bed patient room when someone is discharged or deceased and the other occupant or occupants remain. It is nearly impossible to keep the contact transmission of infectious organisms from virtually any object in the room, such as the IV pump, sheets, bedrails, telephone, overbed table, cubicle curtain, sharps disposal box, computer keyboard, or door handle, just to name a few. These contaminated objects can become the source of infection for another patient, even in cases in which hand hygiene is carefully performed and the same nurse or caregiver is not assigned to the second patient. A casual moment in which a lab coat contacts the same chair that another nurse has touched may be the path for a resistant organism to pass to a new patient. There has been publicity about institutions which have banned the physician's necktie for reasons of infection control.

Florence Nightingale may not have had access to today's science, but she knew that patient health required physical separation, fresh air, and scrupulous cleanliness. Her designs for hospital wards 150 years ago separated patients by physical dimensions not previously respected, and her regimen of well-scrubbed nurses who kept the patients in clean linens made great strides in dramatically improved care (Nightingale, 1859, 1863). If she had access to the current data on infection, resistant organisms, and airborne and contact transmission, as well as knowledge of the available contemporary technology for filtered air and decontamination, she would surely campaign for highly separated (or private) conditions for critical care beds.

Room size

Despite the miniaturization of some equipment components and the integration of information system components with various electronic devices, it appears that optimum patient room sizes could continue to increase (Cadenhead, 2005). Larger room sizes seem to be a result of increasing patient acuity which brings with it more equipment, an increase in the number of diagnostic studies and therapeutic interventions in the room, and the increasing provision of space to accommodate the family's presence in the patient environment. On the other hand, no one likes to hear that more square footage, with its accompanying cost, will be needed.

The 1996 version of the American Institute of Architects' *Guidelines for Design and Construction of Health Care Facilities* required a minimum size of 150 square feet (approximately 13.9 square meters) for a critical care room, with no dimension less than 12 feet clear of any obstruction (about 3.65 m). This minimum standard is clearly inadequate for the ICU of today, much less for the high-tech ICU of tomorrow. The 2006 edition approved a minimum size of 200 square feet clear or 18.58 square meters, with a minimum headwall width of 13 feet per bed or 3.96 m (Facility Guidelines Institute, 2006).

The task force preparing a new edition of the *SCCM ICU Design Guidelines* makes the point that the AIA *Guidelines* (FGI, 2006) are based on a minimum standard to be enforced by the authorities having jurisdiction (AHJ) in most states. The SCCM task force believes that an optimum design would most likely exceed the prescriptive minimum standard and has suggested the use of a performance standard.

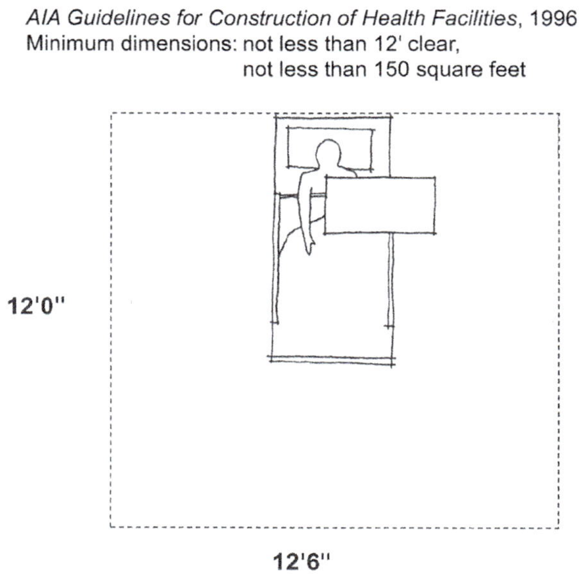

Figure 4.1: *Patient room dimension drawings*

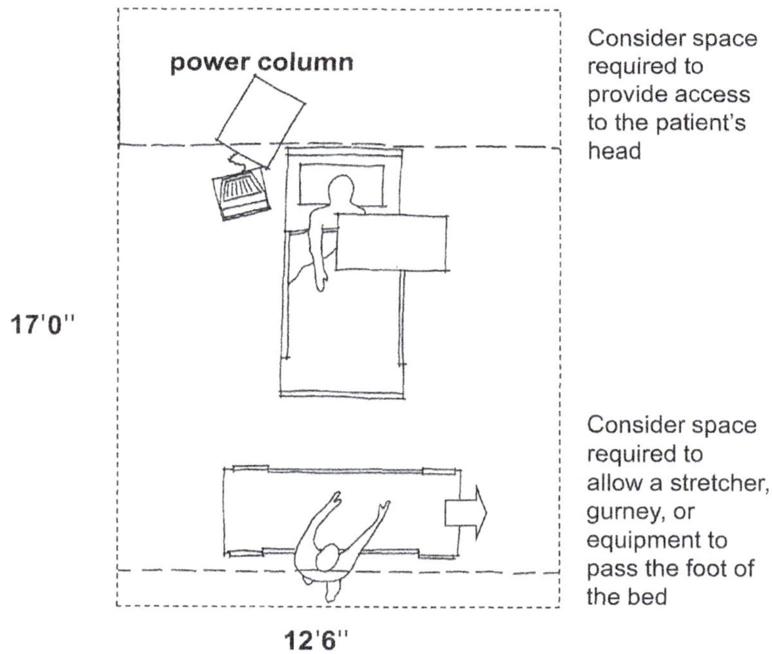

Figure 4.2: *Patient room dimension drawings*

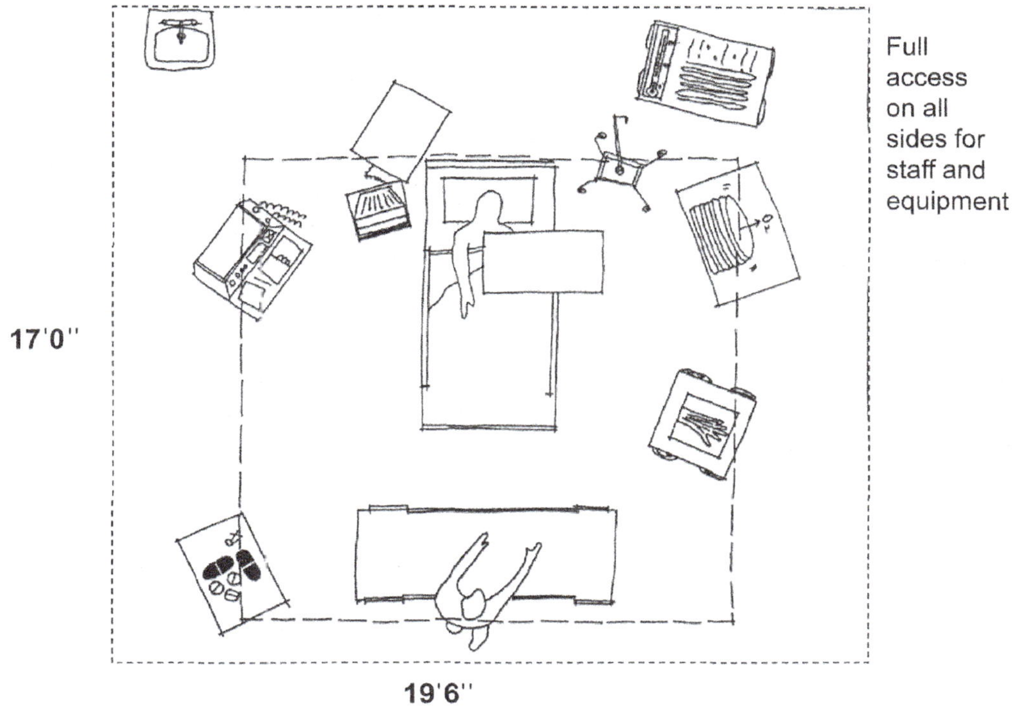

Figure 4.3: *Patient room dimension drawings*

Performance standards

Consideration of a *performance* standard for the patient room size requires a review of the real needs within the room. The ability to readily move equipment past the foot of the bed requires a head-to-foot dimension along the lines of 15 feet (about 4.55 m), given today's typical ICU bed dimensions. This should suffice for a headwall design in which the head of the bed is positioned against the wall and life support systems are accessed from the wall. In the case of planning for a power column design, or to provide continuous access to the patient's head, the head-to-foot dimension for the room becomes 17 feet (4.75 m). Providing access for staff and equipment in the work zone on both sides of the bed would call for a width of as much as 19 feet 6 inches (5.95 m). A room of this size has an area of about 330 square feet or 30.58 square meters, considerably larger than the regulatory minimums and significantly larger than the typical room size today. These dimensions would increase if the size of the typical critical care bed should increase in order to add technical features or to serve bariatric patients, for example. These dimensions could also increase if an area is devoted to accommodating the family in the patient's room, or if the caregiver is given a work zone inside the room.

The modern ICU patient room requires working space for staff on all sides of a larger critical care bed, which is likely to be surrounded by more equipment than ever before. Allowing for equipment and the movement of staff around the room is necessary for efficiency and can be vitally important in a crisis. A larger interdisciplinary team requires space in order to work effectively, especially during a crisis. In some ICU models, the normal nursing support functions and certain high-use supplies are accommodated within the room. In addition, there is a clear trend to provide space to accommodate family within the patient room without creating problems for the staff.

Today's standard for a head-to-toe dimension is in the range of 14–17 feet. A truly flexible room of the future might be expected to be 16–20 feet in the head-to-toe length. Contemporary ICU rooms in the United States are designed with 15–18 feet on the headwall in a side-to-side orientation. The truly flexible room of the future, suited for the highest-acuity patient and multiple equipment items, might need as much as 18–22 feet of side-to-side clearance.

The new *SCCM ICU Design Guidelines* (expected in 2010), if approved as written by the revision task force, will probably be performance-based rather than prescriptive, so they will not describe a minimum dimension. They are likely to suggest an optimum distance of at least four feet from the bed to the wall at the head and foot, and at least six feet of space for staff and equipment on either side of the bed. This is exclusive of space allocated to family and a work zone for clinical staff.

The patient room can also be too big. There are procedure rooms in which it is not possible to reach the patient with equipment that has been plugged into the wall without an extension cord. An oversized patient room can have similar problems. The reach of cords and lines can be exceeded. Distances between the patient and supplies, or between the patient and staff work areas, can be stretched beyond the dimensions associated with optimum efficiency.

Zones of use

Some designers have begun to identify distinct zones of use within the patient room. The concept of a zone allows the designer to consider the performance of the space for specific purposes.

Patient zone

This is the area comprising the patient, the bed, bedside and overbed tables, and the immediate area occupied by clinicians in the act of providing care.

Hygiene zone

This area, usually in a separate room, comprises the patient toilet, sink, and activities associated with maintaining the patient's hygiene.

Staff zone

An area just inside or outside the entry to the patient room that is suited to support nursing and caregiver functions: this can potentially include a writing surface, provisions for hand hygiene, patient information (computer or chart), medication, and supplies.

Family zone

Space dedicated to family use and social support for the patient can include seating, provisions for overnight stay, storage for personal effects, separate lighting, access to the Internet, and a writing surface, among other potential amenities.

Entertainment and display zone

An area can be located toward the foot of the bed, or in the direct view of the patient, intended for orientation and positive distraction, where the patient can see a television, a clock, bulletin board or white marker board, and shelving for flowers or mementoes.

Flexible zone

A totally flexible area might be located close to the patient zone that is dedicated to medical equipment use, or a range of other possible uses that could include anything from an office arrangement for a business-oriented spouse to a crib for the patient's infant child.

Nature zone

A zone in or adjacent to the room for plants and flowers, such as a window box or an exterior balcony and garden, is highly desirable.

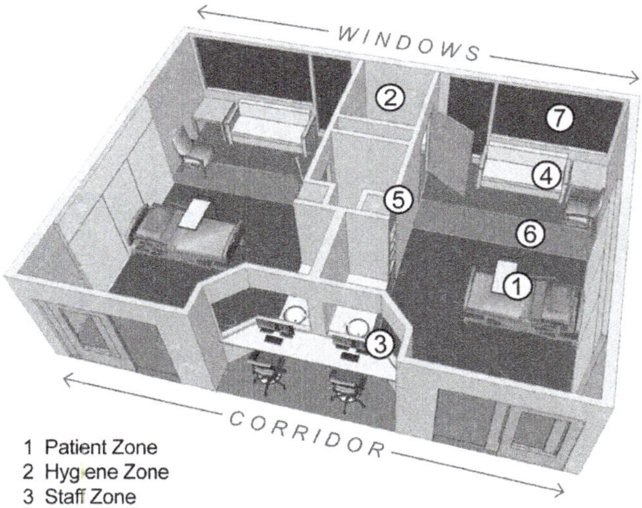

1 Patient Zone
2 Hygiene Zone
3 Staff Zone
4 Family Zone
5 Entertainment & Display Zone
6 Flexible Zone
7 Nature Zone

Figure 4.4: *Zones of use*
Architect: WHR Architects
Drawing: Elizabeth Viets

Observation and privacy

Observation and privacy could be described as incompatible polar opposites. One might be expected to choose one or the other. At one level the discussion about a private room versus a multi-bed room would illustrate the extremes. At another level the degree to which any patient is visible from the corridor is an issue. Is the patient to be in a fishbowl, or are they to be protected from unnecessary public view?

There are, however, gradations of privacy available with the presence or absence of fixed walls, windows of varying sizes with differing types of drapes or blinds, and doors of various sizes, including those with different areas of inset glass. Many sliding doors available for the critical care setting behave like a glass wall, some with an additional ability to swing against a wall, leaving a large open front to the patient room.

Sophisticated monitoring systems provide constant information about critical care patients, but they cannot substitute for caregiver attendance and direct visualization. Direct visual observation remains important to patients and families, as well as to the staff. There is a fishbowl effect created by the all too typical central nursing station, surrounded by open cubicles or rooms with glass walls and doors. The effect is intentional and suits the clinical purpose of a critical care unit.

The clinical case is easily made for a high degree of observation by staff to offer the potential for instant response and patient safety. Many clinicians request a wide-open character in the ICU to allow staffers to know what is going on everywhere, at all times, and to readily summon help in a crisis. There is an obvious need for staff to be able to visually monitor every patient's condition and situation. Similarly, we know that many patients are reassured to see the staff and to know that they are being watched by a skilled professional caregiver (Picker Institute, 1999; Conway et al., 2006; Stichler, 2007).

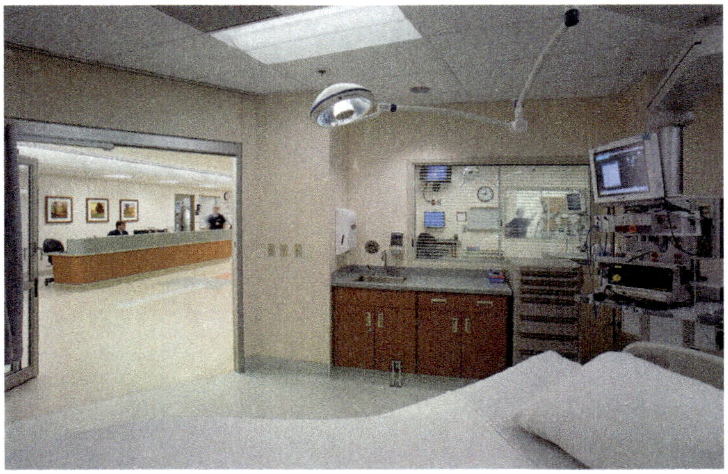

Figure 4.5: *Studies have shown that patients find a view of staff to be reassuring*
Location: Barnes-Jewish Hospital Cardiovascular ICU
Architect: Christner, Inc.
Photo credit: Debbie Franke, photographer

In recognition of the dual requirement for observation and privacy, it seems that good designs should be able to deliver the extremes of both visual observation and protected privacy, as well as various intermediate levels of visual and acoustic privacy. When appropriate, higher levels of privacy can be made available, with walls, doors, blinds, or drapes, in an environment that features enough glass to ensure that clinical observation requirements can easily be met while preventing patients' view of other patients.

Decentralized workstations allow the caregiving staff to remain near the patient. Such an arrangement is reassuring to patients. Windows along the corridor from these decentralized stations maximize the staff's ability to see into the room. Flexibility is provided by drapes or blinds that can be closed when the patient desires privacy, during rounds, or when treatment requires seclusion.

Due to the configuration of some units, constant electronic video monitoring of some or all beds is utilized to satisfy some jurisdictions' regulatory requirement for visual control of all patients from a single point. An effective method of such visual control is electronic monitoring by a group of specialists capable of advising a local team in a timely manner (Breslow et al., 2004). The growing spread of so-called e-ICU units has the same issue, providing constant monitoring by means of a video feed (e.g., Sentara Health, Norfolk, Virginia). Unfortunately, while observation is enhanced for the clinical staff, any privacy for the patient or control of privacy by the patient is lost with this system. For many patients in critical care, depending on their acuity, it could be important to accommodate their need for privacy and respite in addition to the staff's preference for enhanced observation.

Elevated nursing stations have been designed to raise the eye level of the seated observer in the central station (e.g., Mother Frances Hospital, Tyler, Texas). Ramps that provide access for the disabled to such an elevated station require considerable space and even greater length as the raised section rises in height (e.g., University of Cincinnati, Cincinnati, Ohio). Observation suggests that these elevated sections may not be as well utilized as intended. Some elevated sections are designed to allow the "second row" to see over the front counter of the station, permitting some additional observation by a larger number of the staff (e.g., St. Luke's Regional Medical Center, Boise, Idaho).

Decentralized nursing positions

The trend toward higher proportions of private rooms reduces the ability for effective observation from a single central point. The increasing acuity of critical care patients requires nurses and other caregivers to spend greater amounts of time closer to the bedside. A frequent design response to this issue is the creation of nursing positions adjacent to one or two patient rooms or bed positions.

Robust decentralized positions may include provisions for handwashing, documentation, communication, clean supply storage, medication storage, soiled holding, and isolation supply storage. Many will include the ability to directly observe one or more patients. The ability to clearly see the patient's face is important. The design goal for decentralized staff positions is to support the work of the caregiver and to reduce unnecessary work and delays associated with fetching items located at a distance from the patient or returning to a central location in order to document care. Careful design of decentralized positions may save caregiver steps and partially reduce the need for centralized supplies and storage. Decentralized positions can also increase the inventory of supplies and linen, so they must be planned with careful attention to management of the supply chain.

Individualized medication storage

Bedside medication storage or storage just outside the room must be secure. The most frequent model is a unit dose, which provides a full day's prescribed drugs in a cassette or cartridge that enhances the nurse's ability to deliver the correct dosage in a timely manner. Individual storage should also accommodate medications other than unit dose cassettes, as in the case of large items such as syringes or intravenous (IV) bags.

Accommodation of multiple levels of acuity

There is much discussion about ways in which patients can be treated without unnecessary transfers. At the same time, there is pressure to efficiently allocate the human and technical resources of the critical care unit for those patients requiring the most intense clinical interventions, thus moving the most stable and partially recovered to another location.

Acuity-adaptable lessons learned

Terry Ritchey, RN, MBA

Jennie Evans

"Our goal is to work around the patient, rather than have the patient work around the hospital!" *This became the credo for many hospitals and architects that designed universal rooms and implemented the acuity-adaptable critical care model in the late 1990s. Thumbs up were given from boardrooms, patient advocates, and many caregivers—until nurses tried to fit the design model with their care delivery model. Who could argue with a concept that puts patients first, eliminates patient transfers and hand-offs in care with associated safety implications? One of the key impediments to the ultimate success of this breakthrough idea is that operating systems and models of nursing care were not as flexible and innovative as design.*

Definitions for universal and acuity-adaptable rooms vary around the country and are often used synonymously. For purposes of this discussion, the "universal" patient room is a room designed with the sufficient space and infrastructure for critical care equipment, medical gases, and power capacity to provide care to the sickest patient as well as patients with lower acuity levels. The term "acuity-adaptable" room is applied here to a patient room that has the infrastructure (plumbing on the outboard wall, access to additional medical gases and electricity) for future renovation into a universal room.

It is equally important when planning universal rooms to consider the nursing model of care on a particular unit. The model of care for a unit with universal rooms is called an acuity-adaptable model of care. For the model to be successful, staffing ratios and nursing competency must be able to flex and meet all levels of patient acuity. In higher levels of patient acuity, or in a mixed population of high and low patient acuity, nursing competency becomes more specialized, more specialty equipment is used, and often larger waiting room space is necessary. Therefore, planning for universal rooms or acuity-adaptable rooms requires the unit to match the potential function.

In a recent exploratory study conducted by HKS and Herman Miller, five Greenfield hospitals designed as acuity adaptable were assessed for their operational functionality. Initially each hospital's goal was to not transfer patients from ICU to another bed as their acuity improved; however, in all but one of the hospitals the acuity-adaptable model was changed to a more traditional concept of ICU and patients were again transferred to another unit of care as their condition improved.

The study identified several challenges in operationalizing the planned acuity-adaptable model of care which included: 1) difficulty in training and maintaining critical care nursing competencies for an acuity-variable unit; 2) staffing challenges to match nurse competency with patient acuity; 3) recruitment of ICU specialty nurses who wanted to work only in an ICU; 4) physician satisfaction and perception that the hospitals were not serious about critical care; 5) cost of equipping all rooms on a unit with medical gases and sophisticated monitoring technology, and 6) lack of adequate support space for medications, equipment, supplies, and ICU family waiting. While patient rooms were designed to provide critical care, the units themselves typically were not designed for the unique needs of the unit. Security and traffic flow through the unit was also problematic for some hospitals that had patients, family, and visitors walking past emergencies and other life support events. A key lesson learned is that an acuity-adaptable unit should be designed to accommodate the sickest patients, with critical care operations in mind.

The clear advantages of the universal room and the acuity-adaptable unit are the operational flexibility over time. As patient populations and service lines grow, acuity-adaptable units are appealing. The initial goal to work around the patient and minimize transfers and hand-offs in care is just as important today, and many hospitals have had success in creating the acuity-adaptable nursing care model. Operations must be planned and considered along with design. By applying the lessons learned from acuity adaptable-units over the past several years, healthcare professionals and designers are planning more universality to both patient rooms and critical care units.

Terry Ritchey, Vice-President, and Jennie Evans, Clinical Advisor, are members of the Clinical Solutions and Research team at HKS.

Universal room

In a notable attempt to consider flexibility in design, a group of vendors associated with Massachusetts General Hospital in Boston conducted a study of a universal room (Spear, 1997). The concept tested the idea that it might be effective to build every patient room in a hospital with the capacity to treat the most critical patients. The patient room is the most often repeated space constructed in a hospital. The research group intended to explore methods to standardize design and construction at the upper end of a patient room's functional requirements.

The universal room would be sized to meet the needs of a critical care patient and would be fitted with the utilities and life support systems usually found in a critical care room. These additional capabilities might be concealed behind sliding panels until they were required to care for a higher-acuity patient. With this concept, any patient could be admitted to any room in the hospital and would not need to be transferred as their acuity changed. Such a design would reduce the difficulty associated with finding an available bed in the right location. Staff would be assigned to patients on the basis of their diagnosis and clinical needs and would go to where the patient is located, instead of having the patient moved to the unit with appropriate staff. Ultimately the study group determined that it would be too expensive to construct such a room, and the staffing model might not offer the advantages originally proposed.

Acuity-adaptable room

Another model for a patient room that is suited to multiple levels of care was piloted at Clarian Methodist Hospital in Indianapolis, Indiana. In this case the experiment was limited to a single service line. The 56-bed coronary critical care unit had both critical care and stepdown beds under single management. After a bumpy and difficult beginning, the unit became a notable success story, with documented performance improvement, improved clinical outcomes, fewer medication errors, fewer transfers, and significant financial savings (Hendrich, Fay & Sorrells, 2004). Ultimately, due to the opening of four nearby heart hospitals which changed the patient acuity mix, the unit today does not operate as originally conceived and does not include stepdown capability.

The future of intensive care: considerations for acuity-adaptable environments

Ann Hendrich, RN, MSN, FAAN

Joy Kalt, RN, BSN

Gerri Staffileno, RN, BSN, MBA

As we face the current economic crisis and the escalating costs of care in hospitalized patients, it is time to take another look at the value of two levels of specialty care—the acuity-adaptable medical surgical patient and the "super acute" intensive care patient. The greatest single barrier to either reducing the number of critical care beds or assuring minimal "wait" times for the patient who needs a "super" intensive care bed will be our ability to manage the complex medical surgical patient in a safe and efficient environment. The barriers have been cultural, individual, knowledge, and skills. Acuity-adaptable does not mean specialization goes away. In fact, medical-surgical specialization is coveted and concentrated by unit specialty within the acuity-adaptable room.

Over the last 20 years, numerous versions of the ICU of the future have emerged. Many of these designs envisioned a larger, technology-dense environment, with an acute or chronically ill patient who may have implantable devices, and/or transplanted organs that demand concentrated care. Some ICUs have implemented remote monitoring so specialized clinicians observe, intervene, and care for more patients with the aid of technology. As a result, more and more ICU capacity is being added while another population with analogous needs, known simply as the complex medical-surgical patient, has been mostly overlooked.

For more than a decade we have seen the acuity of the medical-surgical patient and the need for transfers to and from an ICU increase, perhaps artificially increasing the number of ICU beds actually needed. A number of demonstration units have been established to transform the medical-surgical room into an acuity-adaptable environment that can accommodate some basic changes in acuity that include simple arrhythmias, temporary ventilator support, titration of drugs, and complex assessments. However, the will and skill to align behavioral factors of change, patient flow and educational advancement for the care team has proven to be elusive. Many of these units have quickly regressed to the familiar model of transfers when change in condition disrupted the expected routine. Patients move from one hospital room to another for primarily two reasons: 1) the technology in the room, and 2) the skill set of the nurses. This transformation of the environment and nursing skills might seem simple, but it is not. However, the opportunity to elevate medical-surgical practice to align with an acuity-adaptable room is a strategic opportunity toward the 'true' hospital of the future.

At Columbia St. Mary's Hospital Ozaukee, a member of Ascension Health, the largest Catholic, non-profit healthcare system in the United States, an up-and-coming demonstration project for the acuity-adaptable room is emerging as a success story.

The unit has a patient room design that accepts all types of patients, including acute, progressive (stepdown) and critical care. At its inception, only 16 of the 32 beds were equipped with beside monitors and the other rooms were supported by mobile monitoring. This required frequent moving of patients from one room to another on the unit and quickly became a dissatisfier to staff, physicians, patients and their families.

The unit is staffed by multi-functional, cross-trained nurses who make up a blended team consisting of progressive care and ICU nurses who flex their assignments in order to move to the patients to meet their needs versus the traditional model of moving patients to units that provide different levels of care.

Most admissions are patients that come from the emergency department or from medical-surgical units following an event whereby their condition becomes unstable or has the potential to become unstable. The acuity of these patients can fluctuate from the most critical to recovery/discharge status. With few exceptions, the patients who start on this unit will stay in one room with the same nursing staff until recovery/discharge. This model replaces the traditional method of moving patients from unit to unit in order to provide varying levels of care. In doing so, there is a reduction of patient transfers and hand-offs, and a reduction in delays with initiation of care for patients whose conditions are rapidly deteriorating.

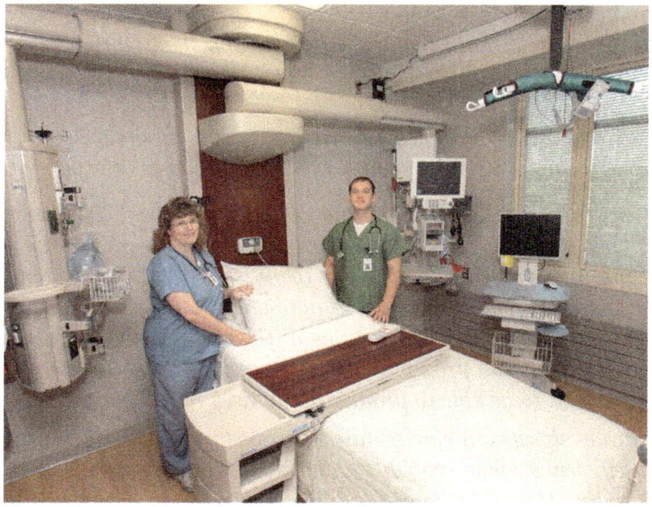

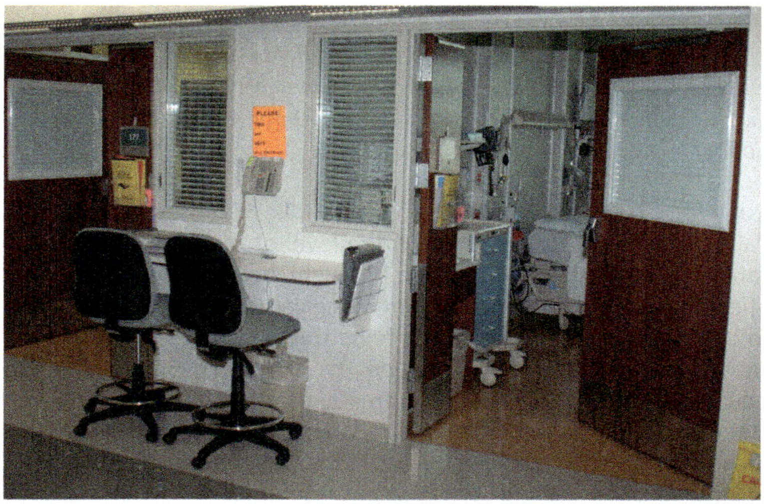

The unit design promotes a decentralized nursing model of care. Nurses view and provide surveillance from outside the rooms through off-set glass windows rather than the traditional "breakaway doors" of ICUs. Wooden doors with small glass windows prevent the patient from being

"on display" to the public walking down the corridors. The nurses are supported with audible and visual monitors that keep them informed about their patients. Early outcomes include:

- *reduced patient transfers*
- *provision of a more healing, peaceful environment*
- *reduced errors caused by repeated hand-offs to new team members*
- *increased satisfaction for patients as they keep the same team of nursing staff*
- *increased efficiencies for MDs as there are reduced hand-offs no transfers and rewriting orders*
- *increased physician satisfaction as they work with a consistent team of nurses*
- *reduced staff time and frustration spent in moving patients and items (packing/unpacking, transferring, reporting)*
- *increased staff satisfaction with the ability to develop therapeutic relationships with patients and families*
- *reduced throughput problems*
- *eliminated costs of replacing lost-in-the-transfer patient personal items*
- *reduced resources required to clean rooms due to turnover at time of transfer.*

The model is patient- and family-centered and visitation is open. Each room has a recliner and a family member is welcome to stay in the room during critical points in the patient's care. At other times, they may stay in the family lounge. The room is large enough to handle patients of all acuity levels, but the increased square footage is not so excessive as to be cost prohibitive. The unit offers special professional growth opportunities in that nurses are exposed to a variety of specialties, including medical-surgical, progressive and intensive care. Nurses partner with each other at the bedside. We are proud to be able to provide a seamless model of care to our patients.

This effort demonstrates significant opportunities to transform a patient environment that can improve patient safety and efficiency while providing a holistic care experience. When caregivers, leadership, architectural design, and technology unite, a different care model emerges. These types of demonstration projects should inform our national efforts in hospital design, caregiver education and leadership roles to respond to the many challenges facing healthcare delivery now and for the foreseeable future.

Ann Hendrich is the Vice- President, Clinical Excellence Operations, for the Ascension Health system. Joy Kalt is the Director of the ICU/Acuity Adaptable Unit at Columbia St. Mary's Hospital Ozaukee. Gerri Staffileno is the Vice-President, Hospital Operations/CSM, and Chief Nursing Officer at Columbia St. Mary's Hospital Ozaukee.

Semantic or substantive differences

Since the physical design of the room itself and the level of technology is the same for both the universal room and the acuity-adaptable room, it might be possible to describe the differences as purely semantic. Why was the universal room perceived as a failure, yet the acuity adaptable-room was shown to be a success? There appear to be three significant differences: 1) the universal room model was originally intended to include every room in the entire hospital, perhaps unrealistically including general acute beds and greatly increasing the capital investment required, whereas the acuity-adaptable model only extended to critical care and associated stepdown beds; 2) the universal room model suggested that any patient could be admitted to any bed in the hospital, requiring specially trained staff to move anywhere in the building to serve a patient, while the acuity-adaptable model was limited to a single service line (cardiac at Clarian) that permitted staffing concentration and consistency along the lines of specialized clinical skills and appeared to require less movement of staff; and 3) the acuity-adaptable model instituted a single manager over the combined critical and stepdown unit to serve a single type of patient, directing which level of staff (critical care or stepdown) should be provided for each patient at any phase of the course of care, whereas the universal room model implied a more difficult hospital wide management task for proper staff assignment.

Design for special conditions

Some critical care units will be customized for a particular clinical specialty. Most could be used for any of several specialties. Exceptions can include the most critical trauma units and burn units, which have different types of equipment that must be accommodated and which may require different kinds of rooms or spaces to house these provisions.

Other special cases call for a very different type of bed, such as a "circular" bed or tilt board in which a strapped-in patient can be carefully rotated to the vertical, or a bed containing an air system to "float" the patient. These unique types of beds may be stored in the building or on the unit, and may be delivered to the room in which they will be used when required. These specialized beds do not need to be used often enough to justify full-time positioning in a room or a group of rooms.

Bariatric considerations

Another type of specialized unit is appearing in the United States: the acute bariatric unit, designed to accommodate obese patients. These units have sturdy oversized beds, ceiling-mounted lifts, floor-mounted toilets of special design, oversized doorways, and other features to address the needs associated with caring for individuals who may weigh anything from 300 to 900 pounds. A question for critical care units is whether the morbidly obese will be present in sufficient numbers in the future to justify the inclusion of some degree of bariatric features in a typical critical care unit.

Critical diagnostic and treatment capacity

Some critical care units may identify the need for diagnostic or procedure capability to be planned near the unit, within the unit, or in the patient room. The goal is to reduce the need to move a patient and to limit the distance traveled when moving is required.

Every critical care patient room should be designed to accommodate portable imaging technologies, including ultrasound, radiography, and fluoroscopy. Additional consideration might be given to specialized imaging capability, such as catheterization or angiography, in close proximity to the patient room, either on the unit or nearby.

A certain number of invasive procedures are predictably performed on critical care patients. These procedures can include line insertions, catheterization, implants, endoscopic examinations, minor surgeries, and interventional imaging, among others. The ability to perform some of these types of procedures in the room can offer a clinical benefit and reduces the need for risky patient transport. Designers may plan dedicated rooms on the unit or nearby to handle instances when a procedure cannot be performed in the patient room. Planners should proceed cautiously, however, when the volume of such procedures is insufficient to support a properly trained and experienced staff. Issues of duplication of space, equipment, staffing, and supplies must be clearly understood before developing such a model.

Special procedure carts

These carts, used in some units, are stocked for a specific procedure and are brought into the patient room, or the procedure room, when required. After use, the cart is disinfected and restocked for the next procedure. These carts can be stored in the clean supply space or another designated location on the unit.

Light

Attention to the role of light and the diurnal cycle is potentially important because of the role it can play when the body's natural rhythms are disturbed. There are many ways in which light can be provided and controlled.

Windows and natural light

Many regulations and building codes require a window in each patient room. These codes originated from early fire safety concerns, in order to provide a window that could be opened to evacuate smoke in the case of a fire. Contemporary fire safety theory and mechanical ventilation have reversed the need to open windows for smoke relief, but the requirement for a window persists in recognition of the importance of natural light and the diurnal cycle on both the physical and psychological state of patients.

The requirement for a window to the outside environment has an important impact on unit configuration. Older units, and some high-acuity units, may contain multi-bed rooms or wards that use a single window to provide daylight to multiple bed positions. Some jurisdictions have permitted the use of so-called "borrowed" light through the use of glass between rooms, allowing the window in the first room to serve as the source of daylight for the second room. In some cases, the ICU has been labeled "ICU/Recovery" in order to avoid the window requirement. St. Luke's Episcopal Hospital in Houston, Texas, used such a windowless unit for patients in the first 24 hours following cardiovascular surgery.

Some clinicians, especially those who work with unconscious patients, feel that a requirement for a window is unnecessary. When the severity of the situation requires heroic measures, they feel that orientation to the diurnal cycle is a minor influence best left to stepdown beds or acute units. Others are convinced that natural light and the diurnal cycle contribute to the patient's sense of place and time while reducing the likelihood of so-called ICU psychosis (Hewitt, 2002). Some feel this may even be the case for an unconscious patient. Others believe the mechanism for regulation based on exposure to light can be abolished by serious injury (Perras, Meier & Dodt, 2007).

European and Scandinavian countries have requirements for natural light and windows in staff work areas. This design is intended to improve the working conditions for employees who spend long hours in the hospital. For this reason, the geometry and configuration of European hospital buildings are often quite different from those in North America. A European hospital, like the Rijkshospital or National University Hospital in Oslo, will have narrower wings and blocks of buildings interspaced with courtyards, in comparison to large artificially lit and ventilated blocks in the United States (Monk, 2004). It is no coincidence that staff satisfaction surveys in the U.S. contain a consistent request for windows.

Artificial lighting

All contemporary critical care units make use of artificial lighting. Unlike an acute unit where most patients sleep during the night and staff interventions are few, a critical care situation often demands activity and interventions around the clock. For most parts of the unit, the purpose is general illumination or task lighting. The most common sources of illumination are fluorescent and incandescent, with a high proportion of installations using fluorescent sources. The choice of fluorescent fixtures is usually based on the ability to provide the intended lumens at low cost and with a relatively inexpensive use of energy. Incandescent fixtures are often used as accents to provide highlights and a warmer spectrum of light, and in some cases as task lighting. The use of mercury vapor lighting is normally confined to storage areas, garages, and outdoor areas.

Many designers try to specify indirect lighting in corridors and patient spaces to prevent patients who are on beds or gurneys from staring up into a harsh or glaring light source. Contemporary best design practice (Fong, 2006) also suggests that lighting should be varied rather than uniform. This means that the lighting in a unit should be bright and effective for work tasks, while general illumination might be more muted and feature spots where the light is brighter or dimmer.

Lighting intensity should be capable of being reduced at night. An interesting side effect of lower light levels is that people instinctively lower their voices. Thus, lowered light levels can also contribute to a quieter unit.

Best design practice for patient room lighting includes general illumination, a reading light for the patient, and an examination light over the bed. Many patient rooms will also have a night light, a light over a sink and mirror, and lighting for a guest seating area. To provide the patient and family with higher levels of choice is a goal of some designs. This implies the ability to vary the level of light from dim to bright and the ability to light selected areas within the room, such as the patient bed, the caregiver's work zone, or the area used by family and visitors.

Studies suggest that natural sunlight and vitamin D contribute to good physical health (Hollick, 2004). Some studies suggest that fluorescent lighting can cause eye strain and lacks the features of natural light that contribute to health (Wilkins et al., 1989). The implication of these studies is that artificial lighting in healthcare settings should attempt to offer a full range of the color spectrum, including the wavelengths available from natural sunlight. Mayer Spivak describes the specular reflection in natural sunlight, with the further implication that full-spectrum artificial lighting should be enhanced with a bit of sparkle from quartz or halogen sources. One could infer that with full-spectrum light sources enhanced with specular reflection, workers might be more productive and patient rooms might contribute to improved patient outcomes. It would be interesting to see the results of a study to test such a hypothesis.

Orientation

The head-to-toe direction of the patient bed varies with room design. In the case of pendant-mounted fixtures on the ceiling, the bed can be oriented a full 360 degrees if obstacles permit. Wall-mounted pendant fixtures have a broad range of orientations, but not as broad as the ceiling pendant allows. Power columns may allow a range of orientations of somewhat less than 180 degrees. Finally, the traditional headwall fixes the location of the bed and offers a minimal or non-existent range of rotation. Some designers and their clinician clients elect to cant the headwall towards the corridor, in order for the patients to be more readily visible to the staff, and others choose to cant the bed towards the window to offer the potential for a view, orientation to the day/night cycle, and to give the illusion of greater privacy from the corridor.

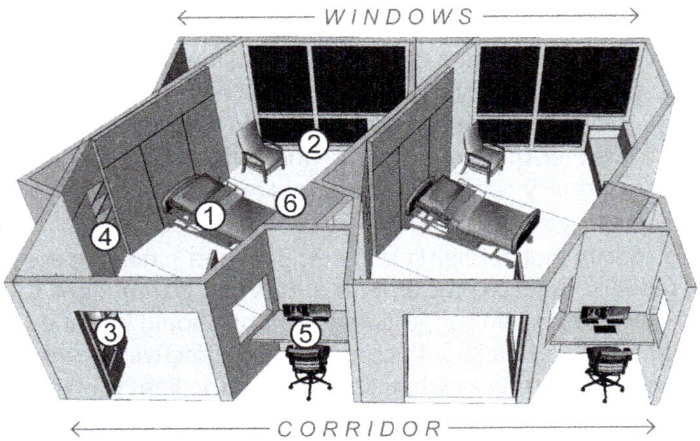

1 Patient Zone
2 Family Zone
3 Hygiene Zone
4 Clinical Zone
5 Charting Sub-Station
6 Swivette or Waste Disposal

Figure 4.6: *Bed canted to corridor*
Architect: WHR Architects
Drawing: Elizabeth Viets

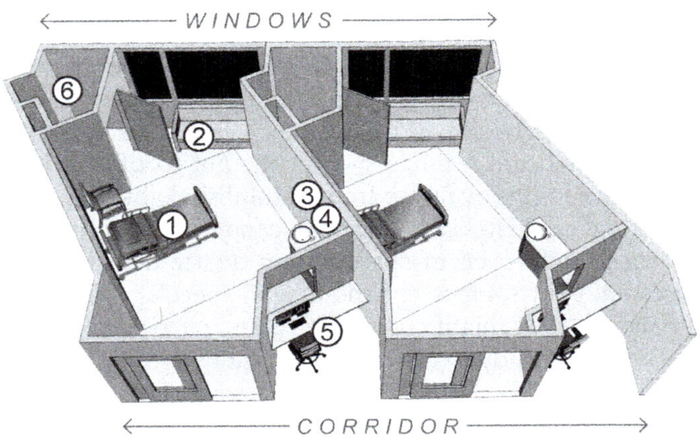

1 Patient Zone
2 Family Zone
3 Hygiene Zone
4 Clinical Zone
5 Charting Sub-Station
6 Toilet Room or Waste Disposal

Figure 4.7: *Bed canted to window*
Architect: WHR Architects
Drawing: Elizabeth Viets

Comfort

The temperature, humidity, and movement of air in the room are generally thought to be the components of comfort for occupants, and comfort depends on their interaction. A properly designed system of ventilation, heating, and cooling will usually go unnoticed, but a system that has problems coping with the external temperatures or that does not respond to the occupant's control is likely to become a cause of dissatisfaction.

Controls and engineering systems

Designing systems for heating, cooling, and ventilating patient rooms is a topic for mechanical engineers and will not be dealt with in detail here. On the other hand, performance specifications for the patient room are within the realm of the user and the designer. Best design practice strives for individual thermostatic control of the temperature for each critical care patient room. Moving the air without creating a draft directly on the patient is important. The engineer must also address the different heat gain/loss condition at the windows. Humidity control is mandatory for the proper operation of much equipment. Control of odors from a toilet or from other parts of the unit is a key to maintaining olfactory comfort.

A plumbing engineer will be responsible for the design of the water and medical gases that are piped to the patient room to accommodate handwashing and toilet facilities. This design may include a connection for the water supply of a dialysis machine, which best practice has begun to place in many critical care rooms rather than have a separate room to which a dialysis patient must be moved. The plumbing engineer is also responsible for designing the sprinkler system required for fire protection.

The electrical engineer designs and locates the electrical circuitry associated with the patient room, ensuring sufficient capacity for the demands of the sophisticated bed, computers, and mobile equipment. Location of some electrical outlets on the wall at convenient heights for nurses, rather than the more frequent practice of locating them near the floor, is suggested. Other electrical needs, such as convenience outlets located for use by the family, will be part of the electrical design.

An important part of the electrical design is the allocation of life safety systems and uninterruptible power. Electrical sockets with red cover plates are generally designated to be on the circuits linked to the emergency generator. The minimum life safety requirements of the patient and ongoing care delivery need to be connected to these emergency circuits.

Today's best practice includes the design of low-voltage electrical systems, which include: telephone, paging, nurse call, and voice communication systems; transmission of monitoring data; wireless transmission; radio frequency transmission; and locator devices. This proliferation of systems and devices has led to an engineering subspecialty.

Patient rooms are generally equipped with a television or entertainment system. In some units new overbed devices that include television, medical information systems, and Internet access are being mounted. Some units will feature telephone, television, and/or Internet access for family members. Commercial television channels are available for closed-circuit delivery. They provide inspirational music and imagery or music composed to offer a soothing, stress-reducing ambiance (i.e., www.healinghealth.com). These systems can include photographs of nature scenes.

4.3 Life support systems

The choice to provide a life support system in the patient room is an important decision that affects design and space. The principal choices today include: 1) a conventional headwall that delivers utilities from connections on the wall, either manufactured or custom-built by the contractor; 2) a power column bringing utilities from the ceiling to connections on the column, either suspended above the floor or fixed to the floor at the base; and 3) a pendant-mounted overhead swivel system bringing utilities from the ceiling to connections on the suspended armature, either in a single or a dual configuration; or 4) a bridge system that spans the head of the bed and may be anchored to the floor or suspended from the ceiling.

The headwall type of life support system is by far the most common in use, having been available the longest. Power columns, developed to provide greater access to the patient's head and airway, are the next most common, now appearing in growing numbers of units. Overhead pendant systems were developed to further increase flexibility of positioning for the bed and utilities independent of the wall. Pendant systems are still less common, having only recently become available, but are also increasing in number. Manufacturers continue to develop new solutions to the important problem of supporting the patient's life and simplifying the work of the clinical staff. Developments on the horizon could include a new generation of highly mobile life support systems that will use the bed as a platform for technology. Such a system might reduce the risks associated with transport of critically ill patients.

Headwall systems

The traditional headwall design has been the standard, from the origin of ICU designs as modified recovery rooms through the mid-1970s (Hamilton, 1999). Medical gases, vacuum, and electrical outlets are mounted on the headwall, behind the patient's head, and are usually distributed as redundant systems on both sides of the patient. Some installations will include wall-mounted equipment, such as blood pressure cuffs, otoscopes, and wire shelving or baskets for supplies. A monitor is normally wall-mounted, on the opposite side of the bed from the door, above the working zone but with reachable controls for staff. Problems occur if the monitor is mounted at a height that cannot be reached by shorter members of the staff.

A variation on the theme is to provide a manufactured or custom installation of devices to conceal the outlets and technology when it is not in use. These may be sliding panels with attractive wooden finishes, or coordinated fabric. Some installations feature artwork that can slide to cover unused technology. These applications are rarely used in high-acuity intensive care settings where the technology may be needed at a moment's notice. They are most likely to be found in coronary units where observation and monitoring are more likely than dramatic intervention, or in stepdown situations where the technology may not be required.

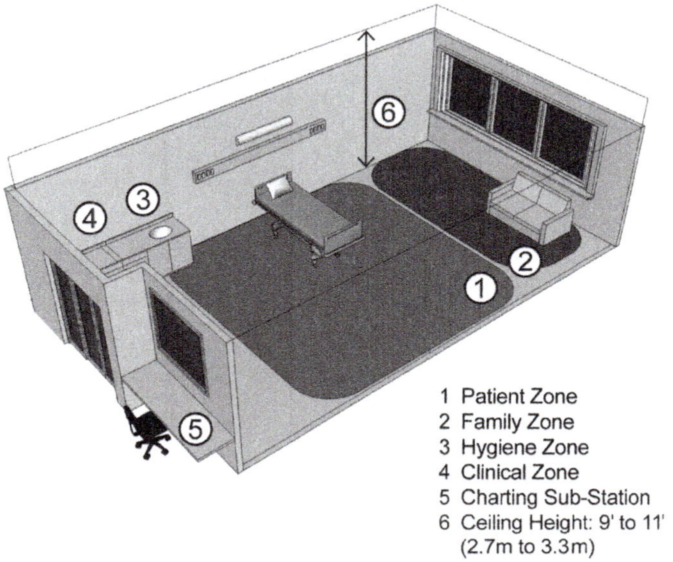

Figure 4.8: *Manufactured rail life support system*
Architect: WHR Architects
Drawing: Elizabeth Viets

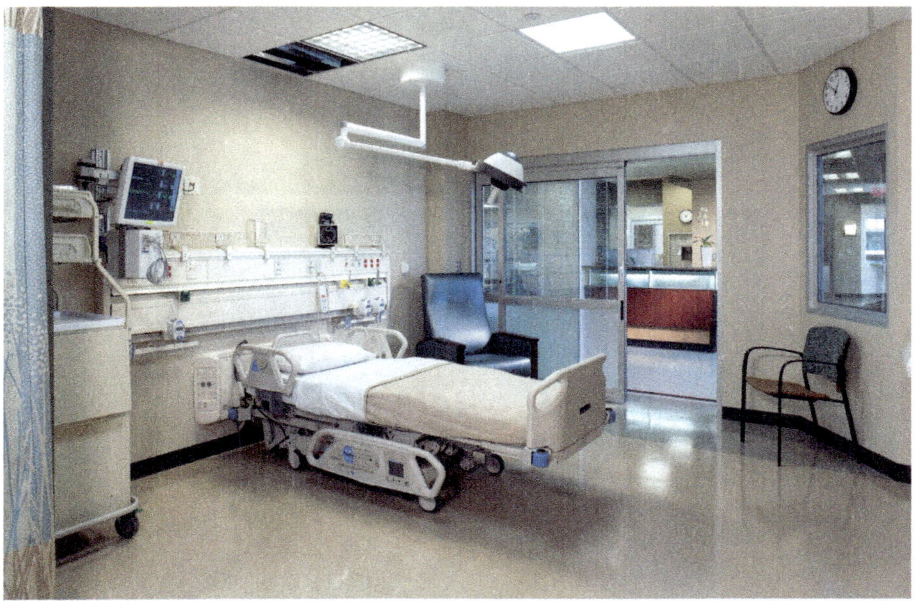

Figure 4.9: *This room illustrates the use of a manufactured life support system on the headwall*
Location: Methodist Mansfield Medical Center
Architect: RTKL
Photo credit: Charles Smith

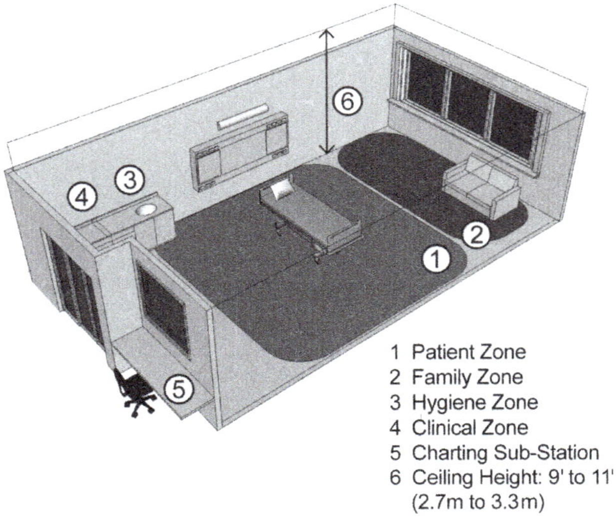

Figure 4.10: *Concealed headwall life support system*
Architect: WHR Architects
Drawing: Elizabeth Viets

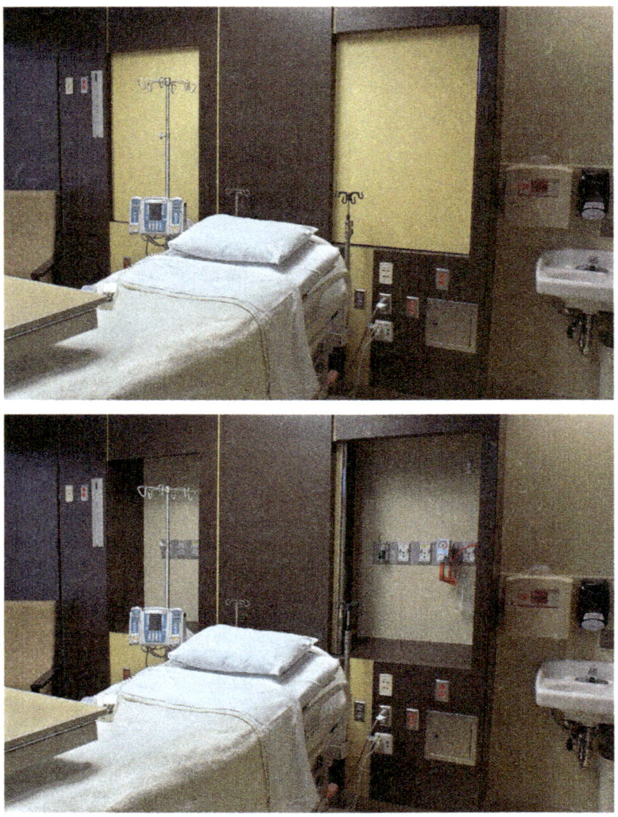

Figure 4.11: *This room illustrates a way of incorporating life support technologies into cabinetry on the headwall*
Location: Central Maine Heart & Vascular Institute: Easter Maine Medical Center
Architect: Morris Switzer Environments for Health
Photo credit: Eric Bauer

Headwalls can be custom-built in the field. The architect specifies the locations of the outlets and mounting brackets to be installed by a contractor. Custom designs are actually significantly more economical than manufactured headwalls but offer less flexibility in subsequent adjustment. Manufacturers have offered a wide variety of factory-built headwall products for the critical care market. As these products have evolved, they have grown to include "rails" to allow horizontal relocation as well as "snap-in and snap-out" features for electrical outlets, medical gas connections, and an assortment of mounts for shelving or equipment. A typical manufactured headwall can be changed easily to a new configuration of gases, utilities, and equipment mounts, although experience appears to indicate that staff makes few changes after the initial setup.

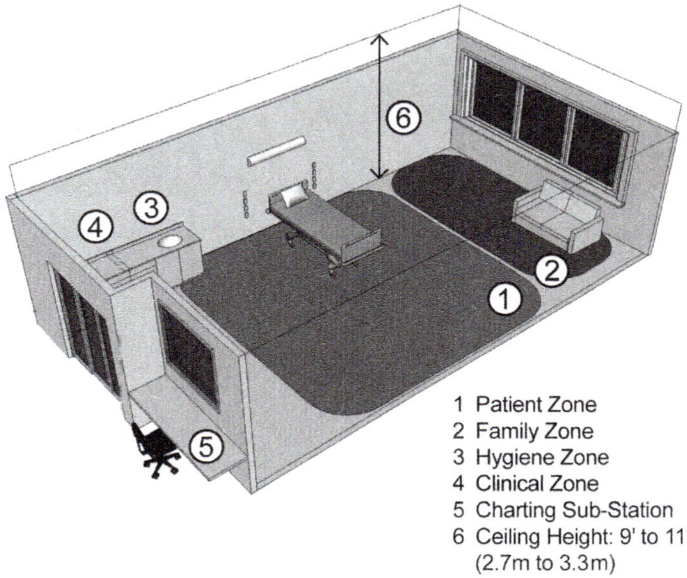

Figure 4.12: *Custom contractor installation headwall life support system*
Architect: WHR Architects
Drawing: Elizabeth Viets

One obvious problem with headwall designs is the requirement in a crisis or code situation to move the bed away from the wall. In an emergency situation, when the team is actively administering intensive care, the bed must be physically relocated to allow access to the patient's airway. The respiratory therapist, nurse, or intensivist must carefully step over the various lines and umbilical connections to life support systems and monitoring interfaces in order to stand over the head of the bed to reach the patient.

The ability to reach the patient's head from behind can be enhanced by raising a step across the headwall, as might be done in an emergency department's trauma room such as the design at Ben Taub Hospital, in Houston, Texas. This feature has been used successfully in the ICU (e.g., University of Cincinnati, Cincinnati, Ohio) with a raised platform, approximately 24 inches deep, along the entire headwall. While this configuration solves a particular problem, it does not enhance flexibility in the room. The bed cannot be positioned in as many different ways, and the relatively narrow width limits the possible uses of the raised area.

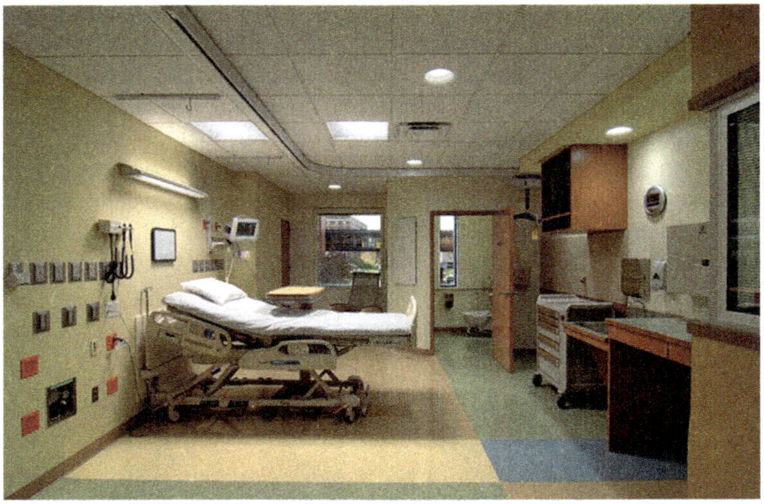

Figure 4.13: *Medical gases and life support utilities are shown in a contractor-built custom headwall*
Location: Summa Health System/Akron City Hospital
Architect: Hasenstab Architects
Photo credit: Scott Pease, Photography

Power columns

By the mid-1970s a few ICUs experimented with an overhead supply for these life support systems (Hamilton, 1999). An early example of a custom design occurred at St. Mary's Hospital in Saginaw, Michigan. In an attempt to solve the problem of access to the head, a 1973 design used the example of operating room overhead connections to anesthesia machines as a conceptual model and custom-built an overhead column for the neuro ICU. The monitor was mounted on the column, along with electrical outlets and gas connections on the sides and bottom. The column did not extend below six feet above the floor. Other organizations were involved in similar experiments, which the industry rapidly converted into the power column concept.

Life support utilities and equipment mounts can now be provided in systems that eliminate use of the wall. The most popular alternative to a conventional headwall system is the power column. The power column is a manufactured utility- and equipment-mounting column fixed at the floor and ceiling that brings utilities from above the ceiling down to the level where they may be effectively used for the patient. It can contain any configuration of power supply, medical gases, vacuum, communications ports, and equipment or monitor mounts. The concept is to allow access to the head of the patient from behind the bed, which is often critical in a clinical crisis or for a neurological patient.

The utilities, monitors, and medical supplies are located on a columnar structure that usually stands diagonally behind the headboard, occupying only about three square feet of floor space (e.g., Swedish Medical Center, Englewood, Colorado; St. Luke's Regional Medical Center, Boise, Idaho). Most contemporary versions of the power column allow some choice in the location of

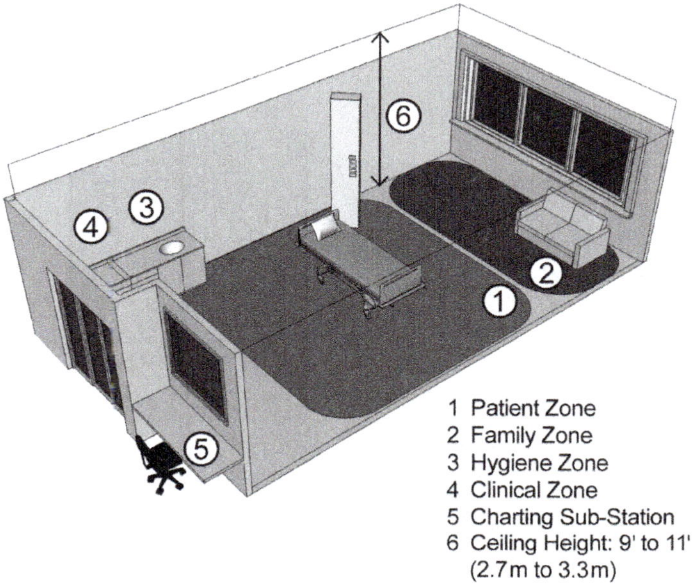

Figure 4.14: *Power column life support system*
Architect: WHR Architects
Drawing: Elizabeth Viets

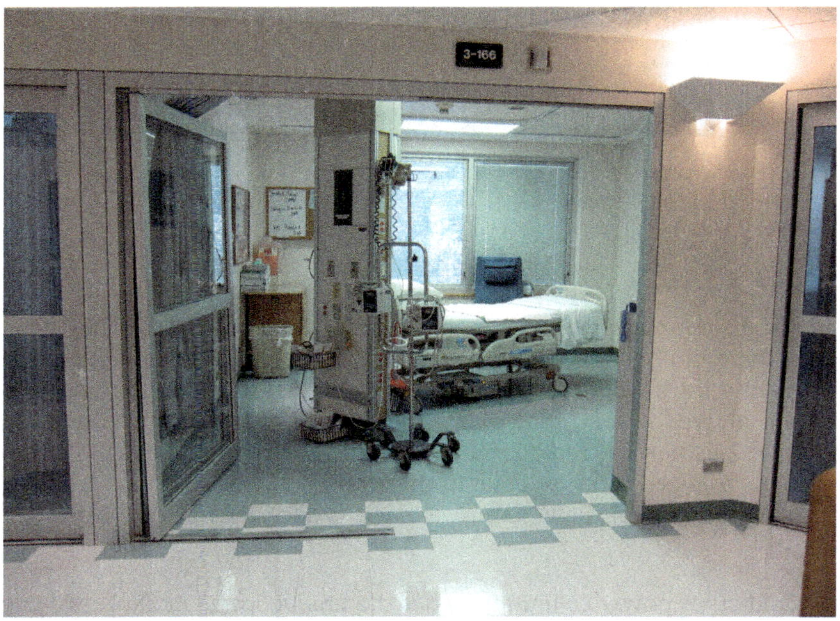

Figure 4.15: *Patient room*
Location: Swedish Medical Center, Englewood, CO
Photo: Charles Cadenhead

components on the column. The principal flexibility associated with a power column is the ability to make major changes in the location and orientation of the bed within the room.

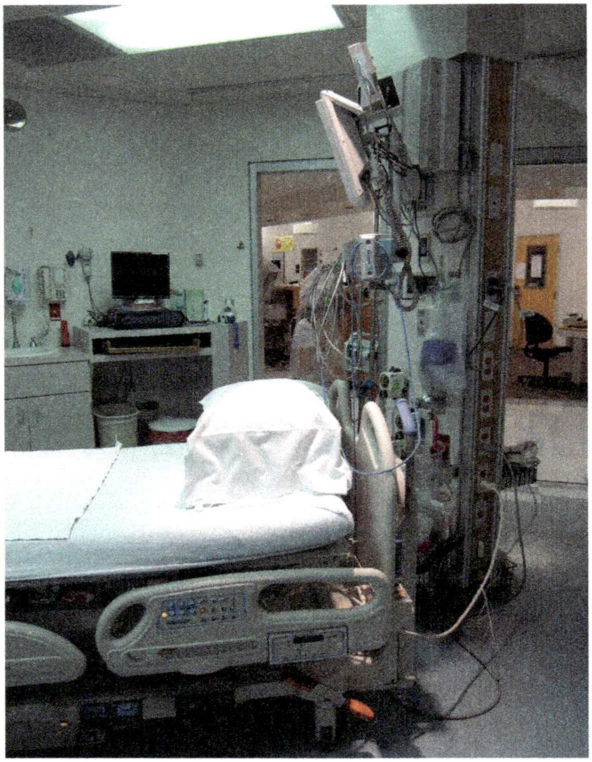

Figure 4.16: *Power column in patient room*
Location: Swedish Medical Center, Englewood, CO
Photo: Charles Cadenhead

These installations are not currently as changeable as headwall products. They have a relatively small footprint in the room and are normally positioned diagonally behind and to the side of the patient's head. Among the advantages of the power column is the ability to position the bed in a variety of locations arrayed around the column's position. In particular, the most appealing feature is direct, continuous unrestricted access to the head of the critical care patient. At least one manufacturer has beta tested a power column that can be swung in an arc to the opposite side of the bed (e.g., Sinai Hospital, Baltimore, Maryland; William Beaumont Hospital, Royal Oak, Michigan).

An interesting variation of power column design is the unique installation of dual power columns in a medical ICU at The Methodist Hospital in Houston, Texas. The concept allows for thinner profiles and smaller footprints for each of the columns while offering positions for utilities on both sides of the bed. Locating utilities on both sides of the patient mimics the convenience of redundant access in headwall designs, without blocking access to the head. One drawback could be that the positioning of the bed is more limited than with a single column. It will be interesting to learn whether there are further advantages to this model and whether other units will adopt a similar configuration.

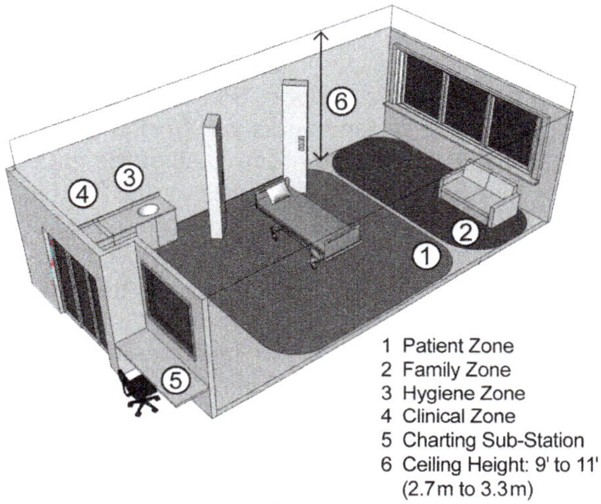

Figure 4.17: *Dual power column life support system*
Architect: WHR Architects
Drawing: Elizabeth Viets

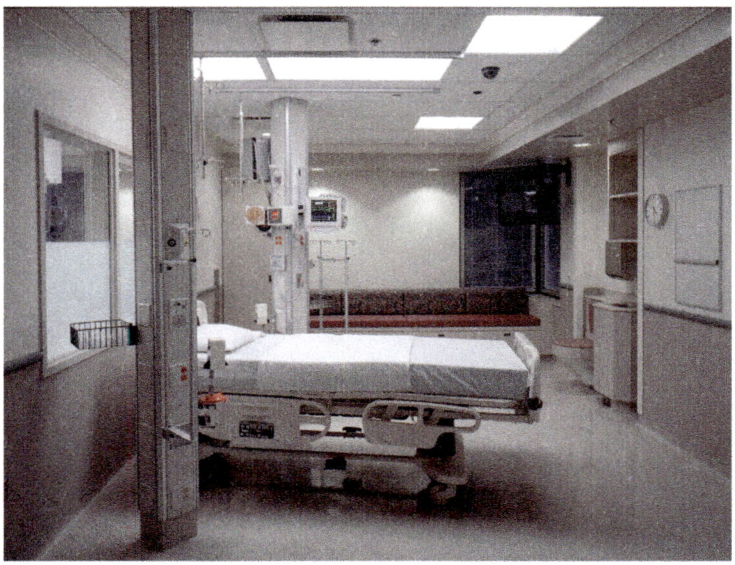

Figure 4.18: *Twin power columns in intensive care unit*
Location: The Methodist Hospital, Houston, TX
Architect: WHR Architects
Photo: WHR

The positioning of the head of the patient's bed away from the wall is one of the major recent influences on the need for a larger room size in critical care. The desirable head-to-toe dimensions changed, from the length of a bed plus six feet to the length of a bed plus six feet at the foot and four to five feet at the head.

Pendant systems

Perhaps the most flexible systems for life support that are available today are the pendant-mounted systems. The design of these systems is derived from the type of overhead utilities and anesthesia services that are available in operating rooms. All of the gases, electrical outlets, monitor mounts, and components that accommodate supplies can be located on pendants suspended from the ceiling, with orbital rotation allowing wide variation in positioning.

Some installations have used dual pendants located to both the left and the right above the headboard of the presumed bed location (e.g., Ryder Trauma Center, Jackson Memorial Hospital, Miami, Florida; Kern Critical Care Unit, Legacy Good Samaritan Hospital, Portland, Oregon). This type of installation appears to provide most of the same flexibility as an overhead system, with the possible exception of freedom to rotate the bed a full 360 degrees.

Pendant systems have been available for more than a decade. The overhead aspect was nothing new. Some clinicians and designers observed that there was no real need for the power column to come to the floor, or to a height that might hit the bed for that matter. Some staffers requested access to the patient from beneath the column. The real innovation in pendant products is the ability to swing the orbiting arm to a variety of locations, improving on the fixed

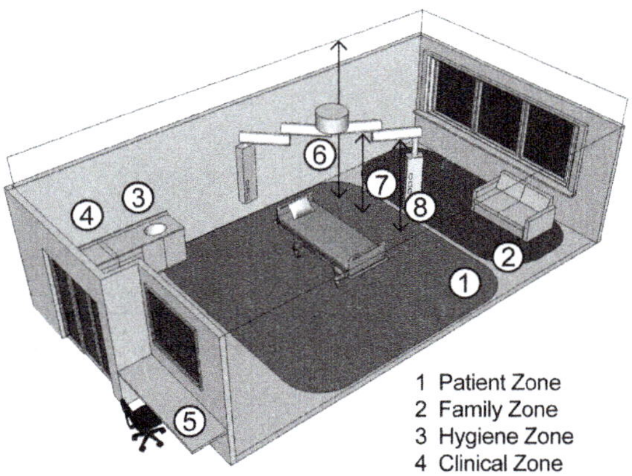

Figure 4.19: *Ceiling-mounted pendant life support system*
Architect: WHR Architects
Drawing: Elizabeth Viets

nature of the more common power column designs. The original designs for these orbiting overhead arms again came out of examples from operating rooms. Very high-acuity settings like trauma ICUs were the first users of these systems (e.g., Ryder Trauma Center, Jackson Memorial Hospital, Miami, Florida).

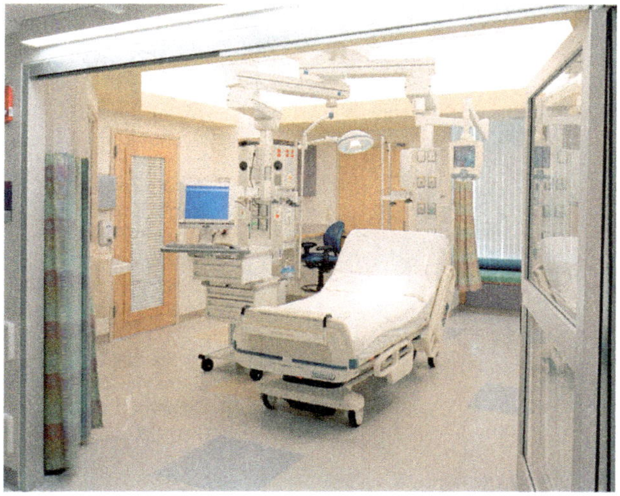

Figure 4.20: *This pendant-mounted life support system utilizes a wheeled cart for supplies and provides access all around the bed*
Location: Children's Hospital
Architect:Shepley Bulfinch
Photo credit: Richard Mandelkorn, photographer

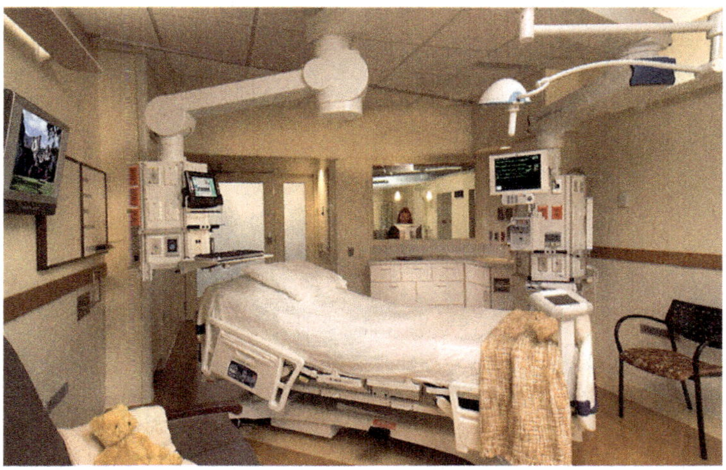

Figure 4.21: *Dual pendant-mounted life support systems provide flexible high-tech support in a room that is capable of minor procedures*
Location: Mercy Medical Center, Cedar Rapids, IO
Architect: HGA Architects & Engineers
Photo credit: Dana Wheelock Photography

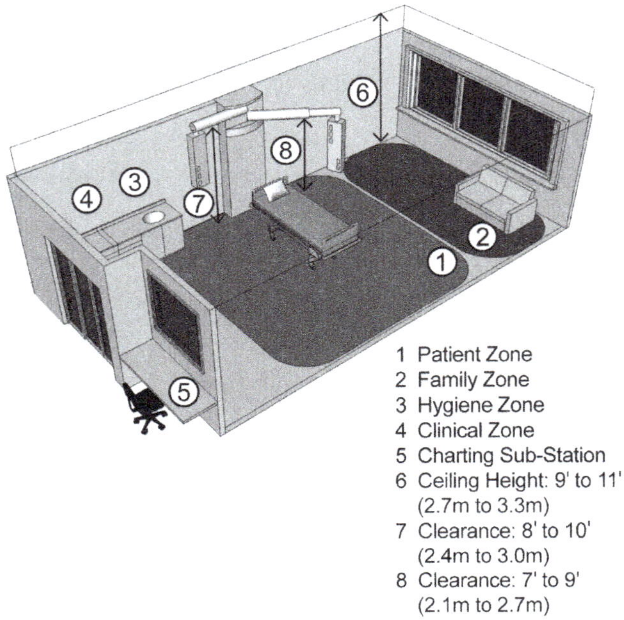

Figure 4.22: *Wall-mounted pendant life support system*
Architect: WHR Architects
Drawing: Elizabeth Viets

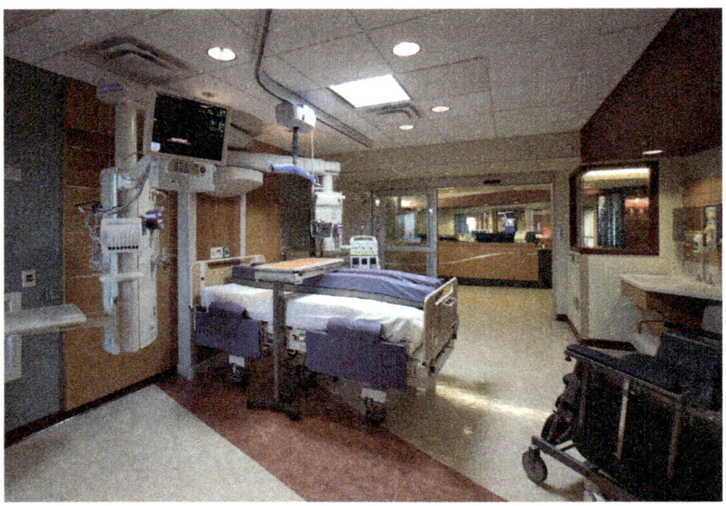

Figure 4.23: *The life support system in this room is wall-mounted and features overhead pendants*
Location: Lancaster General Hospital
Architect: RTKL
Photo credit: Charles Smith

An effective design by Tom Sagerser for the Kern Critical Care Unit at Legacy Good Samaritan in Portland, Oregon, features overhead pendants. This unit is notable for a variety of features and is well worth a benchmarking tour. The twin pendant-mounted orbiting arms allow for a wide variety of bed positions, locations for monitors and equipment mounts, along with outlets for power and gases. Beds can be rotated to face the garden, turned toward the central station, or moved to face decentralized staff positions along the corridor. When a line insertion is performed in the room, the life support system swings away to allow for a portable C-arm fluoroscopy unit, which can support the monitors needed for the procedure's imaging requirements. These pendant devices represent today's most flexible life support systems. The higher cost of such systems may contribute to the relatively slow pace of their adoption.

A possible concern with both the power column and overhead pendant designs is orientation. Studies have shown that some mental health patients can be disoriented in irregularly shaped rooms due to perception difficulty. "Normal" rooms have familiar rectilinear shapes. It is plausible to hypothesize that positioning beds away from the wall and not aligning them in a configuration for a simple rectangular room might cause disorientation in some patients, especially if they awaken for the first time in a confusing situation.

Bridge systems

A European solution to full access is a bridge configuration that spans the head of the patient and offers locations for attachment of pumps, electrical outlets, and medical gas connections. A possible difficulty is the height of the crossbar and the difficulty a shorter staff member might have working with connections.

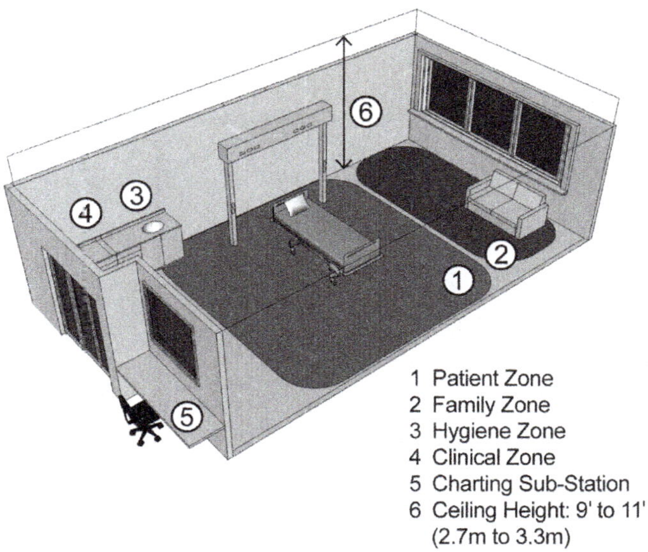

Figure 4.24: *Bridge life support system*
Architect: WHR Architects
Drawing: Elizabeth Viets

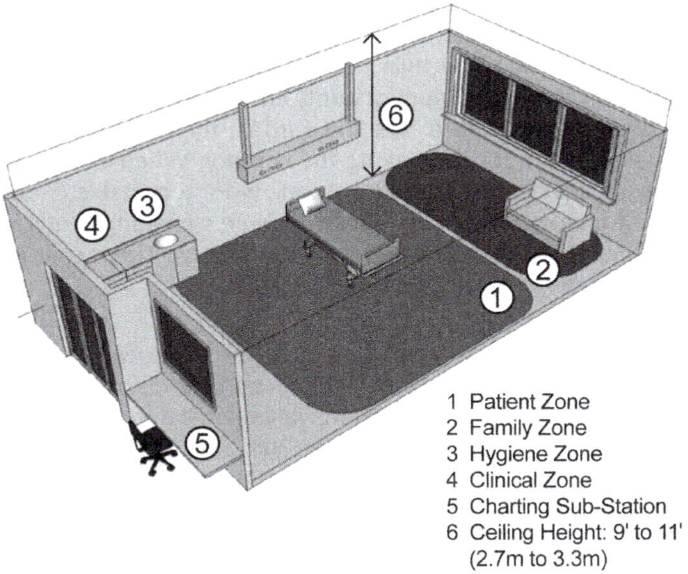

Figure 4.25: *Suspended bridge life support system*
Architect: WHR Architects
Drawing: Elizabeth Viets

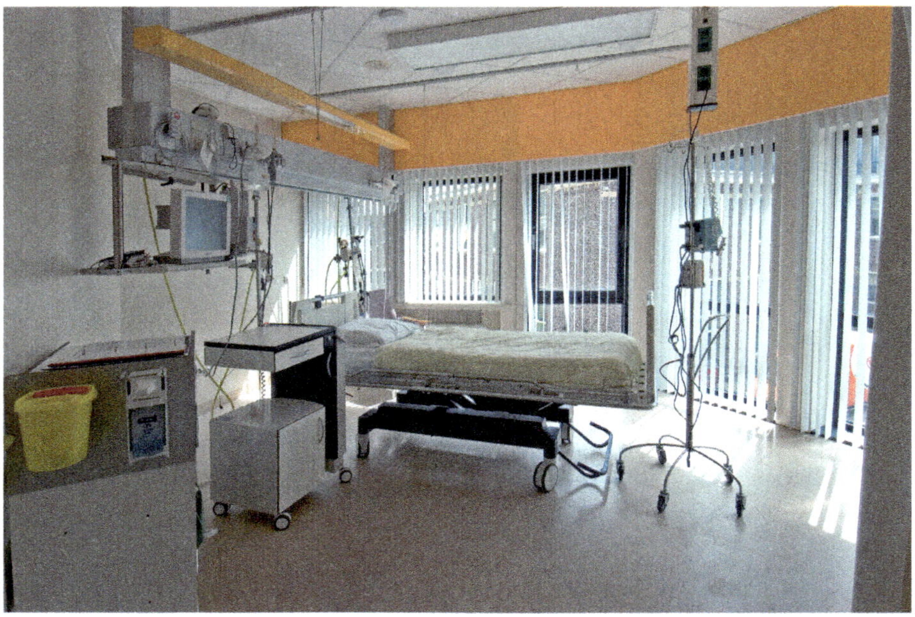

Figure 4.26: *Bridge system*
Location: Groningen Academic Medical Center, The Netherlands
Photo: By permission of GAMC

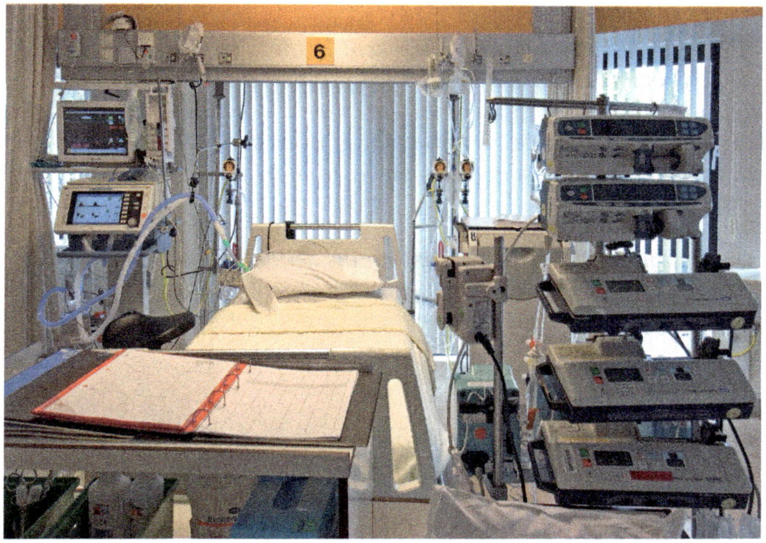

Figure 4.27: *Intensive care unit bed with pump*
Location: Groningen Academic Medical Center, The Netherlands
Photo: By permission of GAMC

Considerations for medical gas delivery system

Jennie Evans, RN

In recent years, several medical gas delivery system options have entered the market. Variations and customizations exist to provide healthcare providers with the ability to optimize teamwork and provide safe patient care. System options that exist are medical gas booms, columns, and headwalls. Although all systems provide staff with the ability to deliver safe, effective care, does one system really outperform the other? Does one particular system provide more opportunity for flexibility, enhanced teamwork, and patient and staff safety? The answer to these questions remain unclear; hence the dilemma for healthcare providers and administrators in choosing a medical gas delivery system.

The workflow within an intensive care room ranges from highly predictable to highly unpredictable—sometimes within seconds. Considerations discussed in this review will assist to identify the challenges with choosing a medical gas delivery system.

Standardization

Standardization of the patient room as well as the medical gas delivery system is a key factor in improving healthcare safety. Medical gas systems should have the same number and type of medical gases in the same location in each room. The number and location of the gases on the system should be decided by a multidisciplinary team consisting of nursing, respiratory therapy, and physicians.

Ergonomics

Repeated stretching to reach gas outlets and cords can cause healthcare provider injury. The boom and the column potentially offer an advantage over headwalls; however, proper installation height and design of the headwall is important to minimize potential for injury.

Flexibility

As patient acuity increases, people and equipment in the patient room increase. Four to six pieces of equipment, of varying sizes, may require a footprint around the patient's bed. The boom and the column provide the caregiver with the ability to locate life-saving equipment and the patient's bed for optimal circulation and access. Observation of intensive care rooms with booms reveals that once a patient is stabilized, the boom rarely moves from its original position.

Equipment/Electrical cords

The location and number of electrical outlets on the delivery system is critical to safety of the care provider and family. Walking over cords causes a potential trip hazard and rolling equipment over cords may cause damage. Simulated patient care scenarios will assist to anticipate all potential requirements.

Intravenous medications (IV)

Placement of the IV medications within the room is dependent upon the workflow of the care providers and the design of the medical gas delivery system. IV pumps can be located on bed poles, the boom, the column, or the headwall (not commonly seen). The workflow requirements of the registered nurse and the respiratory therapist often dictate the location of IVs within the room. Registered nurses (RN) require frequent access to IV medications. Respiratory therapists (RCP) require frequent access to the patient's ventilator. Therefore, if medications are placed in the same location as the ventilator, competition for workspace becomes evident between the RN and RCP.

Circulation

Circulation paths for the movement of people and equipment in and out of the room should be considered for all levels of acuity. Circulation space can be compromised with a boom if the room is not adequately sized.

Patient head access

In respiratory emergencies, easy access to the patient's head is imperative. Booms and columns provide healthcare providers with easy access to the patient's head and access to the airway. A headwall may cause providers to walk over cords and medical gas tubes to access the patient's head. Frequency of required access to the head should be discussed with healthcare providers.

Patient and workflow

The environment must readily adapt when patient acuity rises and emergencies occur. Providing for RN, RCP, physician and other clinician space is important. Consider the locations for patient charting, placement of additional equipment, and how mobile diagnostic equipment will move in and out of the room. In higher-acuity settings, space for surgery teams, their equipment, and their supplies should be considered.

Bed location

The headwall determines the single bed location within the room. The column and the boom offer flexibility for bed location. With booms and some column types, the patient's head could face any direction within the room with adequate access on all sides of the bed.

Family space

Typically, the family zone is provided on the outboard side of the patient room. The placement of the column and the flexibility of the boom within the room have the potential to decrease family space and view to the patient.

> *The success of any medical gas delivery system requires consideration of workflow, patient acuity, types of procedures to be conducted in the room, and the hospital's budget. Advantages and disadvantages exist for all delivery systems; therefore, careful planning and coordination with the architect, intensive care staff, and the vendor will assist to mitigate and provide solutions for the challenges that exist in intensive care environments today.*
>
> *Jennie Evans is Clinical Advisor of the Clinical Solutions and Research team at HKS.*

Mobile life support

The prospect of using the bed frame as a platform for life support, power supply, point-of-care testing, and physiologic monitoring modules is real. These robust, high-tech beds would be designed to dock with utilities in the room and would be self-contained during transport, without disengaging life support and continuous monitoring. They will probably be designed to work with some sort of motorized tug, allowing a single staffer to complete whatever transport assignment is required.

Manufacturers are working on prototypes of life support systems that would be integrated into the bed itself. When and if these types of products are made available to hospitals, there may be an improved flexibility, since the bed itself will carry the capability for life support. This will theoretically eliminate the constraint of umbilicals in the critical care patient room. Critical care will then be available wherever proper staffing and this new type of bed can be found, ranging from the mobile ICU vehicle and helicopter service to the emergency department, trauma service, surgery suite, cath lab, recovery room, and critical care unit. The movement of patients becomes, in theory, less problematic, and critical care becomes defined by the location of specially trained staff rather than as a designated place with an advanced life support infrastructure. Such a definition implies the ability to utilize any patient room of sufficient size for a critical patient, assuming the appropriate staff and critical supplies can be made available. Such a self-contained device will certainly be larger than the traditional ICU bed of today.

Mechanical lifts

An important consideration for safety of patients and reduction of staff injuries associated with moving patients is the provision of devices to assist staff with lifting functions (Joseph & Fritz, 2006; Vieira & Miller, 2008). There are mobile devices which have some problems when not used properly, and ceiling-mounted lift devices. Anyone planning a new unit should seriously consider the possible installation of ceiling lifts and their potential complication of the ceiling space. Ceiling-mounted equipment should be carefully coordinated with the design and installation of the chosen life support system. If mobile devices are chosen, they need to be stored in convenient places and available in sufficient quantities for the staff to use them regularly.

Design for disaster

Each critical care unit should have a disaster plan for the abnormal influx of huge numbers of patients. Such a plan will have a triage model for care of the patients and a plan for accommodation of patients in numbers that far exceed the normal unit capacity. Rooms may be designed for a single patient and family but sized to accommodate two or more patients in a crisis. Equipment rooms might be converted to a ward in a disaster. Anticipation of care positions in the corridor, like those sometimes planned for an emergency department, may be considered. It is important to bear in mind the need for electricity and gases in these locations. The absence of life support technology will mean a number of portable devices, including "splitters" that will allow one service to be provided to a second patient.

4.4 Disposal of human waste

Choosing the correct solution for toileting or disposal of human waste in the critical care unit is a major problem for the design team. There are no demonstrated models that solve all of the potential problems associated with proper hygiene, infection control, disposal of contaminated biological waste, protection of staff who handle waste, convenience for staff, and economy.

Patient toileting options

There are examples of critical care patient rooms with and without toilets. When toilets are present, they may be attached to an individual room or shared between rooms. When a toilet is present, and when the patient is permitted to use it, the issue of distance from the bed is important because monitoring leads are usually connected to the patient and there is usually also a need to move multiline infusion pumps with the patient.

With the exception of medical cardiac patients, the majority of critical care patients do not use a toilet. The majority will be catheterized, will use a bedpan, or will soil an absorbent pad and the bedding. Some physicians have declared that any patient capable of using the toilet should not be in critical care.

There are conventional toilet fixtures, and there are fold-out toilets contained in cabinetry. In nearly every case, the toilets are used most often to dump bedpans, rather than as a site for the patient to use for elimination. Unfortunately none of these devices allows for the disposal to be completely contained. The washing and spraying activity of disposal is a major source of aerosol contaminants and a frequent source of infectious organisms. A paper by Michelle Burrington, RN, (see the Appendix), reviewed the literature and described some of the most common types of problems with organisms and nosocomial infections originating in bedpan disposal and washing (Burrington, 1999).

An excellent alternative to a toilet is a mobile commode chair that contains a bedpan. In a study of cardiology patients at the University of Michigan, surveys indicated that the commode chair was the strong preference for that type of patient (Clipson & Wehrer, 1973). The ability to move the chair directly adjacent to the bed allowed toileting to occur without disconnecting monitoring leads, which contributed to patient confidence. Sitting was preferred over using a bedpan while prone in the bed. One could hypothesize that the result would be similar for any type of ICU patient who is capable of leaving the bed to use a toilet.

The great toilet debate

David R. Vincent, AIA, ACHA, LEED® AP

The dilemma of whether or not to provide either a separate adjacent toilet room or a toilet fixture in the critical care patient room is only partially spelled out in healthcare facility design codes. With the exception of coronary critical care and critical care isolation rooms, the majority of critical care patient rooms are not required to have toilet fixture provisions. Even in the two specific exceptions just mentioned, dedicated toilet rooms are still not necessary because built-in toilet fixtures in casework within the patient room or portable fixtures brought into the patient room can suffice for the functional need.

Why is that the case? Let's examine why a toilet is usually not necessary in conjunction with the critical care patient room. The main reason is patient safety. Critical care patients are too sick, often taking several medications, and are connected to a variety of medical technology devices via tubes and wires. Even with clinician assistance, the likelihood of a critical care patient having a non-eventful and successful journey to a toilet room and back is remote and unnecessary. For many other reasons, as well, portable bedpan utilization is the care provider's option of choice for the critical care patient.

Why is this issue not a simple "over and out" matter and why can't we quickly conclude that toilet rooms don't need to be provided within critical care rooms? In medical facility design, nothing is ever quite that simple. Let's now examine why a provider may want to spend the extra cost to build conventional toilet rooms adjacent to the critical care patient room.

The emptying of patient fluids and other waste, from a bedpan, is a necessary daily function performed by staff members and family. Providing either a nearby toilet or a flushing rim service sink, with a bedpan washer, allows this task to be accomplished efficiently and effectively. The provision of an adjacent toilet room for family use is a consumer convenience and allows the family members to have more vital time close to their loved one.

The variability of architectural and fixture options is broad and diverse. Some cost reduction measures include two- or three-sided toilet alcoves located within the patient room, rotating or swing-down toilets either in casework or wall-mounted in the room, and fixed toilets or flushing service sinks in a corner of the patient room. Unfortunately all the above space saving "economical" approaches inherently have drawbacks associated with them when compared with private toilet rooms. Amongst these negative attributes is reduced privacy, reduced odor control, reduced noise control, and reduced infection control.

When planning for operational and acuity flexibility of the patient care unit over time, one has to consider the probability of whether a future change in patient acuity or service line will necessitate a patient room setting that would require an adjacent toilet room. In universal patient unit and room planning, it has long been recognized that the additional room area, when adapting up from acute or intermediate care, required for critical care must be incorporated into the typical patient room module. Likewise, and when adapting from critical care down to intermediate or acute care, having an adjacent toilet room is a necessity. This approach will best provide maximum flexibility to accommodate the wide latitude of patient acuities and nursing service lines over time, and the increased functionality will be well worth the additional capital expenditure.

David R. Vincent is an Associate Principal of Clinical Solutions and Research group at HKS.

If the commode chair is best for those who can get up, what is the best disposal method for the bedpan, whether used in the bed or on a commode chair? The toilet with an inadequate bedpan-washer spray nozzle is a biohazard to both patients and staff (Burrington, 1999). Conditions can be even worse in the case of a smaller, fold-out version of a toilet in which the toilet bowl size can be mismatched with the bedpan size. The next most frequent choice for bedpan cleaning might be a clinical sink with sufficient size to properly clean a bedpan in a deep bowl. Even such a clinical sink, sometimes called a hopper, produces a contaminated aerosol. The only safe system is a closed system.

Toilets in critical care patient rooms, if they are provided, should assume that every patient is handicapped in some way, even if only temporarily impaired by a regimen of drugs. In the United States, a civil law, the Americans with Disabilities Act (ADA), requires consideration in all public facilities for persons with a disability. It has been up to the courts to decide what that means in normal practice, except in some states, such as Texas, where the expectations have been clarified by other documents. The Texas Accessibility Standards clarify this ambiguous situation for projects in that state.

It would appear that best practice in a critical care patient toilet would include provision of a higher than normal height of the toilet fixture, with appropriate handrails to assist in moving to and from the toilet and sink as well as to assist in rising from a sitting position on the toilet. The standard recommendations for handrails in the United States were promulgated based on the needs of a population of wounded veterans from the Vietnam War who possessed upper body strength. A fragile, elderly woman disoriented by medication is unlikely to be helped by such handrails in rising from the toilet.

One might question whether someone capable of toileting without staff assistance belongs in a critical care unit. It is not often that a critical care patient would be using a wheelchair, and one can expect that a staff member, or members, will be assisting the patient. For this reason, the width of the doorway into the toilet is an issue. A patient being assisted by one or more staff members needs a wider than normal opening to allow for all to move together. Some falls have been documented as a result of staff members' inability to accompany the patient through a narrow doorway; such falls occur when the staff member is "peeled off."

Closed disposal systems

Devices that macerate disposable papier-mâché pans and dispose of the waste inside a sealed chamber have been used in Europe, and are only recently available in North America. The device is about the size of a household dishwasher and may offer an alternative for North American designers interested in a different and safer disposal method. There are currently only a few installations of this technology in the U.S. and Canada.

The design question for a sealed disposal system is whether the device should be provided for every patient room, shared between a pair of rooms (as has been done at the University of Iowa), or provided in a utility room that serves a larger number of beds. The infection control perspective would likely suggest a design that avoids the carrying of soiled bedpans in the corridor. Infection control experts are contending that dumping biohazard waste into a sewer is not a good idea, so there are early explorations of devices to sterilize the waste before it is flushed or macerated.

Selecting a toileting option remains one of the most difficult decisions in critical care design because the options are few, and none seems to solve every variation of the problem. This is a highly important area for further study and innovation.

4.5 Design for isolation

There is a need to design for the capability to isolate certain patients, either to protect the larger population from the patient's known or unidentified infection or to protect the immune-compromised patient from acquiring an infection present in the larger population. The filtered air supply and exhaust from an isolation room should be on a separate system from other spaces on the unit.

Negative-pressure isolation means that the air pressure in the isolation room is negative, or always less than the pressure in the rest of the unit. When the isolation room door is opened, air will move from the unit into the room towards the negative pressure. This protects the rest of the unit from the airborne transmission of pathogens that may be present in the isolation room.

Positive-pressure isolation means that the air pressure in the isolation room is positive, or always greater than the pressure in the rest of the unit. When the isolation room door is opened, air will move from the room towards the lower pressure out on the unit. Positive pressure protects the immune-compromised patient from the airborne transmission of pathogens that may be present on the unit.

Variable-pressure isolation means that the air system design can allow for either positive or negative isolation, as needed or desired. A switch is installed to change the amount of airflow into the isolation room to achieve the desired effect. Such systems are currently not allowed in the United States, unless controlled by an engineer outside the unit, because of concerns about operation and maintenance. It seems that variable systems were subject to error on the part of staff who misunderstood the role of positive versus negative isolation and maintenance personnel who did not understand the clinical importance of the system. The variable system is significantly harder to engineer, as the changes in pressure can alter the overall system balance and result in unintended performance. It appears that properly designed variable-pressure isolation systems will need clearly marked switches and pressure gauges, and should be designed to work without upsetting the balance of the main system.

Use of the ante-room

Standard isolation practice has for many years, since the introduction of mechanical ventilation in hospitals, included the provision of an ante-room between the corridor and the isolation room. The ante-room is generally stocked with a handwashing sink and cabinets for isolation supplies such as gloves, masks, and gowns. In some properly designed air systems, the positive pressure of the ante-room means that no air from the patient room can reach the corridor, and no air from the corridor can reach the patient room. High pressure in the ante-room means air is moving out in both directions, towards the corridor and into the patient room.

Proper ante-room design will allow for the movement of the patient on a stretcher or bed through the doorways and confined space of the entry. The same is required for equipment. Some designs feature an ante-room strictly for personnel, while a larger door directly from the room to the corridor is provided for beds and equipment. This arrangement has the potential to unbalance the positive or negative air pressure relationship.

Fred Ognibene, M.D., an infectious disease expert at the National Institutes of Health (NIH) in Bethesda, Maryland, and the 2007 President of SCCM, has said that the ante-room is not necessary for the care of an isolated patient. Ognibene (2000) surprised a conference audience when he said that effective treatment of the isolated patient can be performed with a properly equipped isolation cart outside the door to the patient room. He is satisfied that a cart and a handwashing area in an alcove outside the patient room is sufficient, removing the need for an ante-room and the complication of extra doors.

Different units manage the supplies for isolation patients in different ways. In some cases, few or no special provisions are made for medication or supplies in isolation rooms. In others, an attempt is made to store an appropriate amount of supplies and linens to serve the patient, in order to reduce the number of trips for the caregiver into and out of the room. When supplies are kept in the room, they may be stored in cabinets or on rolling carts, which can vary widely in size. In a few cases, the nurserver model pioneered by Gordon Friesen is used. It features cabinets that can be loaded from outside the room and accessed by staff inside the room, but it can create problems with fire codes and balancing the air system. Most isolation rooms will have provisions for patient medications to be kept in the room, usually in some form of unit dose cassette.

Projecting the need for isolation is a serious concern. In the United States, it has been standard practice to plan for isolation in 10% of the beds (rounded up to the nearest whole bed) on any given unit (Facilities Guidelines Institute, 2006). As acuity increases, resistant strains appear to persist, and as the threat of epidemic on the scale of SARS or biological terrorism increases, the number of available isolation beds can become a larger issue. The multi-bed settings in the United Kingdom are apparently not effective in defending against the spread of MRSA. It would not be surprising to learn that some future critical care units will be designed for 100% HEPA-filtered isolation. The M.D. Anderson Cancer Center has built a patient tower with 100% HEPA-filtered air, and these units include both acute and isolation beds.

The outbreak of severe acute respiratory syndrome (SARS) in Toronto infected 375 persons, many being healthcare workers and hospital visitors. Forty-four people died. It seems that the Canadian hospitals were unprepared for such a virulent source, and once the source was known the staff may have taken precautions too lightly. If worldwide epidemics and pandemics are going to continue, what facility designs will help reduce the danger of subsequent outbreaks? The prospect of an epidemic raises the question of whether isolation capacity for 10% of the rooms is sufficient. Is there a need to better understand the relationship of design to handwashing compliance? What is the role of HEPA-filtered air systems in the case of an outbreak? Some engineers have suggested that in the case of another SARS outbreak, the air-conditioning and ventilation systems of the hospital should be shut down to reduce the chance of cross-contamination. Today's typical North American hospital is not designed to deal with the absence of mechanical ventilation. In China, where many more have died from SARS, facilities are being built in anticipation of an outbreak of bird flu strains resulting from mutations, or from other virulent and highly contagious organisms. These facilities are designed with exceptionally high rates of fresh, uncirculated air and assume that every patient must be isolated. This may be a lesson for the rest of the world.

4.6 Family features in patient rooms

There has been a proliferation of ideas for family-related features in patient rooms. There has not yet been much research to examine whether any particular feature is effective or significantly influences family satisfaction (Casscells, Kurmel & Ponataski, 2009), but there is fairly wide apparent agreement that the patient environment should accommodate the needs of loved ones and family members.

The most common item that has long been available in most ICU rooms is a visitor chair. These have sometimes been the focus of family complaints, especially if they are uncomfortable or not suited to sleep. The frequently expressed desires of family members include the need for a place to sleep and a place to keep a few personal possessions. A niche in the furniture industry has grown around the design of sleeper chairs and sofas for healthcare. In many situations a single chair or seating option will not be enough to provide for the likelihood of multiple visitors.

Family members want to be able to control some of the room's features, such as lighting, temperature, window shades, entertainment systems, and privacy from the corridor. Other elements that have been designed to serve the needs of family members include separately controlled lighting in the family zone, curtains that can screen the family area, and work surfaces dedicated for the family, many with telephones and Internet connections. Message boards can increase the communication between family and staff.

Some patient rooms have a separate television or the ability to turn it in such a way as to allow viewing without disturbing the patient. There is a need for a television which can also be used for information and training purposes. Some hospitals employ soothing music and images, such as provided by the CARE channel (www.healinghealth.com), which can be played in patient rooms or waiting rooms. The technology is beginning to permit television, closed circuit broadcasts, Internet access, and hospital information systems to be available on the same monitor.

When one of the authors was in the role of family member for Alice, the mother-in-law who was not able to communicate, one of the most helpful tools was the family's boom box CD player which allowed the patient to hear familiar soothing, spiritual, and favorite music selections. This highly personal intervention was not assisted by the design; the boom box was kept on the floor. Nursing personnel indicated that it became their favorite room, as it apparently reduced their stress as well. How does the design allow a family to play CDs, or to allow them to bring their own player?

4.7 Family support facilities

In addition to the family features of a properly designed patient room, critical care units should consider a number of family support elements. The principal activities that should be considered in the planning process include waiting and distraction, information and communication, hygiene functions, consumption of food and drink, storage of personal effects, and sleep.

Since patients with strong social support have better outcomes than those who do not (Brummett et al., 1998), it seems important to design family and visitor facilities that will encourage that kind of strong support for the critical care patient. Widely recognized healthcare interior designer, author, and speaker Jain Malkin has suggested that a good model for the design of a family support space would be an airline frequent flyer lounge, where guests are provided with both relief from the typical stresses of airline travel and a cluster of pleasant amenities that help pass the time (Malkin, 2008).

Family lounge

Every critical care unit has groups of individuals who await news about a patient or loved one. The desire for quality communication about patient status, and what is to be expected, consistently receive the highest responses in surveys of family need or family satisfaction (Press, 2002).

Units can provide receptionists, most often volunteers, to help take messages and pass them on to families. Some units have designed clever message centers with family-controlled passwords as a way to share information. Access to telephones with some level of auditory privacy and access to Internet e-mail are important. Pleasant, nonclinical consultation rooms may be used for discussions with physicians, nurses, social workers, chaplains, and grief counselors.

Organizations most sensitive to family needs usually provide access to some types of food, ranging from cookies baked by volunteers to vending machines or passes to the cafeteria. A coffee bar is almost always a standard feature of any family lounge. In rare instances, the lounge may offer a limited ability for families to prepare something on a hot plate or in a microwave. Planetree facilities may provide a kitchen for family use.

All family lounges provide some sort of access to public toilets. The best examples have convenient access to dedicated family toilets that offer dignity and privacy (by not opening directly into a waiting room, for example) and will have a shower available for those who find themselves at the hospital for the long hours of an unexpected vigil.

Units with accommodations for families in the patient rooms may elect to provide some facility for a family member to sleep over, but in some cases the family member may need the extra rest and respite that a family sleep room can provide. Few institutions have the space and resources to provide this level of amenity, but, recognizing its importance, some have found a way to develop a relationship with nearby hotels. Family members can be convinced to go to a nearby hotel if given some assurance of direct communication through something like a beeper or cell phone. Some hospitals have an attached or proximate guest hotel that is made available to family members.

One innovative solution to breaches in privacy for critical care units is the use of an external perimeter corridor to provide access for family and visitors, as demonstrated at Griffin Hospital in Derby, Connecticut (Werdal, 2000). The elimination of this public traffic from the internal staff corridors reduces the patient's perception of being on display. The loss of views to the outside is an undesirable side effect of this feature.

It is the patient who receives the care and the intensive treatment, making the patient room the locus of patient-centered care. As we learn more about the important supportive roles played by family, loved ones, and close friends, the patient room also becomes the locus of family-centered care.

References

Ulrich, R.S., Zimring, C., Quan, X., & Joseph, A. (2004). The role of the physical environment in the hospital of the 21st century: A once-in-a-lifetime opportunity. Concord, CA: Center for Health Design.

American Institute of Architects. (1996) *Guidelines for Design and Construction of Health Care Facilities,* Washington, DC: AIA Press.

Design of the staff support spaces 5

A portion of the space on any critical care unit will be devoted to the staff and their work requirements. These spaces should be configured to optimize the work process, offer convenient support for the normal activities of the staff, and contribute to the quality of the work experience.

5.1 The staff core

The quality of patient care is thought to improve when delivered by a dedicated team representing multiple disciplines (Hanson & Aranda, 1999; Rainey, 2000). Interdisciplinary team members may include clinical specialists, pharmacists, dieticians, social services personnel, chaplain services staff, case management workers, child life specialists, respiratory therapists, and other therapists.

Historically, centralized critical care nursing station design is a result of dependence on a single paper medical record, the presence of central monitors, and a variety of regulations that encouraged the design of a single centrally located station intended to offer direct visual observation of all beds within the unit. This historic model is most appropriate for designs of smaller units with good visibility of patients from a central position, such as those featuring an open bay design. The numerous factors influencing the design of centralized nursing stations have changed.

Interdisciplinary team center

Interdisciplinary teams are more prevalent, and nursing is moving closer to the bedside. The old nurses' station terminology is therefore less appropriate, as the station serves many others besides the nurse, and the nurse is more likely to spend the majority of their time in decentralized locations. The draft *SCCM Design Guidelines* proposes to use *interdisciplinary team center (ITC)* as a term to describe a location for the centralized activities and interactions of the interdisciplinary team. The task force felt the "nurse station" language no longer reflected the true purpose of the team's principal collaborative work setting.

Emergency crash cart storage

Provisions must be made for the storage and rapid retrieval of emergency life support equipment such as a CPR resuscitation cart or an airway cart. The equipment should be easily seen and identified. If there is more than one ICU, the cart or carts should be housed in the same location on each unit so that personnel will always know where life support equipment is located. An uninterrupted power supply to charge the batteries of the cart's equipment should be provided at the location where the cart is stored. These carts can be in an alcove. They should not be located out of sight, as in a room or behind a door.

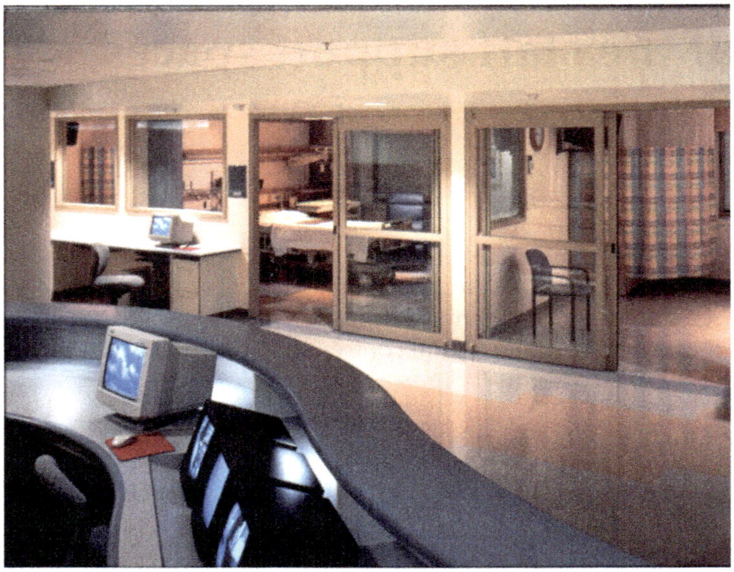

Figure 5.1: *The central position for staff can be seen in the foreground while decentralized positions are also visible across the corridor, adjacent to pairs of rooms*
Location: Suburban ICU
Architect: WHR Architects
Photo credit: Debra Burge

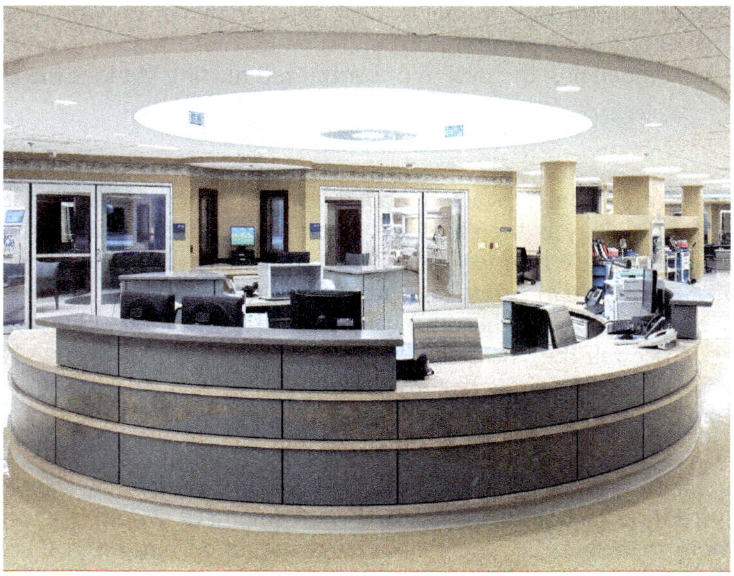

Figure 5.2: *Access to natural light will help mitigate the negative impact of plans that require limited window views*
Location: Floyd
Architect: Artekna
Photo credit: William Montgomery/WM Photographic Services

Medication

Each critical care unit must have a secure medication space, centrally located in an alcove or room. It should have adequate space for storage of medications and needles, a refrigerator restricted to pharmaceuticals, a double-locking cabinet for control of narcotics, and a sink with hands-free faucets. There should be a counter for medication preparation. A disposable sharps container should be provided. If the medication prep area is in a room, windows or glass walls should be considered to allow for visualization of the patient area during medication preparation. A telephone, intercom, or other mode of communication should allow contact with others, including the main pharmacy. The medication space should allow an individual nurse and a colleague to double-check accuracy without interruption of the task. If there is only one such space, it should be located in proximity to the central work zone for the interdisciplinary team. In the case of multiple med prep stations, they should be evenly distributed on the unit to minimize nurses' travel distance.

While medication prep can include the mixing of some IV fluids or other custom mixes of ingredients, preparation generally involves the acquisition and administration of drugs, compounds, and liquids prepared elsewhere. These items can come from the main pharmacy, a satellite pharmacy, or in some cases from a pharmacy outside the hospital. If a satellite pharmacy is nearby and serves the unit, medication prep and storage on the unit may be less extensive.

Automated medication dispensing systems

If automated medication dispensing systems are used, space should be allowed for the computerized device. Electrical outlets and data ports may be necessary. Automated dispensing systems should be centrally located, and, in the case of larger critical care units, strong consideration should be given to providing more than one device.

Charting and dictation

There may be a need to offer a central space for interdisciplinary medical personnel to sit, review cases, write orders, and dictate into the medical record. Such areas should be visually and acoustically private, offering a minimum of distractions, perhaps similar to a library carrel. Such a space is perhaps best located adjacent or proximate to the ITC. It should be equipped with dictation equipment, telephones, and monitors.

Report and conference space

There is frequently a need for a relatively quiet space in which nurses finishing a shift can report to the nurse just arriving for the next shift about the condition of their patients. Sometimes this reporting takes place on the fly, in the patient room, in the corridor, or in a crowded central station. This activity should be focused and thorough, as a lapse in reporting can lead to a deterioration of the patient's condition, and the requirement suggests a distinct room with sound control. A report room can be used at other times for meetings and conferences. Such a room will often have shelving for reference books and a computer intended for Internet searches. At times, this adaptable space will be used as a classroom or training room.

Some critical care units make frequent use of computer-based education modules. Staff members can play a DVD to receive training and educational refreshers. A space specifically suited to this activity might be in the form of a study carrel, which could either be separate or included in a conference space.

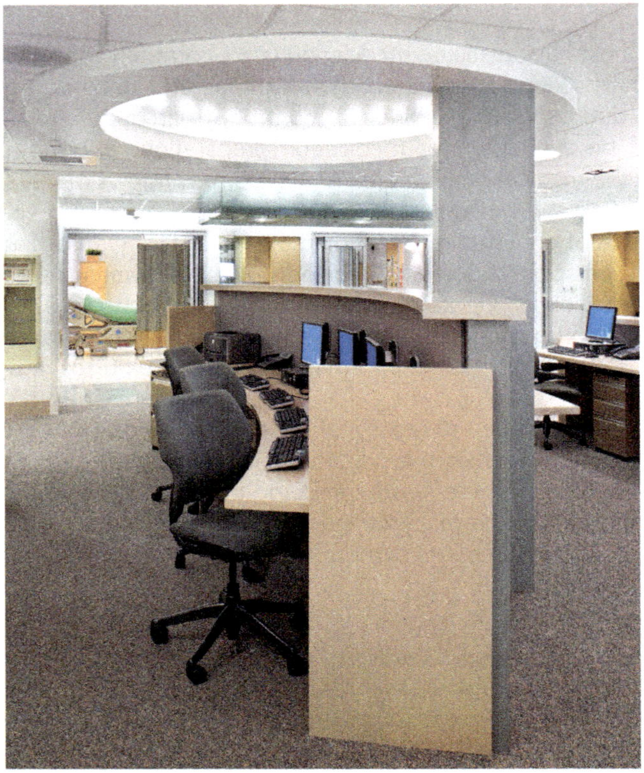

Figure 5.3: *Critical care unit desk for doctor's dictation*
Location: Hoag Hospital, Newport Beach, CA
Architect: TAYLOR and Questar Construction
Photo: Assassi Productions

Diagnostic image interpretation

Newly developed digital technology allows immediate access to medical records and digital imaging. Centrally located computers for reviewing such data should be made available on the critical care unit. If digital review is not implemented, space is still needed for film storage, and multiple locations for film view boxes should be provided.

Phone extensions and computer workstations should be placed in these areas to allow consultations with other medical personnel while reviewing online patient medical data. Patient identification should be carefully protected, and privacy should be maintained during case review discussions. The physical design of these areas should reflect these requirements.

Logistics

To support the immediate functions of the care team, access to supplies and materiel, such as equipment, ice, and food, is required. Similarly, there is a need to dispose of materiel when used or contaminated. Other items will need to be recycled for later use.

Clean utility

The clean utility space is used for the storage of all clean and sterile items. It should be centrally located and easily accessed by the multidisciplinary staff. It provides space for storage of clean supplies, both disposable and reprocessed. It may be supplemented by decentralized locations associated with satellite work locations proximal to patient beds.

Shelving and cabinets for storage must be off the floor and not so high that staff cannot reach the top shelves. The clean utility workspace should contain a work counter, hand-hygiene station, and storage facilities for clean and sterile supplies. Space may be required for rolling carts with clean supplies, including clean linen carts in some cases. The clean utility space is sometimes used for storage of frequently needed and smaller rolling equipment such as IV medication pumps. Security for syringes and sharps should be considered.

Typically the space for clean supplies has been designed as a separate room, but there are also successful examples in which supplies have been placed in convenient and discrete alcoves that offer easy access (e.g., Legacy Good Samaritan, Portland, Oregon). For infection control reasons, this space must be separate from the soiled utility workroom.

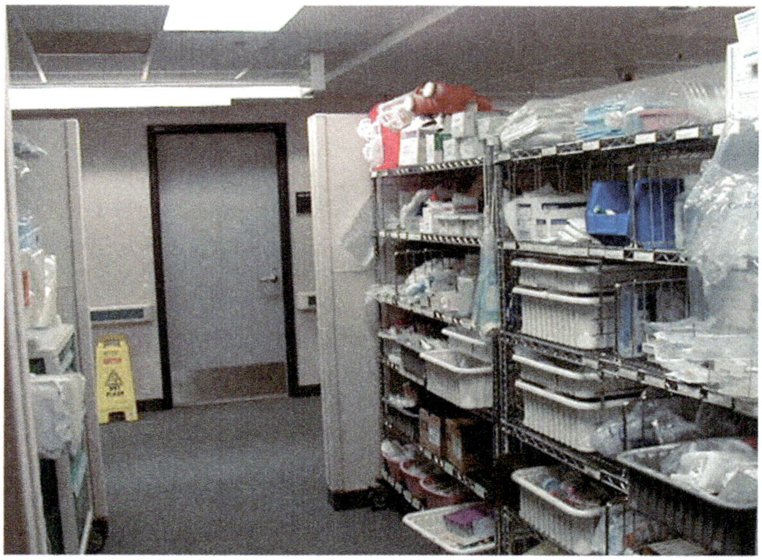

Figure 5.4: *Shelving on carts in an open alcove; walls do not touch the ceiling*
Location: Legacy Good Samaritan, Portland, OR
Photo: Kirk Hamilton

Linen storage

Provisions should be made for the storage of clean linens within the critical care unit. Linens are most often stored on rolling linen carts, with wire shelving to reduce the accumulation of dust. Clean linens may be stored in a separate room sufficient in size to accommodate the required linen carts, or they may be stored in the clean utility room along with clean supplies. If the unit is large or configured in a pod format, decentralized linen storage space located in the pod may be provided. Mobile bedside carts within patient rooms can also reduce clutter outside of the room. Some ICUs feature a cupboard in the patient room, in which clean linens can be stored.

Soiled utility

Proper design and numerous regulations require the provision of a separate space for the preliminary cleaning of soiled items and the holding of large quantities of waste products. This space is most often called the soiled utility room or soiled holding. Its purpose is to provide a place to clean and briefly hold used items to be reprocessed, and to safely hold soiled goods and trash until they are removed from the unit. A soiled utility room will contain multiple containers, cans, bins, bags, or hampers to collect several categories of soiled materials, especially hazardous waste.

The soiled utility room must be designed to accommodate large quantities of waste. Space should be allocated for separate covered containers for soiled linen and a variety of waste types. Bagged trash is often stored in these rooms until it is removed by housekeeping or environmental services staff. If a trash chute is available, this may reduce storage needs.

The soiled utility room must be separate from the clean utility room to reduce the potential for cross-contamination. For infection control purposes, a sink for hand hygiene is required. A means for the disposal of liquid waste should be available, such as a large clinical or flushing rim sink. This room is where preliminary cleaning or disinfecting of items takes place before they are reprocessed, sterilized, and returned to the critical care unit. There should be a work counter for sorting instruments and preparing trays to be sterilized.

Soiled utility rooms are often used to disinfect items that are returned to clean storage. The room should have space to store cleaning items used for such purposes. A bin, a cart with wire shelves, or other means to collect and transport such items should be considered to avoid further contamination of items set on countertops or on the floor. Proper storage can reduce workplace hazards.

Disposal

Categories of waste have been developed to identify many of the types of waste that might be found on a critical care unit (Bencko, Kapek & Vins, 2003). The complexity of today's hospital requires more precise definitions of waste than simply "trash".

The disposal of hazardous waste has become very expensive and shows signs of becoming an even more serious problem due to cost and diminishing landfill areas (Lee, Ellenbecker & Moure-Ersaso, 2003). Steps should be taken in the healthcare field to reduce the overall quantity of waste and to ensure that only truly hazardous waste is included in that category, either by selective handling or by onsite treatment to lower the rating of waste to non-hazardous waste.

Storage of hazardous waste

The holding of materials, such as "red bag" biohazard waste, sharps, and radioactive materials, should be planned. Removal of these items from the bedside to a separate location for disposal reduces risk to the care providers and to the patient. Policies and procedures for the institution should direct the disposal and storage of such items.

As the intended point of initial disposal, the soiled utility room should contain separate containers for many categories of waste, which, other than human bodily waste, may include many of the following items: soiled linens, soiled bandages and dressings, sharps and needles, hazardous or potentially contaminated biohazard waste, white paper waste, colored paper waste, various types of plastics, clear glass, colored glass, aluminum cans, metals, oil or petrochemical products, pathological waste, or radioactive waste. Each of these categories must be handled in its own way, with hazardous, pathological, and radioactive wastes requiring the highest level of care and expense.

Nourishment

There is a need for space on the unit to provide nourishment (ice, food, drink, utensils) for patients, with minimal facilities for preparation. The level of patient nourishment items provided should be based upon the populations served. In addition to a sink with hot and cold water, automated, self-dispensing ice/coffee machines should be readily accessible and conveniently located. Adequate refrigerator-freezer and storage space should be provided. A microwave oven may be useful. Depending on the method of food service deliveries, the nourishment space may need to be planned for the presence of dietary carts and their electrical requirements.

The presence of food items and moisture require that appropriate infection control measures be taken in this communal area. Countertop designs with openings to garbage bins below may reduce one path for the spread of germs, while designs that decrease the likelihood of standing water will reduce another. Choosing antimicrobial materials may also be helpful. Space for recycle bins should be considered.

Dietary carts

Patient meal trays that are not collected by dietary personnel are often placed in soiled utility rooms until the next meal delivery. A tray storage cart may need to be housed in this room to collect such meal trays, or space may need to be provided for dietary carts to be held while on the unit between distribution and collection. If the soiled utility room is not intended to serve this function, other space should be planned. Dietary carts should not routinely be found parked in the corridors of the unit.

Equipment storage

The storage of equipment on critical care units is a persistent problem. Multiple areas should be dedicated for the storage of nonemergency equipment such as specialty beds, stretchers, wheelchairs, isolation carts, IV pumps, ventilators, traction devices, and the like. Each space for equipment should be capable of being secured. Since storage of mobile electrical equipment is common (e.g., transport monitors, IV pumps, etc.), adequate electrical capacity for recharging batteries should be planned.

Equipment rooms should be readily accessible and generous in size to allow for easy retrieval of items as well as for future upgrades in medical equipment. Storing items to keep them out of ICU corridors improves aesthetics and can help to enhance the retrieval of equipment in emergency situations. Unfortunately it is common for users to sacrifice adequate storage when faced with budget dilemmas during design. Similarly, equipment space may be converted to other functions in subsequent renovations. These persistent tendencies explain why storage is at such a premium on nearly every critical care unit and why every effort to maintain storage space in the design stage will be important.

5.2 The departmental support zone

Many functions on a critical care unit are required to support the direct caregiving activity. The spaces that accommodate these support functions are important to the efficient operation of the unit.

Clinical support

A variety of satellite functions of the larger hospital can often be justified in the critical care setting, especially if the hospital department is not close by.

Respiratory satellite

The frequency with which a respiratory therapist is required on the critical care team is very high. Use of respiratory equipment and supplies on a critical care unit is constant, and in some cases there is a high usage of mechanical ventilation. This is why it is essential to provide space for the storage of respiratory equipment and supplies on the unit, or immediately adjacent to the unit. In many cases there will also be a need for an office for the therapist or therapists.

Satellite pharmacy

A critical care unit is likely to be one of the biggest customers for the hospital pharmacy. The growing importance and complication of pharmacological interventions in critical care has led to a much higher frequency of pharmacists rounding with physicians. A facility response to these trends is the location of a satellite pharmacy in close proximity to the critical care unit. A pharmacy expert has suggested that a satellite pharmacy can be justified to serve as few as 12 high-acuity patient beds (Anderson, 2000).

Satellite laboratory

A major element in the decision-making process for patient care and treatment is the data from laboratory tests. Most critical care units depend on a clinical laboratory for the accurate performance of these tests that have been ordered by a physician or intensivist. In some cases the hospital laboratory may need to send the sample to an outside reference lab. The physician and interdisciplinary critical care team, on the other hand, want immediate turnaround of results so that appropriate care can proceed as soon as possible. In a crisis, any delay can be life threatening. This dilemma has led to the installation of satellite laboratories, often called a stat lab, in close proximity to the critical care unit or units. Such a lab may have the ability to perform the most often needed tests for the critical care team with a more rapid turnaround of results.

Point-of-care testing

As devices for clinical testing become miniaturized and portable, the next logical step beyond a satellite laboratory is the adoption of point-of-care testing (POCT) on the unit. This has happened for many years with, for example, simple dipstick urine tests and more recently with countertop blood gas analyzers The difference today is that many of the other important lab tests can be accurately performed with equipment suited for use at or near the bedside. The useful emerging technology of point-of-care testing offers simplicity and immediate reporting of results. The speed with which these results can influence a patient's care plan is why the use of point-of-care testing will increase in high-acuity units. When this type of testing is used, appropriate space should be allocated for the point-of-care devices. Planners must recognize that multiple devices may be required to protect patients from cross-contamination and exposure to infection.

Point-of-care testing in critical care

Neil A. Halpern, M.D.

Introduction

Critical care medicine focuses on expediently identifying and correcting acute laboratory abnormalities. This requires rapid laboratory evaluation of blood samples taken from intensive care unit (ICU) patients with quick turn-around of data back to the ICU bedside. Laboratory testing may be performed in a traditional central hospital laboratory or within a STAT laboratory located within the central laboratory. This approach requires specimen transport systems, either by transporters or pneumatic tubes, and a central laboratory staff and analyzers responsive to the sometimes emergent needs of critically ill patients. Alternatively, laboratory testing may be performed locally within the ICU environs, either in an ICU-based STAT laboratory or at the patient's bedside. Locally-based laboratory testing, in any environment, is commonly referred to as point-of-care testing (POCT). Other terminologies include near patient testing, decentralized testing, ancillary testing or alternate site testing. POCT is real-time near the ICU patient, thus minimizing the need for specimen transport and empowering the bedside care team to obtain the sample, run the necessary tests and gain immediate access to the results. Thus, POCT facilitates diagnosis, therapy, and ongoing monitoring.

Typically, ICU-based POCT testing profiles include blood gases, electrolytes, cardiac markers, and hematologic and coagulation parameters. POCT devices are commonly known as analyzers or monitors. Analyzers measure analytes on whole blood permanently withdrawn from the patient. In contrast, monitors evaluate blood not permanently removed from the patient.

POCT analyzers employ biosensor technology and are classified by dimension, weight, portability and complexity, and type of the testing platform. There are three types of analyzers: benchtop, mid-size, and hand-held. The benchtop units are normally set permanently in one location, usually in a central or STAT laboratory, and are complicated devices that require sophisticated support. Mid-size units have replaced many of the benchtops in central or STAT laboratories, but mid-size devices can also be mobile, rolling on carts to various hospital areas as required. Hand-held devices, available as both non-disposable and disposable, are small and lightweight and can be easily carried from bed to bed. The operative testing platform in all analyzers consists of four essential components: a sample entry port, sensors, reagents and a waste receptacle. The packaging of these components, however, differs per type of analyzer. The components may be stand-alone within benchtops, disposable multi-use cartridges (with variable day limits) in mid-size devices, or very small single or multi-use cartridges in the hand-held units. Additionally, some of the hand-held units now also employ on-board strip readers for laboratory tests not programmed onto the cartridges.

Two types of POCT monitors have been used in the marketplace. The first is the intravascular (in-vivo) monitor where blood is analyzed by a multi-array probe that is inserted into the artery. The second is an extravascular (ex-vivo) device where the blood from the artery or vein is temporarily aspirated by the POCT device into tubing with an indwelling sensor array. The blood is then returned through the tubing to the patient. Only ex-vivo systems are commercially available today. These devices, although logically conceived, have been quite expensive to introduce to the marketplace due to the cost of the single-patient use testing arrays as well as the array's sensitive nature that necessitates frequent replacement.

Quality control (QC), otherwise known as quality assurance (QA) or quality improvement (QI), is a necessary step in the monitoring of POCT devices and for the maintenance of device and personnel certification. In the past, QC was performed manually by laboratory technicians or other users. Fortunately automatic QC is now available from most POCT vendors. As such, the automated

QC systems may be programmed to test the analyzer elements on a regular basis, transmitting data and messages to device managers, disabling poorly performing sensors as needed, and storing data and generating reports.

Data management systems (DMS) are required to handle the large volume of data produced from POCT devices. Such data includes laboratory testing results, QC data, and sensor and cartridge control data. Either POCT vendor-specific proprietary DMS or commercially available non-vendor-specific DMS may be used. DMS servers can reside locally near the POCT devices or anywhere on the hospital network. DMS can be programmed to forward laboratory results to the hospital's laboratory information system (LIS) and to the electronic medical record (EMR) or hospital information system (HIS), and onto the Web or to mobile devices. DMS with bi-directional capabilities may electronically or by scripted interface place orders for POCT. Permanently-based POCT devices are usually wired to the network. Mobile POCT devices are connected by wired or wireless systems. Of course, both wired and wireless connectivity demand network infrastructure. Wired systems require data jacks or docking stations near the devices, whereas wireless systems require both device and hospital-based wireless transmitters. Of note, sophisticated DMS exist for POCT analyzers. In contrast, DMS has never been a priority for the POCT monitors.

Over the years, POCT vendors have attempted to connect POCT devices to the ICU bedside physiologic monitors using various approaches. Such connectivity would permit POCT data to be presented on the bedside monitor alongside other patient data (heart rate, blood pressure, etc). The most common methodology was to connect the POCT devices to ports within the physiological monitoring racks, or to multiport concentrators associated with the monitoring network. The POCT devices, just like mechanical ventilators or infusion pumps, would be identified to the monitoring network through the use of device identifying cables or attachments. The second technique was to construct a POCT module that would fit into the module rack of the bedside physiological monitor, similar in style to the manner in which blood pressure or pulse oximeter modules slide into these racks. Presently, to my knowledge, the modular approach has been abandoned. For the most part, POCT devices are now functioning independently of bedside monitoring systems, although if properly configured, POCT lab data can still be transmitted to the bedside monitor jumping from the hospital network to the monitoring network.

Implementation of POCT systems requires a familiarity with laboratory regulation and certification bodies. The main national players include the Clinical Laboratory Improvement Amendments (CLIA) program of the Centers for Medicare and Medicaid Services (CMS), as well as The Joint Commission. State and local health departments may also play significant roles depending on the hospital location. Additionally, there must be a general recognition and understanding of the political landscape and the potential minefields within the hospital setting when it comes to introduction, ownership, monitoring and control of POCT programs.

In closing, commercially available POCT technologies have improved over the last two decades mainly with smaller, more efficient analyzers, broadened testing profiles, automated QC, better data management and connectivity, and enhanced cost controls. The future of point-of-care testing in the ICU will certainly include further stepwise improvements in the current platforms, but hopefully will also include entirely new systems with easily implantable probes, nano-technology, and other technologies that can raise POCT to include genomic testing.

Neil Halpern, M.D., is chief at Critical Care Medicine Service and Medical Director of Respiratory Therapy Department of Anesthesia and Critical Care Medicine at Memorial Sloan-Kettering Cancer Center. The ICU at Memorial Sloan-Kettering Cancer Center was the winner of the 2009 Society of Critical Care Medicine National ICU Design Citation.

Emergency eye wash

Healthcare workers in the ICU are frequently exposed to many body fluids, increasing their risk of contact with infectious agents. Despite proper universal precautions, splashes of chemicals or bodily fluids can occur, and can be devastating. An emergency eye-wash station should be located on each intensive care unit to provide rapid treatment. The station could be located in a clean utility space or other designated area. If a floor drain is provided, it should be fitted with a drip mechanism to ensure that the plumbing trap does not dry out.

Satellite materials management

A critical care unit has a need for a constant flow of supplies. In most cases, a central department keeps a standard amount of supplies in one or more clean supply rooms on the unit, replenished daily by a par stocking in which a standard level of supply items are replenished, or by an exchange cart method in which a new cart with the standard set of items replaces the partially used cart. In some cases, however, the ICU staff chooses to hoard supplies on the unit to avoid problems with slow deliveries from a central materials management department. In either case, there can be a call for a stat item to be delivered immediately from the central source.

One solution to the dissatisfaction often associated with supply availability is to have a satellite materials management service located in proximity to the critical care unit or units. Stanford University Medical Center in Palo Alto, for instance, instituted a satellite system that featured supply clerks who were part of the critical care unit staff, and a materials management storeroom near the ICU. Using this system, the medical center reported exceptionally high availability of supplies. They maintained greater than 97% item compliance within three minutes of ordering (Radl, 2000). In the Stanford University example, the satellite service was part of a larger successful hospital wide supply chain initiative.

Staff support

Some functions require spaces that serve the staff. These must also find a place on the unit.

Staff offices

If a critical care unit has individuals who are permanently housed there, as in the case of a unit manager, intensivist, advanced practitioner nurse, respiratory therapist, and even a pharmacist, they need to have some kind of office space. The unit manager needs a place to meet privately with members of the care team. As budget pressures occur in the planning process, these offices typically risk being eliminated. While these offices are clearly not patient care spaces, the individuals who occupy them play an important role in the smooth operation of the unit. They may be provided with offices elsewhere in the complex, but this increases the risk that these individuals will not be readily available to the full team at potentially important times. In some cases, shared space may suffice.

Staff lounge and lockers

The staff of a critical care unit should have a place where they can take a break from the activity of the unit and the stress of their work. Many units have combined a lounge function with a report room. While this configuration saves space, it also means that the lounge function is not actually available for a percentage of the time, and lounge activity may be constrained by the dual role of the space.

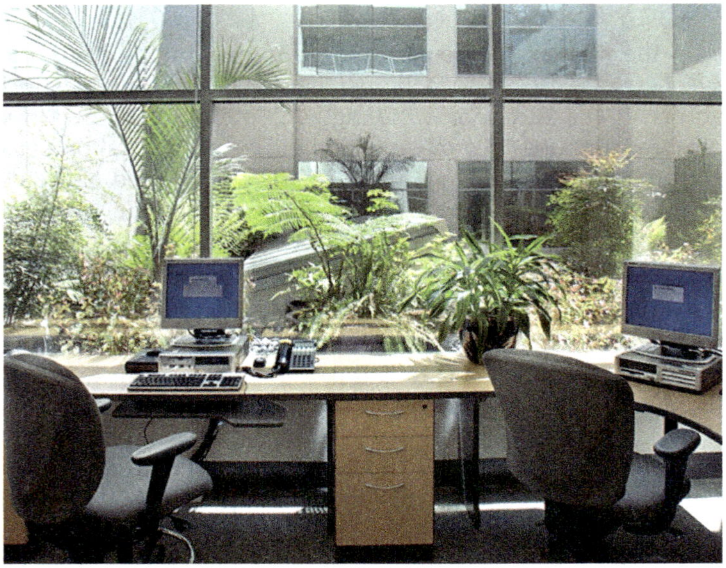

Figure 5.5: *Uninterrupted views of nature may impact stress levels*
Location: Grossmont Hospital
Architect: The Design Partnership
Photo credit: Dennis Sullivan

The lounge space should be a place of retreat from the unit, out of view of patients, family, or visitors. It should have seating appropriate for relaxing and a place to eat. A good lounge will include a coffee bar and refrigerator. Some lounge spaces may include a staff kitchen with a microwave, a range, and a dishwasher.

Staff lockers should be provided for secure storage of personal items. Depending on the climate, the lockers should be sufficiently large to store boots and winter coats. While lockers are often located in the lounge space, it is recommended that they be placed with some visual and auditory separation from lounge activity.

Staff toilets

The staff members on critical care units are exposed to pathogens on a regular basis, and one way in which they attempt to minimize their risk is to avoid the use of patient or public bathrooms. For this reason, the staff on these units will likely insist on having separate toilets available for use only for the staff. Design of these staff toilets should include provisions for visual and auditory privacy so that they do not open directly into the lounge or other frequently occupied space. Because leaving the care setting for any period of time is often difficult, staff toilets should be conveniently located close to the maximum traffic for staff members and/or evenly distributed across the unit.

On-call rooms

A frequently disputed issue in ICU design is the provision of suitable space for staff members who may need to be available at all hours of the day or night but who are not actively working continuously during those hours. These individuals, including intensivists, critical care physicians, advanced practitioner nurses, and respiratory therapists, will frequently request that the design include sleep rooms for staff members who are on call. This issue is particularly important for teaching institutions in which members of the house staff may be assigned to the unit for extended periods of time.

Those with administrative responsibility for construction budgets may consider a sleep room to be a convenience rather than a necessity, and may attempt to strike these spaces from the program. In other cases, rather than completely eliminate these rooms, administrators offer to provide less costly space in another part of the complex. In many situations, however, the requirement for key personnel to be immediately available in the case of a crisis is an issue of safety and clinical quality, and therefore proximal on-call rooms are indicated.

An on-call room need not have much in the way of size or furnishings. It might simply provide a single bed, a small desk with a bookshelf, a single chair, and a telephone. A room that is seven feet by seven feet can meet that requirement. A toilet and shower should be available adjacent to the room or nearby. Dormitory style accommodations may be less than satisfactory as people need to come and go at all hours; they are also less than ideal when one person needs to be awakened and others are disturbed, or when someone's snoring disrupts the sleep of colleagues.

5.3 Equipment and technology considerations

A variety of hospital systems will need to be connected to the critical care unit. Other systems will originate on the unit.

Hospital systems

Information systems

Computerized hospital information systems are an absolute requirement of the contemporary critical care unit. The range of system capability is quite varied, and the prospect of a paperless record is remote for some. For others, the paperless record, or a very near equivalent, is available today.

In addition to basic information in the hospital system and management of the patient's medical record, some systems provide dictation, transcription, laboratory test results, and transmission of digital images. Some facilities have installed decision support software that can include a variety of capabilities. One of the most interesting examples of this technology is a software program that offers alternative choices for medication, pricing information, and alerts for contraindicated prescriptions based on patient characteristics, allergies, or drug combinations.

Planners of critical care units must prepare for a variety of information devices, including both fixed and portable computers. Conditions to support fixed computers should take into account the issues of glare and visibility of the screen as well as the ergonomic characteristics of the work position. In the case of portable systems, the design must account for data-port connections and/or wireless capabilities in all required work locations. Experts predict that the next generation of physicians will have used computers continuously in their education and training, and will be completely comfortable with using powerful personal computing devices similar to today's widely available PDA.

Physiological monitoring

The physiologic monitor is one of the most crucial elements of contemporary critical care. In some cases continuous monitoring has been part of the description of what constitutes critical or intensive care. Today's sophisticated monitors have many more capabilities than their predecessors. The first monitors simply reported on cardiac parameters. Contemporary monitor designs allow for multiple parameters to be tracked simultaneously, and for continuous automated reporting directly into a hospital information system that can instantly show trend lines and other important comparisons.

The monitor itself is located in the patient room, readily observable to any clinician entering the room, and positioned so that it can be effectively read by the team during a crisis response or code situation. It should be mounted above most daily activity, but at a height allowing the shortest nurse to operate its features.

The readings from physiologic monitors are intended to be viewed at the bedside by team members in the room, but they may also be relayed to other positions, such as a central station, a staff lounge, or another critical care unit. At William Beaumont Hospital in Royal Oak, Michigan, for example, a central team observes all patient information relayed from monitors in the critical care units as well as portable monitors which may be located in any patient room in the hospital. Monitor technicians are able to alert team members in the case of alarms. In the case of an e-ICU model, as at the Sentara system in Norfolk or the Memorial Hermann system in Houston, the monitors can be read at a location removed from the unit where specialists are available to advise the local team. The e-ICU model has been shown to be effective and to reduce the cost of care (Breslow et al., 2004).

Provision for major diagnostic technologies

Development of new diagnostic devices continues without a foreseeable end. These devices include mobile technologies that are often employed on critical care units. At some hospitals, critical care units may have access to an adjacent procedure room, operating room, angiography suite, or catheterization lab. In these cases, the patient must be moved to take advantage of the available technology.

Mobile imaging

Among the most important requirements of a critical care unit is the ability to produce accurate and timely diagnostic imaging. Such imaging can take the form of ultrasound studies, conventional radiography, fluoroscopy, computerized tomography (CT), or magnetic resonance imagery (MRI). In some cases the imaging devices are so expensive and complex as to be available only in the imaging department, thus requiring transport of critical patients. In some cases the technology is available in a mobile form and may be used on the critical care unit. Ultrasound, radiography, and fluoroscopy (C-arm) are all readily available portable technologies that are frequently used on critical care units.

While these portable technologies are usually available, their accommodation is not trivial. There is a need for ample floor space in the patient room as well as electrical circuits capable of handling the added load. Consideration should be given to the radiation exposure of staff members and others in the case of devices that produce radiation.

In some situations, such as implanting pacemakers or inserting central lines, the patient room may need to be prepared for a minor procedure, which may include the use of sterile drapes and alternate levels of lighting. Some units will have a procedure room where such activities take place, but the critical patient must be subjected to the risk of a move to take advantage of the capability.

Computerized tomography (CT) and magnetic resonance imaging (MRI) are less readily available mobile technologies, although portable versions of both are being introduced to the market. Because these devices offer the prospect of superior image clarity and tissue definition, one should expect that there will be growing pressure to use them onsite in critical care units. As the devices are improved and costs come down, more units will have access to these advanced technologies. Again, use of these mobile technologies requires ample space in the patient room and sufficient electrical capacity.

Mobile diagnostics

The critical care unit has a need for many diagnostic devices other than imaging equipment. Fortunately, these other technologies are much more portable than imaging devices.

Cardiac information is vital to the care of the critical patient. The standard physiologic monitor can record electrocardiogram patterns and trends, and may also provide data on oxygen levels in the blood. Mobile EKG machines can be brought to the bedside for special studies.

There are mobile systems for pulmonary function testing, and the physiologic monitor can track a patient's breathing. Mobile oxygen systems, inhalation therapy devices, and mechanical ventilation can be brought to the bedside as needed.

Sleep function testing and mobile EEG devices can also be brought to the patient room. In addition, a growing assortment of laboratory tests can be accomplished in the room.

Fixed equipment

There are times when the use of mobile equipment may be challenged. In some cases the accuracy and reliability of results from a portable device may be questioned when compared with a similar fixed device, such as an imaging device in an imaging department. The critical care unit may not have specially trained equipment operators and technicians available. Due to its portability, mobile equipment may not always be available in its expected location. It can lose calibration as a result of frequent movement or bumping against objects, and it may not be used often enough to justify its expense.

For any of these reasons, the choice to install a piece of fixed equipment in a critical care unit can be important. A crucial factor in the decision is the intention to prevent the transport of unstable patients who are at highest risk, but for whom the diagnostic procedure may be the most critical. A fixed device in a procedure room on the unit may still require patient transport, although it would be a significantly shorter distance and duration than a trip to another department. At the time of writing, the most likely technology for such an installation might be a C-arm fluoroscope. The near future may see multislice CT for critical care usage.

The installation of an open MRI device for critical care patients may eventually be practical. In the case of fixed magnetic resonance devices, shielding could be easier to accommodate than with a portable device, and the room might be easier to keep clear of ferrous materials.

Integration of therapeutic technologies

The array of technologies that can be found in a typical critical care room is daunting. One can expect to encounter IV pumps, often in multiple or ganged configurations, along with machines to heat or cool the patient through hyper- or hypothermia, oxygen pumps and inhalation therapy devices, mechanical ventilators, dialysis machines, and even heart pumps. Design considerations include provision of floor space for a likely combination of machines, along with the appropriate electrical, medical gas, plumbing, and communications connections to permit their effective functioning. As new devices reach the market, more of them will have an integrated capability to communicate directly with monitors, with the health information system, and with other devices.

Technologies to save labor and reduce injury

Given today's persistent shortages of qualified critical care personnel, there is a vital need to stretch the capabilities of individual workers through the use of technology. Similarly, technology that offers to reduce injury-related loss of work time can be important.

The use of computers for documentation is an example of a labor-saving technology. While some individuals have resisted the introduction of computers in the workplace, there are many anecdotes describing painful returns to manual documentation during computer downtime that testify to the effectiveness of well-designed software for clinical documentation. Such technology can include devices that report results directly into the patient record, bypassing the time-honored tradition of quickly jotting and abbreviating notes or recording data on a sleeve.

Other types of labor-saving devices include automated systems, such as robotic carts to deliver supplies or robots that pick medications for unit dose cassettes. In addition, if a nurse can use a point-of-care testing device to quickly make a determination for the physician, treatment can proceed more rapidly, perhaps preventing a decline in the patient's condition that would require much greater effort to reverse. Analysis of medication administration along with observation of nurse travel patterns might lead to investment in an automated drug-dispensing device that can help save costly time and steps.

A ceiling lift for the movement of patients is an example of an injury-reducing technology. Ceiling lifts have been shown to cut the incidence of back injuries in staff (Joseph & Fritz, 2006). To reduce push/pull injuries associated with moving heavy critical care beds, an electric tug can also be employed.

5.4 Space for teaching

In the case of an academic medical center or a teaching hospital that features a medical rotation in the critical care unit, some provision should be made for the presence of students and house staff. The attending physicians will be teaching resident physicians and students. The conversations required for this instruction should not occur in hallways, where patient privacy is easily compromised. There are few good examples of provisions for teaching, as it is inconvenient to observe a patient, retreat to a place for a private conversation with the group, and return to the patient room to commence treatment. Nor is it convenient to round with students on a series of patients, returning to a central classroom between each one.

One possible recommendation to accommodate teaching activity is to design decentralized alcoves near clusters of rooms, with the ready availability of hospital information systems, diagnostic image viewing, and lab results. These alcoves might be in addition to a central classroom or conference room, and may have the ability to project digital imagery on two screens for comparison purposes. Another concern for teaching institutions is to provide a place for the students to work and store possessions, such as a residents' workroom with lockers.

5.5 Design elements

The design of a critical care unit is composed of a set of materials—visible and invisible. Behind the surface of the wall and above the ceiling there are structural elements, engineering systems, infrastructure elements, and miles of wiring. The visible materials include floors, walls, ceilings, furnishings, and every item chosen by the design team. Many decisions are required to properly specify what is needed, as well as some things which are not so much needed as wanted.

Communications

Unit efficiency, staff productivity, and patient safety depend on effective communication. Communication equipment on the critical care unit includes telephones, wireless phones, pagers, intercoms, nurse call systems, e-mail, facsimile devices, pneumatic tube stations, dumbwaiters, status boards or screens, and other systems.

Selection of building materials

Each space in the unit—along with every element of each space—is composed of materials that must be specified by the design professional. Exposed materials in a space are called finishes. Final design plans will include some type of schedule for the finishes in every space. Each space is identified, usually with a number that is cross-referenced on the floor plan, and a matrix is completed to specify the type of flooring, ceilings, walls and wall coverings, doors, and interior and exterior windows, as well as any item deserving special mention.

Flooring

The first choice in flooring is whether to have a hard surface, a rubberized surface, or a fabric surface (carpet or modular flooring). Hard-surface flooring is used in areas where liquids are commonly in use and spills can be expected. Rubberized flooring materials offer a combination of cleanability and impact reduction for falls or walking. Fabric-based flooring is used in areas where noise control, protection from falls, cushioning for walking or standing workers, and/or a non-institutional character might be important.

Hard-surface flooring can be used in the area beneath a patient bed, a bathroom, or a utility room. Examples of hard-surface flooring are terrazzo, ceramic tile, vinyl composition tile (VCT), and sheet vinyl. Rubberized flooring comes in various forms of rubber tiles or sheeting. In addition to cost, performance, maintenance, and infection, control characteristics should be considered. An important issue with hard-surface flooring is the treatment of seams, as any seam presents an opportunity for migration of moisture beneath the flooring material. Cleaning methods are of particular concern, as all too often the cleaning method defeats the intended model of infection control.

Carpet or modular flooring is suitable for areas such as corridors, nursing positions, conference rooms, lounges, and waiting rooms. The mythology associated with carpets, as they were never specified in the early recovery-style ICUs, is that they harbor pathogens, cannot be cleaned, and cause problems with rolling equipment. Each of these myths has at one time or another been refuted (Bakker & Faoagali, 1977; Anderson, Mackel, Stoler & Mallison, 1982). There is a huge difference between the older broadloom carpets installed in early, less successful experiments and contemporary modular carpet tiles that integrate antimicrobial agents. Larger wheels are a simple solution to the rolling resistance. This does not imply an obvious solution as there are still negative reports on carpets.

Flooring choices will ultimately depend on an organization's ability to properly clean and maintain the selected product, as well as their capability to select appropriately sized wheels for all equipment. Barring other criteria, noise reduction on a unit is an important reason to seriously consider carpet as a flooring choice. Another consideration is the potential psychological impact of a less institutional ambiance for a high-stress setting.

Ceilings

For noise control the choice of ceiling materials is more important than the choice of flooring. The principal choice in a ceiling is whether it should be a monolithic and cleanable surface, or whether it can be a less costly method of tiles dropped into a suspended aluminum grid. In the United States the choice is usually between a monolithic ceiling of gypsum board with a painted surface, often epoxy-based for cleanability, and a suspended ceiling featuring lay-in acoustical ceiling tiles. In other parts of the world it is common to find various types of cleanable metal, ceramic, and plastic panels used in hospital and critical care ceilings.

A monolithic ceiling might be used in an area in which contamination or a large amount of moisture is expected, such as a soiled utility room, a bathroom, a tub room, or an isolation room. The purpose of such a ceiling is to minimize the joints or seams through which a pathogen might migrate to other areas or be harbored and cultured in a largely inaccessible location. Many critical care units have chosen to use a monolithic ceiling in every patient room.

The suspended ceiling with lay-in acoustical tiles may be the most commonly used ceiling type in critical care units. While not recommended, when used in spaces like patient rooms, bathrooms, utility rooms, or areas containing hazardous materials, ceiling tiles should be washable. Acoustical tiles are available in multiple forms with varying characteristics of sound control and cleanability.

Walls and wall coverings

The walls in North American and most European hospitals are composed of metal studs (normally aluminum) covered with a wall board, usually with a gypsum composition. The cavity created by the width of the metal stud contains the conduits for utility distribution (electrical, communication, plumbing, and medical gases), and often is packed with insulating material for sound absorption. A major difference in construction technique occurs in most other parts of Asia, Africa, South America, and the developing world. In these areas, hospital interior walls are most often constructed of masonry blocks covered with plaster. Space for distribution of utilities can be carved out of these walls and subsequently covered over, or utilities can be surface-mounted. The difference in construction technique appears to be that in developed economies, construction materials are comparatively cheap and labor cost is quite high, while in the developing world labor is cheap and industrialized construction products such as aluminum studs are exceptionally expensive.

What is more important than the inner composition of the wall for infection control, maintenance, durability, sound absorption, and aesthetic appearance is the choice of outer surface material. Wall board accepts other applied materials more easily than plaster, but in both cases the wall covering may be as simple as paint. Other choices include vinyl wall covering or hard surface coverings composed of plastic or metal used as a wainscot to protect against bumps from beds, heavy equipment, or carts.

Doors

A variety of door types are used in most critical care units. The most common in North America, other than those for patient rooms, are wooden, often with coverings of wood veneer or plastic laminate. Metal doors are not very common. All doors are permitted to have a glass view panel. In the United States, building codes, especially the exiting requirements of fire codes (National Fire Protection Association, 2009) specify that doors be hinged to swing, and have a positive latch. In many other parts of the world, and especially in Japan and other parts of Asia, sliding doors are equally acceptable.

In the case of doorways for critical care patient rooms, the key elements are high visibility, rapid access, and large openings to accommodate equipment. The typical North American solution has been the glass sliding door, modified with a "break-away" feature to meet the fire code requirement. Some of these sliding doors employ an entire wall of transparent glass on the corridor wall of the patient's room. A curtain may be hung just behind such a glass wall for control of the patient's privacy when appropriate. Another solution is to omit a door altogether, making the patient room into an open cubicle facing the corridor. In the U.S. these solutions are possible in a suite design, in which, according to the current Life Safety Code, suites of 5000 square feet or less are exempt from the requirement that corridors be of 1-hour fire-resistive construction. At the time of writing, increasing the size of allowable suites to 7500 or 10000 square feet is under consideration.

Windows

The American Institute of Architect's (AIA) *Guidelines of Design and Construction of Hospitals and Health Care Facilities* (2006) and hospital licensing regulations in most states require that every critical care patient room have a window. Windows provide natural daylight, offer a view to the outside world, and allow for an experience of the diurnal cycle. When originally written and first adopted, fire codes specifically required operability, so that the windows might be opened to evacuate smoke in the case of a fire. This is no longer the preferred method of evacuating smoke as nearly all hospitals utilize some form of mechanical ventilation, so most contemporary designs specify windows that cannot be opened except with a special key for cleaning purposes.

The window is a source of heat loss or heat gain, depending on the climate and season. For this reason, most contemporary designs use a double-pane insulated assembly. Such windows can reduce the heating or cooling loads on the hospital's power plant. In severe climates, such as in Scandinavia or Alaska, triple-pane windows are used.

In addition to the requirement to include windows in the patient room, windows are recommended in any space where staff or visitors must spend large amounts of time. Designs to accommodate many windows will have a larger perimeter and be relatively shallow in distance from the exterior wall.

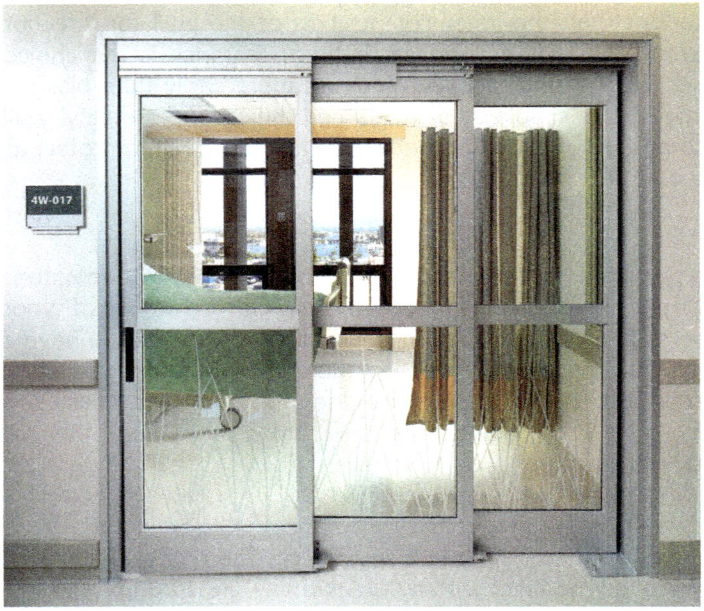

Figure 5.6: *Patient room with sliding glass doors (closed)*
Location: Hoag Hospital, Newport Beach, CA
Architect: TAYLOR and Questar Construction
Photo: Assassi Productions

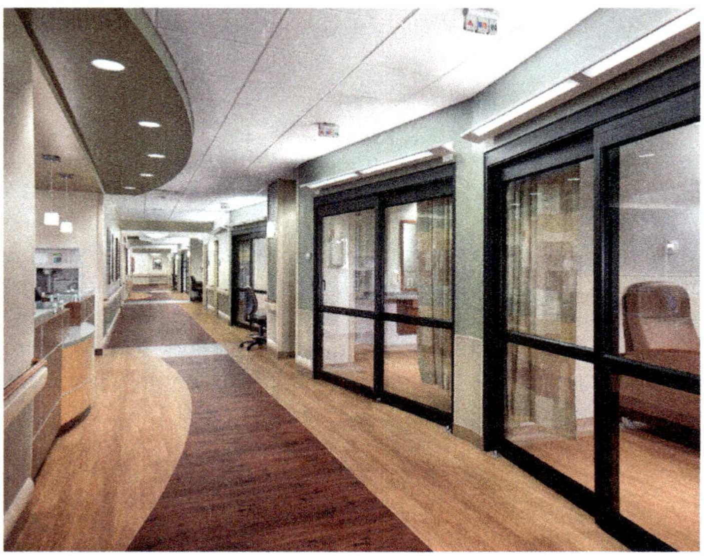

Figure 5.7: *Slight angles on the ICU room glass sliding doors reduces reflections and glare contributing to improved visibility*
Location: Littleton Adventist Hospital, Littleton, CO
Architects: Earl Swensson Associates
Photo credit: Ed LaCasse/LaCasse Photography

Interior windows are used to increase visibility and observation on critical care units. These windows can be strategically placed so that views are available from frequently used staff positions. In the case of interior windows, double-pane assemblies may be used to reduce sound transmission. Double-pane assemblies may also be fitted with internal blinds, or curtains may be hung, to offer control of privacy. Curtains must have antimicrobial characteristics and be subject to cleaning or disinfection between patient admissions.

To address the issue of privacy, manufacturers have created window glass that can be turned opaque with the flick of a switch. Running an electrical current through the glass causes molecular elements to align in such a way as to convert transparent glass into a frosted version; when the current is removed, it once again becomes transparent. One manufacturer has ceased to make the product, and some users of another version have been less than satisfied (McKahan & Hamilton, 2006).

Skylights

When possible given the hospital's roof design or the ICU's position within the larger building complex, skylights can provide natural daylighting. The Kern critical care unit at Legacy Good Samaritan in Portland, Oregon, designed by Tom Sagerser, and the new ICU at Saddleback Hospital in Laguna Hills, California, designed by TAYLOR, are two examples of designs that employ skylights. While similar to those for windows, issues of heat loss and heat gain are sometimes more serious if skylights are located in areas that receive longer exposure to sunlight. On the other hand, in northern climates, the natural light from a skylight can be especially welcome. To accommodate such placement, designs call for double- or triple-glazed skylights. Variations on the skylight can include clerestory windows, north-facing light monitors, and light wells that penetrate more than a single floor. Since a skylight involves penetration of the roof, it is important to be especially careful with the installation design to prevent leaks.

Comfort control

The design of heating, ventilation, and air-conditioning systems (HVAC) for critical care units falls to an experienced mechanical engineer familiar with hospital requirements. The concept is to provide control over temperature, humidity, and the ventilating flow of conditioned air in the critical care environment. Even in hospitals that do not feature complete air-conditioning, the critical care unit or individual patient rooms are normally artificially conditioned.

Engineers have several options when choosing systems to serve hospitals. Generally, the engineering design will feature accommodation of heat loads around the perimeter of the building, with a different system used for internal spaces. Engineers divide the capacity being delivered to the entire hospital into zones usually based on the area a single air handling machine can serve. In the case of critical care, the unit has a need for more frequent air changes and higher levels of filtration than most other hospital departments.

There appears to be a growing trend to provide individual thermostats in every separate patient space. As the move toward providing private rooms continues to expand, this practice seems to increase.

Noise control

The patient's inability to control exposure to noise in the critical care environment is a major source of stress. The presence of hard surfaces that enhance reverberation, the voices of multiple staff members, noise from unfamiliar equipment, overhead paging, the speakers of a neighbor's television, and frequent assorted alarms are just a few of the sources of this stress.

The now quaint signs suggesting that passers-by should be quiet in a hospital zone are obsolete, as the typical ICU is often more noisy than the average city street. The desired goal is to significantly reduce the noise on a unit, dramatically reducing stress levels, allowing patients to experience uninterrupted sleep, and decreasing staff fatigue.

Furnishings

The furniture on a critical care unit, particularly in the patient room, must meet higher standards than ordinary residential or office furniture. The everyday intense wear and tear to which these items are subjected demands a high standard of durability. Patient safety issues prompt the need to control infection and reduce the spread of pathogens. Materials, therefore, must be readily cleanable with harsh chemicals, may need to have antimicrobial characteristics, or must be treated with antimicrobial coatings.

The requirement for life safety must be considered in the selection of furnishings. Fire safety is generally regulated by the authorities having jurisdiction (AHJ), based on codes that require compliance with laboratory-verified flame-spread ratings.

5.6 Design issues external to the unit

Some ICU design decisions are based on the unit's external relationships. No critical care unit exists in isolation from the other services of a hospital.

Earlier discussions of the patient environment mentioned procedures that might be performed in the room, within the unit, or near the unit, including line insertions, pacemaker implants, and relatively sophisticated imaging. Should these capabilities not exist in the patient room or within the unit, planners may wish to consider whether they should be located near the critical care unit.

Emergency and surgery

The design of any critical care unit should take into account the unit's relationship to the emergency department and the surgical recovery room, or post anesthesia care unit. Both of these areas frequently transfer patients to the ICU, so it is important that designs consider reduced travel distances along with safe and rapid patient transport. The transport situation should be evaluated on the basis of the speed with which patients can be transferred from one destination to the other, as well as the safety of the patient while en route. There is evidence that transfers are associated with an increase in major negative consequences (Ulrich & Zhu, 2007).

Major diagnostics

It is often not practical or feasible for hospitals to have more than one of certain diagnostic devices; others cannot be provided on a portable basis within the critical care unit. Such devices include imaging technologies such as magnetic resonance, cardiac catheterization, interventional radiology, angiography, and the like. When critical care patients need one of these technologies, the proximity relationship which governs the length and duration of travel for patients at risk is important. A design consideration for critical care is the distance and time required to transport patients in critical condition to the imaging department, catheterization lab, or location of the relevant technology. Hospitals are increasingly building high-tech interventional suites in which varied combinations of imaging, endoscopy, laparoscopy, and surgery are combined. The design of these suites should also consider the transport of critical care patients.

When laboratory work is ordered for the critical care patient, it is frequently a matter of extreme urgency. The increasing use of point-of-care testing has been mentioned earlier in this chapter. For tests that are not performed on the unit, speed of delivery and rapid turnaround of results are significant design considerations. The method of specimen transport should be clearly identified, and criteria for turnaround time should be considered in the design phase. In the case of the laboratory, transport of the patient is not the issue, but proximity in the context of obtaining specimens, performing tests, and reporting results may influence design decisions.

Pharmacy

Pharmacological interventions are crucial to the delivery of proper care in the critical care unit. As patient acuity and complicated drug regimens have increased, the role of the pharmacy in critical care has become even more important. The concept of pharmacists participating in rounds as part of an interdisciplinary team and the use of satellite pharmacies is spreading.

Proximity to the hospital's main pharmacy, its methods of receiving shipments, and replenishment of pharmaceutical stock on the critical care unit are all factors relevant to the unit's location. Methods of delivery for pharmaceuticals should be understood, especially in the case of stat orders.

Materials management

Another important consideration for the design of a critical care unit is the relationship to materials management and the need for delivery of a constant flow of supplies. Design solutions can range from just-in-time deliveries from vendors directly to the unit, to more typical arrangements of hospital loading docks, receiving functions, and storerooms. Deliveries are usually made on some type of par-level replenishment stocking system or with fully stocked carts simply exchanged for partially depleted carts on the unit.

A properly designed materials management system within an organization's coordinated supply chain should make routine items continuously available to the critical care staff. Such a system must also have a method to provide those items that are used less often, as well as a method to rapidly deliver items requested on an emergency basis. Important elements for the development of a successful system are a careful assessment of the unit's supply usage, the development of standard lists of supplies, and the elimination of unnecessary duplications. The critical care unit's measures for evaluation of its flow of materials are: (1) percentage of routinely required items available at all times, (2) time for delivery of routinely requested items, and (3) time for delivery of stat requests.

Some hospitals have developed the concept of dedicated satellite supply locations staffed by materials management employees. These satellites serve a specific set of patient units. Those that are designated to serve critical care units have been reported to increase the availability of items and dramatically reduce the time for stat deliveries.

Food service

Generally the dietary department is responsible for delivering meals and supplying the pantries or nourishment kitchens, as well as maintaining a cafeteria and dining facilities for staff and visitors. Many critical care patients do not consume typical hospital meals, but some, such as coronary care patients, are likely to be eating normally, although they may be on special diets. Many hospitals have begun to serve hospital meal trays to the families of patients who may be in the patient room.

The dietary department should have access to the critical care unit to allow for relatively rapid and discreet movement of food carts. The hospital's food service, cafeteria, snack bar, or coffee shop should be convenient for staff and family access. Many members of the critical care staff take only abbreviated breaks for meals and prefer to be close to the unit in the case of an emergency. Family members can experience increased stress while away from the unit for meals, especially if the distance is great.

Operations and management models

The organization's operational model can have an impact on the design of a critical care unit. If the unit is under its own independent management, the design could be different from a model in which several units are under a common management structure.

The operating model will have an impact on the need for and location of offices for managers, educators, and clinical specialists of various types. The organization might be operated with centralized or decentralized patterns for meeting rooms, education spaces, on-call rooms, housekeeping or environmental services, and so forth. The ultimate design must take into account each of these separate operating decisions.

Part Three: Research on Persons and Environment

The purpose of Part Three of this book is two-fold. Firstly, it provides a summary of theories and studies which are related to the design of intensive care units. Secondly, it interprets these findings, many of which are from disciplines not specifically linked to architecture and interior design.

The information is organized into three chapters. Chapter 6 provides an overview of theories drawn primarily from the field of environmental psychology. Chapter 7 addresses literature describing the experience of participants in the ICU environment, and Chapter 8 addresses some of the basic activities within the ICU.

Creating therapeutic environments for critical care

6

Many professionals have expressed the need for quality research (Marberry, 1996), although there is a lack of clarity regarding the definition of design research and a lack of consensus concerning which type of research should receive priority. This recognition, however, of the importance of evidence-based design is a huge step forward. Twenty years ago, architects would have been strongly discouraged from pursing graduate research degrees ("I could pay you an extra $10000 per year if you had spent those last four years behind a drafting table!"). Today, however, health design doctoral students are generally welcomed into private practice.

What type of research is being done? In addition to studies on safety issues, such as infection control and falls, the research that has been most useful to designers has focused on therapeutic environments. Malkin (1992, 2008) incorporated research and methods from diverse sources to develop design guidelines for creation of therapeutic environments for specific patient groups.

The purpose of therapeutic environments is to support the caregiving process, in particular the reduction of stress (see Section 6.1 below). The next section discusses the implications of stress, as well as the psychological factors which contribute to or mitigate the negative aspects of the healthcare experience: choice and control, privacy, personal space and territoriality, and social support (Section 6.2). One approach to reducing stress in the environment has been to create positive distraction. Positive distractions such as music, art and nature are briefly described here as well (Section 6.3). The role of sunlight in reducing pain and increasing mental health is discussed in Section 6.4. Lastly, in the context of stress, noise is a primary contributor and one of the most thoroughly researched topics. Therefore a literature review on noise is included in Section 6.5.

The more things change, the more they remain the same

Jain Malkin,

As I visit newly opened hospitals, I am often stunned by the appearance of the critical care rooms. Long ago we learned that patients should be able to look out the window to "experience" natural light, changes in the weather, to "see" sunshine and to receive the hormonal benefits of circadian rhythms stimulated by observing changes from day to night. Yet many of the rooms I visit have the window behind the patient's head and, despite rotating columns for medical gases and monitors, the width of the room makes it unlikely the bed will be rotated to place the patient parallel to the window.

In these rooms I often see white floors meeting white walls and a white ceiling, which means the patient is in effect visually "floating in space." There is no separation between these three planes to orient the patient or to provide a place for the eye to focus. Patients in a critical care setting can become disoriented due to the effects of general anesthesia—especially the elderly—sleep deprivation, and from narcotic pain medication side effects that may cause hallucinations. This condition alone may sometimes extend the patient's length of stay because to discharge a patient who is experiencing hallucinations is a safety risk. These hallucinations (e.g., seeing a fleet of insects running up the wall or mice running across the ceiling) are very real and terrifying to those who experience them. This condition is often referred to as ICU psychosis (Justic, 2000). The built environment can be an intervention if it provides a way to "anchor" the patient's visual field: by creating a distinction or color difference between the floor and wall, and the wall and ceiling; by providing a view of the outdoors; and by placing an object such as a piece of art on the wall where the patient can see it.

I look at these environments that have been created for some of the sickest, most vulnerable patients and wonder why they are so stark and lacking in color? In these same hospitals one might see color on walls of medical/surgical rooms, but not in critical care. Yet color is the elixir of life, it has a powerful psychological effect as a mood elevator which may benefit family members as well as staff.

A suggestion for a color palette that can be used effectively in any patient room to create a sense of harmony consists of three colors based on a triadic color relationship (Albers, 1971; Itten, 1970; Sharpe, 1974). This, incidentally, creates a triad consisting of a long-, medium- and short-wave length color analogous to the concept of full spectrum lighting. Think of an equilateral triangle placed on a color wheel. As the triangle is rotated, any three points or colors will provide the aforementioned relationship. That is not to say that any three of these colors will be appropriate for a patient room, but that's where the skill of the designer comes into play. The saturation of the colors is a key factor, as is the value (lightness or darkness). The only caveat here is to make sure the color will not reflect on the patient's skin and contribute to an incorrect diagnosis.

How is it that today we see what appears to be a lack of awareness about certain design issues that have been in existence for 20 years? This reminds me of that quotation: the more things change, the more they remain the same *although I am pleased to say that for every critical care unit that fits this description, there is one that makes real strides in planning and design.*

Other important considerations are privacy, reduction of noise, proper accommodation of families, lighting and positive distraction.

Issues of privacy are always a trade-off with visibility of the patient. Interestingly, a number of new facilities currently in planning are doing away with break-away glass in order to provide more privacy. This helps with acoustical privacy as well. The best way to reduce noise is through the use of a high NRC (noise-reduction coefficient) acoustical tile in nurse stations and corridors surrounding patient rooms. Look for a rating of .95 NRC. In space planning, carefully consider locations of noisy equipment and use techniques to isolate vibration. Think about locations of doors so that a door to a noisy room does not align with a door to a patient room.

It is surprising that we are still fighting the battle on some fronts about whether family is welcome in the patient room (Molter, 1994). Certainly there are times when family sleepovers may not be appropriate, and the clinical staff can make that determination. However, we still have nurses with the attitude that families get in their way and the less they visit the better. This writer has sat in numerous user-group meetings discussing features of the patient room without once hearing a nurse ask, "What would be best for the patient?" *That consideration doesn't enter into the conversation as bedside cabinets are tossed out because "they get in the way of the nurses and patients can store everything they need on the overbed tray table." Anyone who has been a patient can refute that. And what about architects who plan patient rooms with no space for the clean and soiled hampers, making them a focal point for the patient and, rather than placing them close to the entry to enable housekeeping staff to access them without traversing the room? Unless the room is quite large, these cannot always be accommodated in casework.*

Research on family needs goes back to 1979 when Nancy Molter developed the Critical Care Family Needs Inventory (Molter, 1979; Molter, 1994). It was a landmark study intended to effect change in the care of families of ICU patients. Research since that time has further defined these needs and the Institute for Family-Centered Care is a wonderful resource (www.familycentered-care.org). The confines of this commentary do not permit a detailed discussion of the research, thus a few general comments will be offered.

In our fervor to care for a technologically-demanding patient, we sometimes overlook the trauma of the family who are often on the brink of emotional exhaustion (Harvey et al., 1993). Research shows that how a family responds to a crisis actually influences the patient's recovery. The family lounge environment and amenities influence a family's ability to function and to make some very critical decisions that affect the patient's current well-being and future status. Needless to say the room(s) should have natural light and a variety of areas that allow individual families privacy and the ability to meet a number of needs that change during the day. Family members may, at various times of the day, require a private space where one can vent anger or cry; a kitchen where they can warm comfort foods brought from home; social space for working a puzzle; a meditation room; an office for a chaplain or social worker near the unit; a waiting area that is more like a living room with an assortment of comfortable seating that can be moved around to accommodate family groups and achieve some degree of privacy—a place where a TV does not dominate the room; a private room or lounge with subdued lighting and several recliner chairs where a family member can enjoy a restorative nap.

Would it surprise you to learn that families who are asked to give consent for organ donation respond affirmatively significantly more frequently when they are asked in a room that is comfortable and private, as opposed to one that does not have those qualities? Can we afford to not *consider the comfort and needs of family when it is they who are actually the experts in what the patient would want, should he or she be unable to speak for themself? The mere presence of a family member can reassure a patient in what is surely one of the most threatening and unfamiliar environments that one can ever experience—the critical care setting. Critical care nurses are often task-oriented. Patient safety and survival are their principal objectives. Observing monitors and recording data sometimes take precedence over meeting the family's needs for information, reassurance, and comfort.*

Have you ever experienced a great "first class lounge" in an international airport? It's a good model for critical care. There are showers and well-appointed bathrooms, lockers, wireless Internet access, places to recharge all types of electronic devices, food and drinks, a variety of chairs and sofas in varying levels of privacy, serene sleep rooms for a quick nap and, upon entry, one is provided with a kit containing a toothbrush, toothpaste, razor, mouthwash, lotion, and other toiletries. Despite the volume, they manage to keep it clean and fresh. It truly feels like an oasis in an otherwise chaotic environment.

A few words about lighting are in order. Provide for several conditions: examination/dressing changes/procedures, reading, low level ambient light, charting. One cannot be prescriptive here as the locations of casework, charting and handwash sinks will differ. Putting the very intense examination light on a timer makes sure it will not be left on to disturb the patient after clinicians leave the room. The color temperature and color-rendering index (CRI) of the lamps is important. A lamp with 4100 Kelvin color temperature and CRI of 85 or higher will be appropriate for clinical tasks yet provide a pleasant room ambience.

It would be remiss to not mention the importance of positive distraction, which could take the form of a carefully placed back-lit transparency of a nature scene or the TV monitor may carry a closed-circuit program like the C.A.R.E. channel (www.healinghealth.com) with 60 hours of non-repetitive images of nature accompanied by soothing music. As the patient becomes more outwardly-oriented, the nurses can decide when this amenity would be most therapeutic.

In closing, as design professionals we must be ever more vigilant about our specifications and design in terms of infection control. A recent article (Hota et al., 2009) poignantly highlights this. An outbreak of Pseudomonas aeruginosa *colonization and infection was traced to "imperfect intensive care unit room design" and 71% of the 36 affected patients died. The source of the problem was traced to hand hygiene sink drains where biofilms containing viable organisms were found. Testing revealed that drain contents splashed at least one meter from the sink onto surrounding surfaces when hands were washed. Strategies for preventing this are discussed in the article and these are clearly design issues.*

Jain Malkin is an interior designer, author and speaker. She has also written numerous articles on the psychological effects of healthcare environments.

References

Albers, J., 1971. Interaction of Color. Yale University Press, New Haven, CT pp. 41–42.

Harvey, M.A., Ninas, N.P., Alder, D.C., et al., 1993. Results of the consensus conference on fostering more humane critical care: creating a healing environment. AACN's Clin. Issues Crit. Care Nurs. 4, 484–549.

Hota, S., Hirji, Z., Stockton, K., et al., 2009. Outbreak of multi-drug resistant *Pseudomonas aeruginosa* colonization and infection secondary to imperfect intensive care unit room design. Infect. Cont. and Hosp. Ep. 30 (1), 25–33.

Itten, J., 1970. The Elements of Color. Van Nostrand Reinhold, New York, pp. 72–73..

Justic, M., 2000. Does 'ICU Psychosis' really exist? Crit. Care Nurs. 20 (3), 28–37.

Molter, N.C., 1979. Needs of relatives of critically ill patients. Heart Lung 8, 332–339.

Molter, N.C., 1994. Families are not visitors in the critical care unit. DCCN 13, 2–3.

Sharpe, D., 1974. The Psychology of Color and Design. Nelson-Hall Co, Chicago, IL pp. 119–121.

6.1 Stress

Integral to a discussion of therapeutic environments is the role of stress. Stress is thought to undermine the immune system, and experienced designers and medical staff have concluded that an inappropriate physical environment can create unnecessary stress for patients, family, and staff. The primary goal of therapeutic environments, therefore, is stress reduction.

Stress can be thought of as a stimulus, a response, or the interaction between a stimulus and a person (Brannon & Feist, 2000). Evans and Cohen (1987) provide a definition of stress that is particularly useful. They note that most environmental psychologists define stress as an experience that results when an individual decides that the environmental stimuli exceed that person's ability to cope.

Research suggests that the immune system may be compromised by psychological distress. These immune system changes, in turn, are thought to result in disease (Brannon & Feist, 2000). Evidence exists to support a relationship between stress and disease, although correlations between stressful life events and biological disorders have yet to be fully established (Brannon & Feist, 2000). Stress, however, is considered to be a risk factor for headaches, infectious diseases, and possibly hypertension; it may also be a factor associated with diabetes, asthma, and arthritis (Brannon & Feist, 2000).

Stress is known to influence physiology, task performance, personal behavior, and adaptive behavior (Evans & Cohen, 1987). In terms of physiological implications, Evans and Cohen (1987) mention the increase in hormones such as epinephrine, which cause secondary changes in the activation and arousal of specific organs. Also noted are increases in blood pressure, skin conductance, respiration rates, muscle tension, and heart rate. The two significant elements that affect physical health are reduced immunological resistance and cardiovascular disorders. Task performance, personal behavior, and adaptive behavior may also be impacted.

Nelson et al. (2001) found that inability to communicate, sleep disruption, and limitations on visiting were especially stressful for ICU patients. Other sources of stress included malfunctioning personal relationships, the breakdown of familial relationships, lack of privacy, noise, inappropriately high or low sensory simulation, and lack of information about health status. Most of these conditions are related to lack of control, and are likely to occur in hospital settings. Patients in intensive care units are particularly susceptible to these conditions. Summaries of literature on the needs of patients, family, and staff appear in Chapter 7 of this book.

Conclusions and design implications

A small, but convincing, body of research exists suggesting the relationship between the physical environment and stress. Based on our current knowledge of the impact of design on stress levels, Ulrich (2001) suggests a strong possibility of achieving stress reduction through environmental interventions. Specific design recommendations are provided in the following sections.

6.2 Control and choice, personal space, privacy, territoriality and social support

Designers who are informed about the relationship between stress and control and choice, personal space, territoriality and privacy, and social support have a higher chance of success when devising appropriate healthcare environments.

Control and choice

Control and choice are central themes in environmental psychology. An individual's ability to control privacy and social interaction dramatically influences their sense of well-being (Zimring, 1981). When entering a medical setting, patients are often forced to surrender control of their personal space, and even the intimate space of their bodies. Poor wayfinding, physical barriers, lack of privacy, and poor communication (common characteristics of healthcare environments) all exacerbate feelings of lack of control. Researchers know that lack of control may result in increased blood pressure, suppressed immune system, depression, and passivity (Ulrich, 1991). Providing a sense of control is one of the four primary health facility design guidelines recommended by Ulrich (1997, 1999, 2000, 2001), who points out that control is an issue for staff as well (Ulrich, 2001).

Regarding the impact of control, researchers widely believe that instilling a sense of efficacy in patients helps reduce their stress. The issue of control has been specifically addressed when considering responses to noise. Topf (1984) hypothesizes that providing patients with instructions on how to control aversive stimuli (such as noise), combined with certain of their own personal characteristics, will result in less stress and a quicker recovery. Hansell (1984) proposes that sensitivity to noise is also influenced by an individual's ability to control the noise. Topf (2000) recommends several ways to return cognitive control to patients, including informing patients about what various sounds mean, explaining the purpose of such sounds, and offering options which will enable patients to reduce sound levels. Patients can be taught progressive muscle-relaxation techniques; given access to music, white noise, or earplugs; empowered to make verbal responses to quiet others; and given sleep medication. A broader discussion of noise is provided later in this chapter.

An excellent way to combat lack of control is to provide an individual with choices. While the choices may not be ideal, the fact that alternatives are available will help to improve the individual's sense of independence.

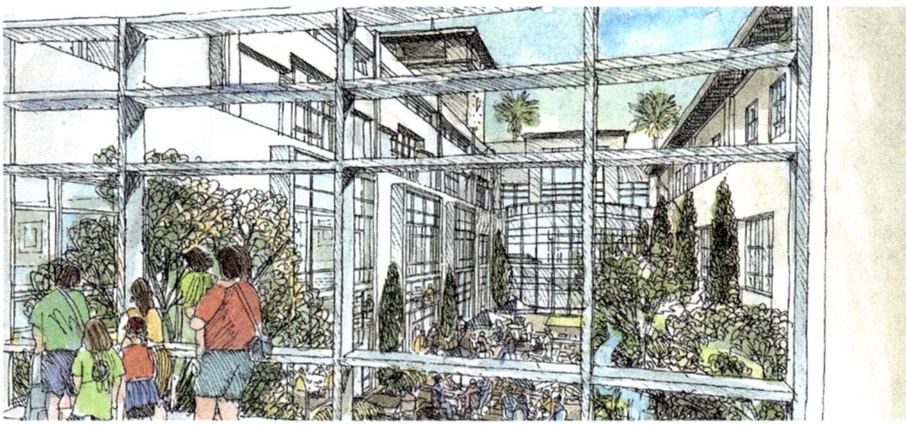

Figure 6.1: *An interior courtyard supports wayfinding, which in turn supports sense of control*
Location: Santa Barbara Cottage Hospital: Santa Barbara, CA
Architect: Lee, Burkhart, Liu
Illustrations by: William Block, Project Vignettes

Personal space, territoriality, and privacy

The concepts of personal space, territoriality, and privacy are the core of much of the research conducted in the field of environment and behavior. While these three terms are related, they are not identical.

Robert Sommer was among the first researchers to explore the intricacies and implications of "personal space." According to Sommer (1969), personal space is an area which surrounds the body into which those who are not invited may not come. Gifford (1987) expands on this by describing personal space as "the geographic component of interpersonal relations" (p. 96). Personal space is related to proxemics (Hall, 1963), which is generally broken into the following four categories of distance between people: intimate, personal, social and public.

Intimate space activities are performed at extremely close range (such as the close distance between mother and child during a care routine). *Personal* space behaviors are conducted between individuals who are well known to one another, and normally take place within a few feet. *Social* space behaviors are conducted between acquaintances at a range of three or more feet, while *public* spatial behavior requires significant distances (such as those that would be appropriate between presenter and audience during a lecture). Using the ICU as an example, a patient's intimate personal space is likely to be violated during normal nursing procedures. In other words, the nurse (who is essentially a stranger) would have to invade the space that previously was only available to the individual's family and closest friends. Routine care protocols may create discomfort for the patient, as patient and staff perceptions of personal space may differ (Edwards, 1998).

Gifford (1987) defines territoriality as a "pattern of behavior and attitudes held by an individual or group that is based on perceived, attempted, or actual control of a definable physical space, object, or idea that may involve habitual occupation, defense, personalization, and marking of it" (p. 120). Sommer (1969) bases his definition of territory on that of Heidegger and describes it as a place that is made distinctive and defended by the owner. Territoriality is expressed by patients, for example, through displays of photos and the arrangement of movable furniture. Families in waiting rooms may express territoriality by reconfiguring furniture arrangements or draping belongings over chairs and tables. The establishment of territory in an ICU setting was demonstrated in Fournier's 1995 study, in which families in ICU waiting rooms created boundaries with furniture to identify personal turf. In an anthropological interpretation of the use of space and touch on an inpatient ward, Edwards (1998) noted that staff and patients sometimes had different interpretations of what constituted personal space.

For more than 40 years, medical staff/researchers have acknowledged the important role of patients' territorial behavior (e.g., Esser et al., 1965). Nurses in particular have been aware that personal space, territoriality, and privacy are critical dimensions in healthcare settings (Kerr, 1982). Allekian (1974) and Santa Maria-Punongbayan (1982) found that anxiety was significantly related to intrusions on territory. Sawada et al. (1996) recorded 95 personal and territorial space behaviors in an analysis of 80 critical incident reports from an inpatient unit. The researchers noted that many of these incidents undermined the personal space and territory of patients. Differing perceptions may account for these variations in spatial behaviors.

Bullock-Loughran (1982) points out that the critical care patient, "because of his illness, is unable to lay territorial claim" (p. 21). She notes that the provision of territory can make the difference between a sense of identity and a loss of identity (see Figure 6.2).

Several suggestions have been made to promote a sense of territoriality, such as knocking on a patient's door before entering, not leaving the patient's body exposed, and arranging the room as the patient desires. Patients may feel like intruders in the nursing unit and wish to establish a territory of their own (Esberger, 1982). Placek (1977) notes that in order to maintain the nurse as

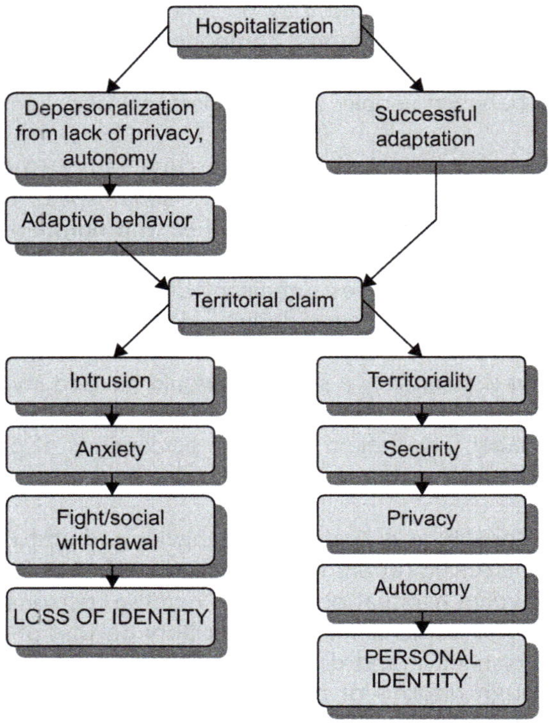

Figure 6.2: *Relationship between territory and identity (Bullock-Loughran, 1982)*

an ally, the patient must transform from an independent individual to a dependent and "meek" patient, which automatically means the surrender of territory.

Regarding privacy, Gifford (1987) provides Altman's definition, which describes privacy as "selective control of access to self or to one's group" (p. 172). Privacy is related to personal space in that private exchanges may take place within one's intimate personal space bubble. On the other hand, privacy can be invaded without an intrusion on intimate personal space. For example, a patient and a family member could be engaged in intimate conversation, but the appearance of someone on the other side of the room could result in an invasion of privacy.

Loss of privacy results in loss of control. "Privacy is sacrificed. . . when patients sleep in rooms with strangers, triage takes place in public areas, financial information is gathered in public, or patients are left waiting on gurneys in corridors" (Shepley, Fournier, & McDougal, 1998). In the case of the ICU, for example, if the curtains were not fully drawn while a catheter was being inserted, the patient would certainly feel violated.

While writing this book, one of the authors visited a friend whose mother had been admitted to an ICU. The waiting room was very small (approximately 200 square feet) and half the seats were filled and arranged in a sociofugal pattern. (Sociofugal seating arrangements are oriented in such a way as to impede conversation, usually in linear patterns as commonly seen in airports.

Sociopetal seating supports conversation, as would be achieved when seats are next to one another at right angles. See Hall, 1963.) We decided to stand in the corridor outside the room, rather than sit where others could overhear our conversation. After 30 minutes or so, we tired of standing and, rather than be forced into a public space, sat on the floor. I believe this behavior was not unusual. The need for privacy may exceed the need for comfort in an ICU setting.

Social support

Although many designers are inclined to believe that the physical environment can cure all ills in a healthcare situation, research indicates that appropriate social support plays a significantly more dominant role in patient recovery. Studies have found that those individuals with a large number of social ties tend to have higher health status (Ulrich, 1999). Research suggests, for example, that one reason women may live longer than men is because women are more socially interactive and therefore have stronger interpersonal networks (Brannon & Feist, 1997). Berkman and Syme (1979) conducted a nine-year mortality study on 6928 adults in California and found that people who lacked social contacts were more likely to die in a nine-year study than those with more extensive ties. The nature of the link between social support and improved health status, however, is unclear (Ulrich, 1999).

When recovering from illness, the average child and many adults would rather be with their family and friends in a homecare setting than in a highly sophisticated technological environment. Social interaction is the objective, and architecture can impede or encourage social opportunities.

The heart of social support lies in family-centered care. Family-centered care may include extended family and close friends. Malkin (2000) identifies the following categories of support for families: reassurance and social support, access to information, easy access to patients via proximity, and good wayfinding and diversions. All of these activities can be supported by the physical environment. A detailed summary of family needs is provided in Chapter 7.

Sometimes the needs for social support, which are addressed through family-centered care, create conflicts with other objectives. A family-centered care program may transform an inpatient unit into a highly populated environment and result in intrusions on privacy and territory (Shepley, Fournier & McDougal, 1998). The various environmental needs must be carefully balanced.

Conclusions and design implications

Control and choice

Control and choice can be provided in small ways, ranging from providing the patient with bedside switches that control window coverings, light levels, and temperature, to giving the patient the opportunity to select room décor such as curtains, posters, and bedspreads. Providing access to medical records also conveys a sense of control by reducing the number of unknowns for the patient. Positioning the bed in such a way that it can be rotated to have a view of the corridor or a view outside is another way to provide patients with choices. Some ICU patients will not be able to take a proactive role regarding their environments; however, families can intercede to meet their needs.

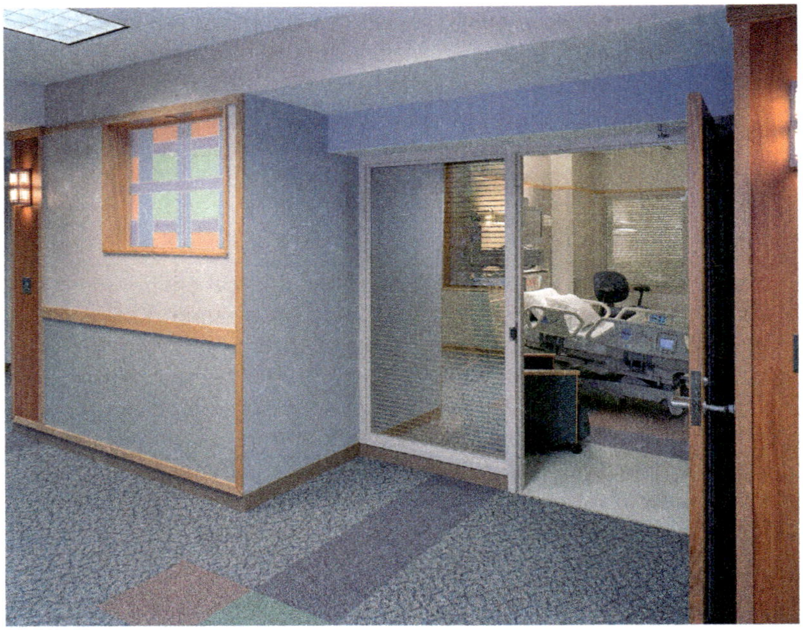

Figure 6.3: *The semi-public space provided by alcoves/entries off of the corridor serves to define the patient's territory*
Location: King's Daughters Medical Center-ICU: Ashland, KY
Architect: Karlsberger Architectural Group
Photo credit: Robert Benson, photographer

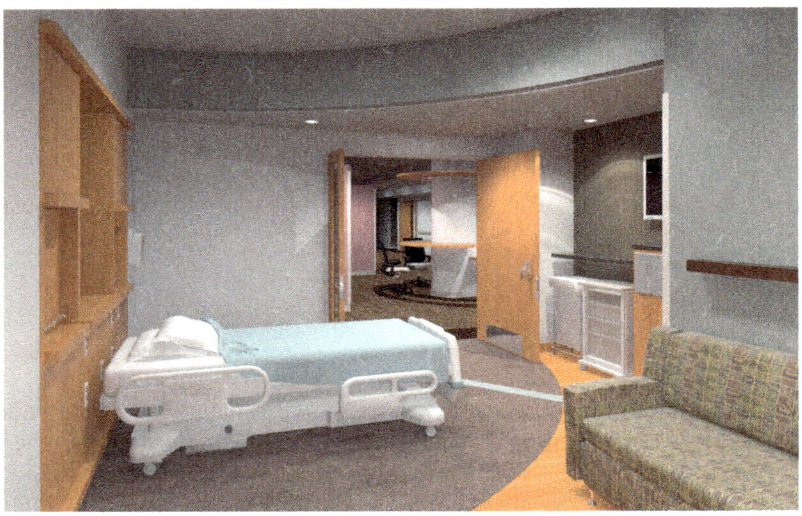

Figure 6.4: *Floor and ceiling patterns create separate zones of semi-private space within the patient room*
Location: Dublin Methodist Hospital, Dublin, OH
Architect: Karlsberger Architectural Group
Photo credit: Robert Benson, photographer

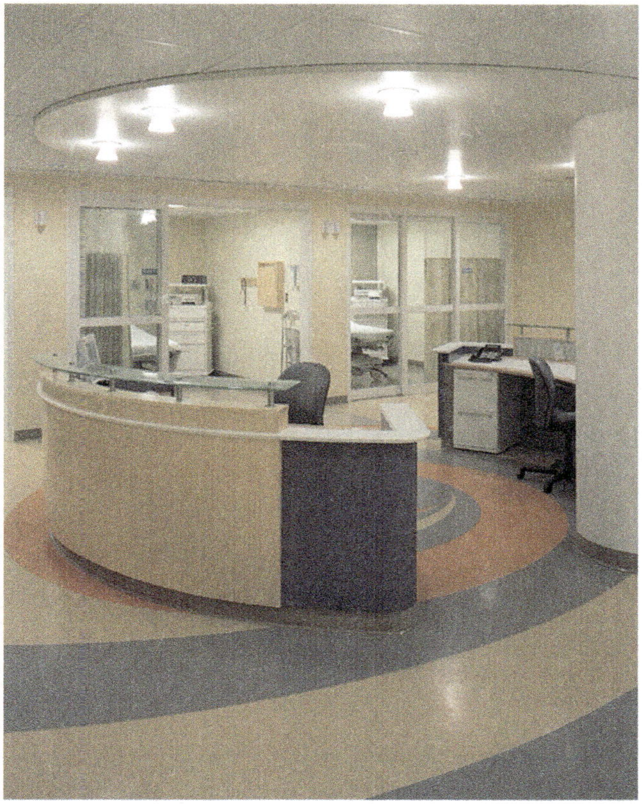

Figure 6.5: *Floor, lighting and ceiling patterns help to define the territory associated with staff functions*
Location: Swedish Orthopedic Institute, Tower 105, Seattle, WA
Architect: NBBJ
Photo credit: Farshid Assassi, photographer

Personal space, territoriality, and privacy

The distance between the patient and room furnishings such as curtains and chairs should be flexible in order to respond to variable personal space requirements. It is helpful to provide patients with opportunities to mark territory using articles that personalize space. Regarding privacy, single-occupancy rooms are a must, and curtains should be used when direct supervision through glass walls is not necessary. Other recommendations include:

- provide clear, redundant wayfinding
- avoid hierarchies suggested by barriers, such as nurses' stations
- provide enough space to keep population densities down
- ensure patient privacy during financial transactions
- provide sufficient space so patients are not left to wait in corridors (Shepley, Fournier & McDougal, 1998).

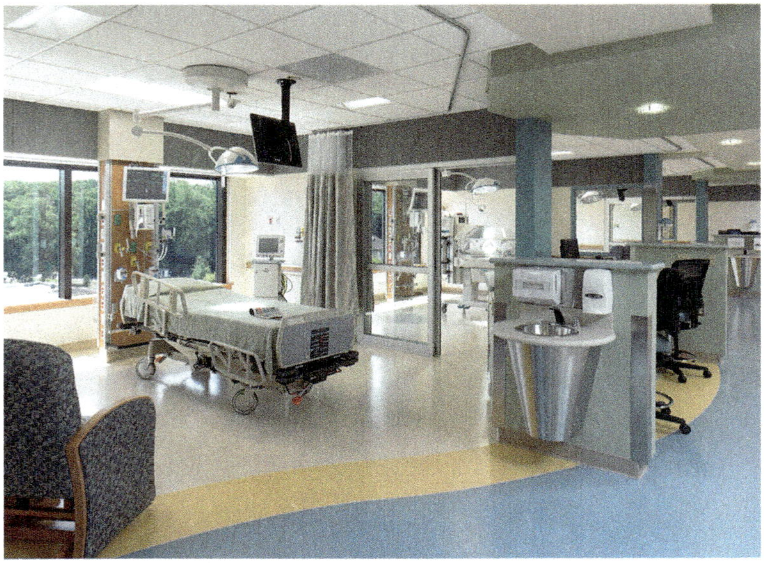

Figure 6.6: *Floor patterns and fixed casework help to define the boundaries of open patient rooms*
Location: Alfred I. duPont Hospital for Children-CIC Unit: Wilmington, DE
Architect: ARRAY Healthcare Facilities Solutions
Photo credit: Jeffrey Totaro/Esto, photographer

To support the need for establishing territory, designers suggest providing bulletin boards, tack strips (strips of material which allow for pinning up pictures and notes), and storage areas for personal belongings (Duffy & Florell, 1990). In an ICU, this may be more for the benefit of the family than the patient, who may not be conscious. Planetree (a patient-centered philosophy and program—see Frampton, Gilpin & Charmel, 2003) proponents support the personalization of space by allowing patients to select their preferred curtains, bedspreads, and artwork.

Social support

Malkin (2000) recommends the following environmental amenities for families:

- therapeutic chair with psycho-acoustic music (involving sound and vibration)
- foot massager
- massage pad for recliner chair
- closed-circuit TV with uplifting messages or nature scenery
- aromatherapy diffusers
- access to telephone
- private room for napping
- multiple styles of chairs
- waiting rooms broken into small-group areas

- diversions such as aquariums, fireplaces, interactive sculptures, or water amenities (e.g., fountains, ponds)
- options for sitting, watching TV, working on puzzles, or using computers
- reference library
- access to drinks and snacks
- clean bathing facilities
- access to newspapers
- live plants
- storage lockers
- social spaces for interactions with other families
- bulletin boards for messages between family members.

Drawing upon the work of multiple authors, Shepley, Fournier and McDougal (1998) identified several other design emphases regarding family-centered care:

- provide sufficient space so family members can be with the patient and not interfere with the activities of staff
- provide spaces that promote visitation
- promote rooming-in (sleeping in the patient's room) by providing appropriate furniture in the patient room
- provide locations for conversations between staff and family members
- provide access to computers to enhance communication opportunities for families.

Social support can also be provided by other patients. The movement to provide single-occupancy rooms will impact the opportunities for this to take place so patient gathering spaces (for those who can ambulate) should be considered.

6.3 Positive distractions

Ulrich (1999) defines positive distraction as an environmental feature that generates positive feelings and maintains attention without creating stress. By so doing, the distraction deflects troublesome thoughts. The primary instruments of distraction related to healthcare environments are art/graphics, music, television/video/virtual reality, and nature. Other factors, such as recreational therapy, humor, and pet therapy, are more program- or socially-focused.

Distraction amenities have been explored in multiple studies, and researchers are attempting to identify their relative effectiveness in promoting healing. For example, what type of art is most therapeutic—abstract or representational? What type of music is most appropriate—classical or contemporary? What type of nature views are preferred—natural or highly "manicured?"

Access to distractions is also important to staff. Cooper Marcus (1999) quotes a nurse as saying, "I work in ICU, which is like a hell hole. For the first four hours I just run. Sitting out in the warm sun is like therapy to me. I can relax, gather my thoughts. I feel like I have my head screwed on straight." A more in-depth discussion of staff needs occurs later in this book.

Most research on positive distraction has focused on the role of art, nature, and music in healing environments.

The environment and pain

Roger S. Ulrich, Ph.D.

Pain is a serious and costly problem in ICUs. Therefore it is noteworthy that a growing body of scientific evidence strongly suggests that characteristics of healthcare physical environments influence pain, and that appropriately designed patient care surroundings can produce significant pain reduction (Ulrich et al., 2008; Ulrich, 2008). The increasing scientific quality of the research on environment–pain relationships is underscored by the fact that several studies are randomized controlled trials published in international medical journals. The strength of evidence also has been enhanced by advances in understanding the mechanisms by which design can affect pain. The credibility of the notion that designed surroundings influence pain has increased to the point where a leading scientific pain research journal recently published an article emphasizing the importance of creating healthcare settings to expose patients to nature, light, and other positive environmental factors found by studies to alleviate pain (Malenbaum et al., 2008).

Pain researchers have proposed that exposure to nature may reduce pain through different mechanisms, including by reducing stress and distracting persons away from focusing on their pain (Ulrich, 2008). According to distraction theory, pain draws considerable attention, and as the amount of attention a patients directs to pain increases, the intensity of pain worsens (McCaul and Malott, 1984). However, if attention is diverted or absorbed by an emotionally pleasant external distraction such as a nature view or garden, distraction theory holds there is less conscious attention focused on sensations of pain, and experienced pain therefore diminishes (Ulrich, 2008; Ulrich et al., 2008). Other research has linked higher stress to elevated pain. Because much evidence has shown that nature can produce substantial recovery from stress, it follows that another mechanism by which nature in healthcare settings should alleviate pain is stress reduction.

Consistent with the predictions of pain theories, several rigorous studies have found that exposing patients to real or simulated nature reduces reported pain intensity and intake of analgesic doses. A well-controlled study compared the recovery records of surgery patients who had been randomly assigned to a bedside window view of nature (trees) or a brick building wall (Ulrich, 1984). Findings showed that the nature view patients suffered significantly less pain, as indicated by needing fewer injections of potent narcotic pain drugs than the wall view patients. As another research example, a randomized prospective study in a hospital by Tse and colleagues (2002) found that volunteers had greater tolerance for pain and a higher threshold for detecting pain if they were assigned to view a nature videotape in contrast to a blank display.

Other studies suggest that nature exposures involving both sound and visual stimulation may tend to be more engrossing than visual distraction alone, and hence more effective in alleviating pain. For example, a randomized controlled trial of patients undergoing colonoscopy found that those viewing nature experienced less pain than patients viewing a blank screen, but that a more diverting combination of visual and audio distraction (nature scenery + classical music) outperformed viewing nature alone (Lee et al., 2004). Findings from another randomized controlled trial suggest that patients undergoing painful bronchoscopy experienced less pain when they were assigned to look at a nature scene and listen to sounds recorded at the nature setting (moving water, birds) than a control group who looked at a blank wall during the procedure (Diette et al., 2003).

In contrast to the pain-reducing influences of viewing nature, a few studies have shown that many abstract pictures or artworks elicit emotionally negative reactions in patients and can worsen stress (Ulrich, 2008). Limited evidence raises the possibility that viewing certain abstract pictures may elevate pain. Pain theory and research strongly imply that healthcare design should minimize well-documented environmental stressors such as noise and lack of privacy, in order to enhance pain control.

In addition to nature exposure, higher daylight in patient spaces appears to alleviate pain. A possible mechanism for pain reduction is that daylight exposure increases serotonin, which may inhibit pain pathways. A well-controlled prospective study found that surgery patients admitted post operatively to bright rooms reported less pain and took substantially fewer patient-controlled analgesic doses than those admitted to shaded rooms (Walch et al., 2005). Additionally, many randomized controlled studies have found that exposing patients to light—daylight or bright artificial light—is effective in reducing depression, including for patients suffering severe depression (Golden et al., 2005). A few retrospective studies suggest that hospitalized patients with severe depression have shorter stays if they are assigned to sunnier rooms in contrast to rooms that receive less daylight (Beauchemin and Hays, 1996; Benedetti et al., 2001).

Design implications

The developing research on environment and pain implies that architectural design and siting decisions should make it possible for bedridden patients suffering pain to look out onto sunny nature spaces. Attention also should be given to installing art or pictures depicting representational nature in patient rooms, procedure spaces, and examination rooms where pain and stress are problems. Evidence also supports providing technology such as flat screens and VR displays to simulate nature views and sounds in spaces where it is not feasible to provide real nature. Pain theories and research strongly suggest that patients should not be placed in spaces that lack nature distraction and daylight but contain environmental stressors such as noise, because pain will likely be intensified (Ulrich, 2008; Ulrich et al., 2008).

Roger S. Ulrich is professor of Architecture at Texas A&M University.

References

Beauchemin, K.M., Hays, P., 1996. Sunny hospital rooms expedite recovery from severe and refractory depressions. J. Affect. Disorders 40 (1–2), 49–51.

Benedetti, F., Colombo, C., Barbini, B., et al., 2001. Morning sunlight reduces length of hospitalization in bipolar depression. J. Affect. Disorders 62 (3), 221–223.

Diette, G.B., Lechtzin, N., Haponik, E., et al., 2003. Distraction therapy with nature sights and sounds reduces pain during flexible bronchoscopy: a complementary approach to routine analgesia. Chest 123 (3), 941–948.

Golden, R.N., Gaynes, B.N., Ekstrom, R.D., et al., 2005. The efficacy of light therapy in the treatment of mood disorders: a review and meta-analysis of the evidence. Am. J. Psychiat. 162 (4), 656–662.

Lee, D.W.H., Chan, A.C.W., Wong, S.K.H., et al., 2004. Can visual distraction decrease the dose of patient-controlled sedation required during colonoscopy? A prospective randomized controlled trial. Endoscopy 36 (3), 197–201.

Malenbaum, S., Keefe, F.J., Williams, A.C., et al., 2008. Pain in its environmental context: implications for designing environments to enhance pain control. Pain 134, 241–244.

McCaul, K.D., Malott, J.M., 1984. Distraction and coping with pain. Psychol. Bull. 95 (3), 516–533.

Tse, M.M.Y., Ng, J.K.F., Chung, J.W.Y., Wong, T.K.S., 2002. The effect of visual stimuli on pain threshold and tolerance. J. Clin. Nurs. 11 (4), 462–469.

Ulrich, R.S., 1984. View through a window may influence recovery from surgery. Science 224, 42–421.

Ulrich, R.S., 2008. Biophilic design of healthcare environments. In: Kellert, S., Heerwagen, J., Mador, M. (Eds.) Biophilic Design for Better Buildings and Communities. John Wiley, New York, pp. 87–106.

Ulrich, R.S., Zimring, C., Zhu, X., et al., 2008. A review of the research literature on evidence-based healthcare design. Health Environ. Res. Des. 1 (3), 61–125.

Walch, J.M., Rabin, B.S., Day, R., et al., 2005. The effect of sunlight on post-operative analgesic medication usage: a prospective study of patients undergoing spinal surgery. Psychosom. Med. 67, 156–163.

Art and color

Awareness of the role of art in hospitals has become mainstream in recent years (Shepley, 2006b). Ulrich and others have examined the use of art in healthcare environments. Ulrich (1986) found that psychiatric patients preferred representational pictures dominated by nature, rather than abstract works. Ulrich found similar negative responses to abstract art in other patients (Ulrich, 1991, 1999). Does this mean that patients of all ages, including children, prefer more representative art? There is research to the contrary demonstrating that young children do not have a preference for one genre over the other (McGhee & Dziuban, 1993).

A discussion of art often includes questions about the role of color. Ireland, Warren, and Herringer (1992) found that anxious individuals had less preference for highly saturated colors. This finding together with the concept that adult patients favor less abstract work suggests that pale palettes and representative genres are less likely to overstimulate or disturb adult patients and their families. Marberry and Zagon (1995) recommend a full-spectrum color palette. In other words, a component representing each major color in the spectrum should be included at least in a minimal way. Although this approach makes intuitive sense, it has yet to be corroborated through research.

The Center for Health Environments Research (CHER) has recently published a literature review to identify color research that is useful to designers of healthcare settings, and which may lead to grounded theories and help create an agenda for research. An additional study, partially funded by the AIA Graduate Fellowship in Health Facility Planning and Design, addresses pediatric color preferences (Park, 2007).

Color preferences in healthcare settings

Jin Gyu Park, Ph.D.

Very little research has been conducted in healthcare settings in terms of color effects. Although the topic of my recent research focuses on pediatric patients in outpatient and acute care settings (Park, 2009), it involves a useful context for adult populations in intensive care settings.

The purpose of this study was to investigate the value of color as a component in a healing environment for pediatric patient rooms. It consisted of two phases: a pilot study and a main study. The pilot study investigated healthy children's most-preferred colors from each of the five hue families defined by the Munsell color system. The result indicated that red (5R 7/8), yellow (5R 9/8), green (5G 7/8), blue (5B 6/8), and purple (5P 7/8) were the most-preferred colors by healthy children. Using those five colors and a white color (N 9.5/), the main study measured pediatric patients' color preferences and then compared them to healthy children's, to investigate group and gender effects.

Environmental elements that produce positive feelings can reduce patient stress (Ulrich, 1981). If environmental colors can have positive impacts, it is possible that those colors may add to the comfort of a patient, thus reducing stress. Although previous color studies are suggestive, none has focused on healthcare settings for the pediatric population. Sick children may not perceive their surroundings in the same way as healthy children. More specifically, patients in negative emotional states have a tendency to develop their emotions in negative ways (Carpman & Grant, 1993). This study addressed a gap in the body of knowledge regarding how children's color preferences change in response to health status.

A simulation method was used in order to investigate the value of color in real contexts and controlling confounding variables. Previous color preference studies typically have been done with small colored chips or papers, which are visually different from seeing a color applied on wall surfaces. In addition, they failed to control confounding variables such as color attributes and light sources (Child, Hansen, & Hornbeck, 1968; Meerum Terwogt & Hoeksma, 1995).

There were no significant mean differences among healthy children, pediatric outpatients, and pediatric inpatients. All three groups showed similar color preference patterns, except for yellow. Both pediatric outpatients and inpatients showed higher preference for yellow than healthy children did. However, the healthier group showed higher mean scores of color preferences: healthy children, pediatric outpatients, and pediatric inpatients respectively. Even though this observation was not statistically significant, it calls for further investigation about whether intensive care pediatric patients respond differently to colors than healthy children do. Gender effects indicated that girls preferred red and purple more than boys did. Regardless of gender effects, blue and green were the most preferred colors by all three groups and white the least.

Suggestions for color in an adult ICU

Although contradictions exist in the literature, a consistent trend is that blue is one of the most-preferred colors across age and gender (Eysenck, 1941; Guilford & Smith, 1959; Valdez & Mehrabian, 1994; Park, 2009). White is pervasive in healthcare facilities, but is the least preferred by healthy children, pediatric patients (Park, 2009), and adults (Park, 2007). A trend in emotional associations with color has also been identified; brighter colors are associated with positive feelings, in contrast, darker colors evoke negative feelings (Boyatzis & Varghese, 1994; Hemphill, 1996). It has been observed that males consider the range of cool colors the most pleasant, whereas females consider the range of warm colors the most pleasant (Helson & Lansford, 1970).

While previous findings are suggestive, long-term effects for intensive care patients are inconclusive. (The study described here did not include intensive care patients.) Single colors, especially white, or a monotonous color scheme throughout the unit may be perceived as institutional and boring. A balance of both color and light in the elements of the unit is suggested. One way to achieve harmony in colors is to use color samples in different brightness or saturation from a single hue family. Brighter primary colors are recommended as main theme or accent color since those are associated with positive emotions. There may be a multitude of equipment and furniture essential to the function of the unit; blending them within the overall color scheme can help make the space seem less disturbing.

Light sources are also critical to retain quality of color. Under incandescent or florescent lighting, color can be distorted due to the unequal spectrum of wavelength. Therefore, full-spectrum light sources would be beneficial to get the best results of color effect.

Jin Gyu Park is Assistant Professor of Architecture at University of North Texas.

References

Boyatzis, C.J., Varghese, R., 1994. Children's emotional associations with colors. J. Genet. Psychol. 155 (1), 77–85.

Carpman, J.R., Grant, M.A., 1993. Design that Cares: Planning Health Facilities for Patients and Visitors. American Hospital Publishing, Chicago, IL.

Child, I.L., Hansen, J.A., Hornbeck, F.W., 1968. Age and sex differences in children's color preferences. Child Dev. 39 (1), 237–247.

Eysenck, H.J., 1941. A critical and experimental study of color preferences. Am. J. Psychol. 54 (3), 385–394.

Guilford, J.P., Smith, P., 1959. A system of color preferences. Am. J. Psychol. 62 (4), 487–502.

Helson, H., Lansford, T., 1970. The role of spectral energy of source and background pleasantness of object colors. Appl. Optics 9 (7), 1513–1562.

Hemphill, M., 1996. A note on adults' color-emotion associations. J. Genet. Psychol. 157 (3), 275–280.

Meerum Terwogt, M., Hoeksma, J.B., 1995. Colors and emotions: preferences and combinations. J. Gen. Psychol. 122 (1), 5–17.

Park, J. (2007). Environmental color for pediatric patient room design. Unpublished doctoral dissertation, Texas A&M University at College Station.

Park, J., 2009. Color perception in pediatric patient room design: healthy children vs. pediatric patients. Health Environ. Res. Des. J. 2 (3) in press.

Ulrich, R.S., 1981. Natural versus urban scenes: some psychological well-being. Environ. Behav. 13 (5), 523–556.

Valdez, P., Mehrabian, A., 1994. Effect of color on emotions. J. Exp. Psychol. Gen. 123 (4), 394–409.

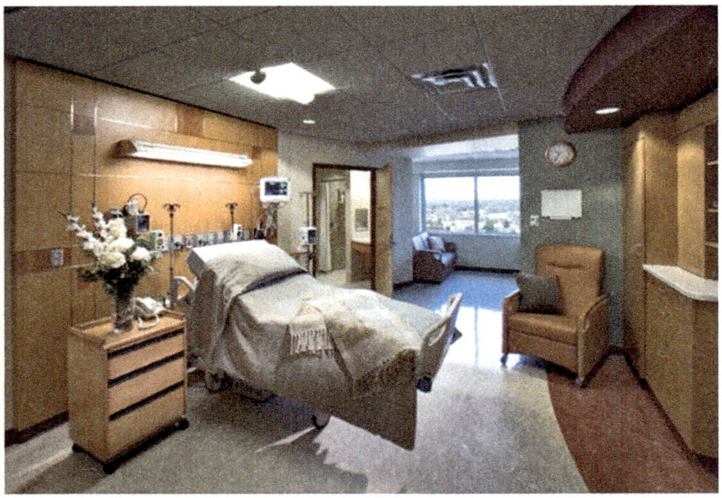

Figure 6.7: *Wall and floor colors reinforce spatial definitions of patient and family spaces*
Location: Lancaster General Hospital: Lancaster, PA
Architect: RTKL
Photo credit: Charles Davis Smith AIA, photographer

Nature

Views of nature have been shown to positively impact health outcomes. In his seminal study, Ulrich found that patients with a view of nature requested less pain medication and had shorter lengths of stay than patients with views of a building (Ulrich, 1984). In a study of patients who were shown nature and abstract pictures while recovering from open heart surgery, Ulrich, Lundén and Eltinge (1993) found that patients who viewed nature pictures had less post operative anxiety than subjects who viewed abstract art, and control conditions. Tse et al. (2002) studied the response of healthy subjects to pain induced by a tourniquet, and noted that pain threshold and tolerance was higher when the participants viewed natural scenery, as opposed to a blank wall. In a recent study at Johns Hopkins University, researchers found that patients who listened to nature sounds and viewed a landscape mural during bronchoscopy procedures reported that pain control was good or excellent, compared to patients in the control group (Diette et al., 2003). In *Healing Gardens: Therapeutic Benefits and Design Recommendations*, Ulrich provides an excellent summary of the research that has been conducted on the impact of nature on health outcomes in *Gardens in Healthcare Facilities* (Cooper Marcus & Barnes, 1995).

Music

Music has been employed as a stress-reducing or noise-mitigating strategy in several ICUs (Coughlan, 1994; Elliott, 1992; Henry, 1995; Johnston & Rohaly-Davis, 1996; O'Sullivan, 1991).

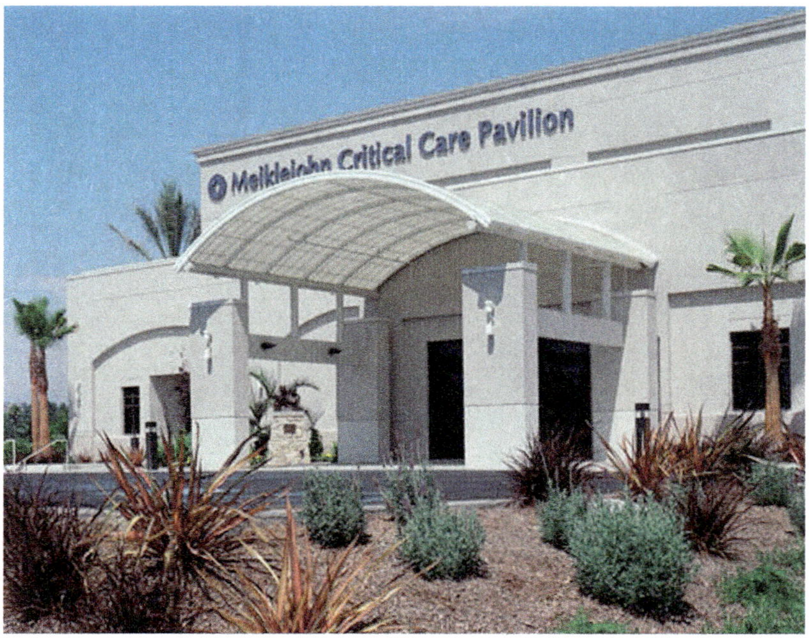

Figure 6.8: *Nature, particularly indigenous plants, should be introduced at the entrance to a facility*
Location: Saddleback Memorial Medical Center—Meiklejohn Critical Care Pavilion: Laguna Hills, CA
Architect: TAYLOR & Associates Architects with Questar Construction
Photo credit: Assassi Productions, photography

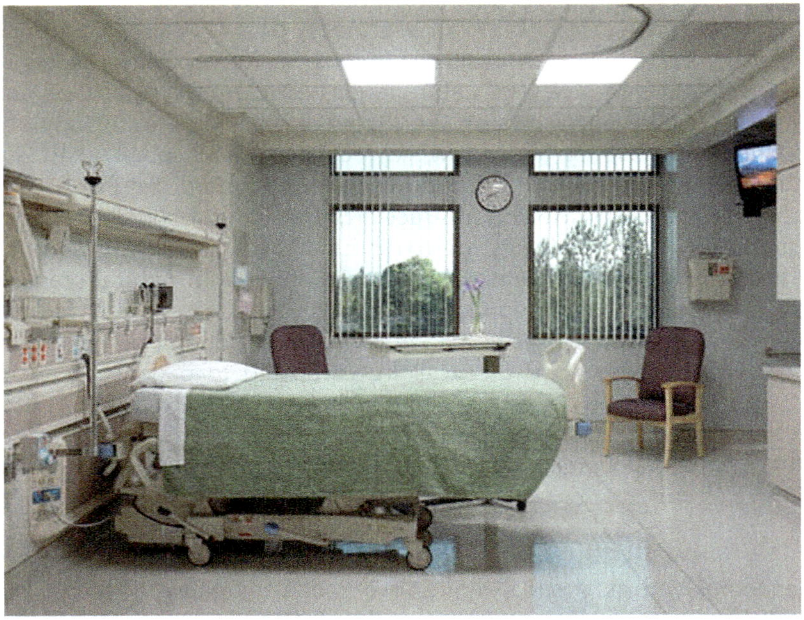

Figure 6.9: *Nature also has a roie in the patient room*
Location: Saddleback Memorial Medical Center—Meiklejohn Critical Care Pavilion: Laguna Hills, CA
Architect: TAYLOR & Associates Architects with Questar Construction
Photo credit: Assassi Productions, photography

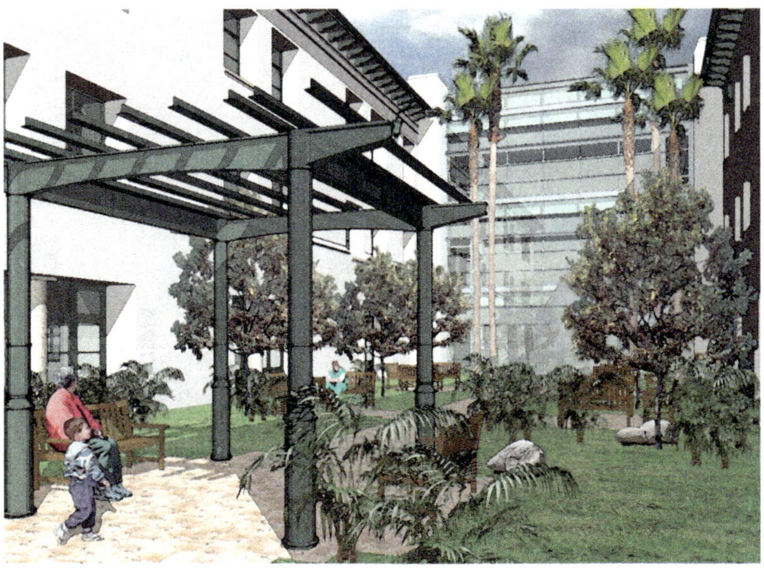

Figure 6.10: *Courtyards with seating and wandering paths provide an opportunity to interact with nature*
Location: Santa Barbara Cottage Hospital: Santa Barbara, CA
Architect: Lee, Burkhart, Liu
Photo credit: Courtyard Watercolor2: Lee, Burkhart, Liu

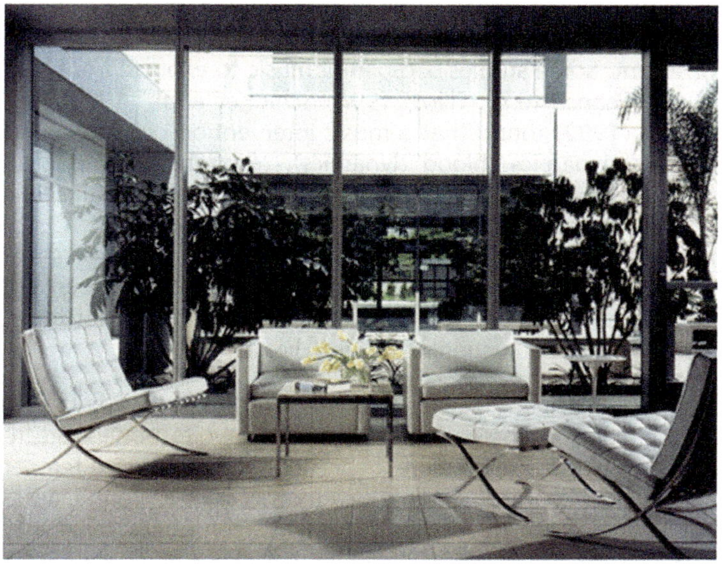

Figure 6.11: *Views into courtyards from waiting areas could have stress-reducing qualities*
Location: Valley Presbyterian Hospital-Lobby: Van Nuys, CA
Architect: Lee, Burkhart, Liu
Photo credit: ©Erhard Pfeiffer 2004, photographer

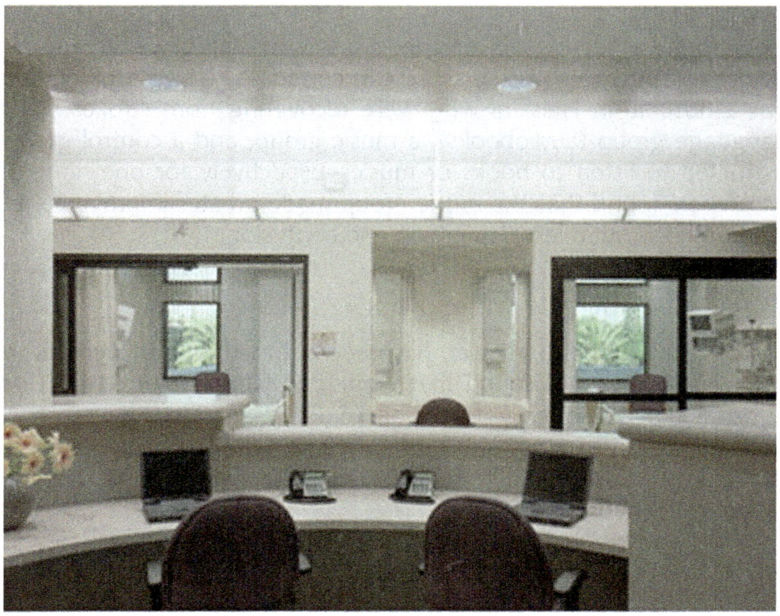

Figure 6.12: *Well-defined lines of sight will enable both patients and staff to enjoy views of nature*
Location: Saddleback Memorial Medical Center—Meiklejohn Critical Care Pavilion: Laguna Hills, CA
Architect: TAYLOR & Associates Architects with Questar Construction
Photo credit: Assassi Productions, photograph

Studies on the impact of music in these settings are varied in their conclusions. While subjects generally report the experience as being positive (Neuhof et al., 1980), physiological responses to music are not consistent. Some studies comparing music to expected outcomes have not demonstrated statistical significance (e.g., Elliot, 1994; Schinner et al., 1995). For example, Heitz, Symreng, and Scamman (1992) found that a music intervention did not impact pain level, morphine requirement, hemodynamics (blood dynamics), respiration, or length of stay. Subjects exposed to music, however, waited longer before requesting analgesia and perceived their experiences as more pleasant. Most recently, Chlan et al. (2007) studied 10 ICU patients who were receiving mechanical ventilation. Of the four physiological measures of stress response which were measured, there were no statistically significant differences between patients listening to music and those who rested for 60 minutes. The authors concluded that the results might have been confounded by endotracheal suctioning and medications.

Other researchers (e.g., Zimmerman, Pierson, & Marker, 1988) have produced more encouraging results. Coronary care patients exposed to either music or white noise were reported as having improved outcomes in terms of blood pressure, heart rate, and digital skin temperature. Statistically significant impacts have been found regarding lowered heart rate (Bonny, 1978; Byers & Smyth, 1997; Guzzetta, 1988; White, 1992, 1999; Zimmerman, Pierson, & Marker, 1988), decreased blood pressure (Byers & Smyth, 1997; Updike, 1990; Zimmerman, Pierson, & Marker, 1988), reduced respiratory rate (White, 1992, 1999), decreased myocardial oxygen demand (White, 1999), decreased perception of noise-annoyance (Byers & Smyth, 1997), decreased galvanic skin response (Guzzetta, 1988; Zimmerman, Pierson, & Marker; 1988), increased pain relief (Bonny, 1978; Good, 1995; Menegazzi et al., 1991;Nilsson, Rawal, & Unosson, 2003; Zimmerman et al., 1996), and lowered anxiety/depression (Bonny, 1978; White, 1992, 1999).

Music has also been found to reduce self-reported stress levels in ICU waiting rooms (Routhieaux & Tansik, 1997). More recently, Särkämö et al. (2008) conducted a single-blind, randomized study on patients from a hospital in Helskini who were recovering from strokes. The subjects were divided into a language group (audiobooks), a music group, and a control group. The first two groups were instructed to listen to books or music, respectively for one hour per day for two months. The researchers found that the music group made greater improvements in verbal skills and attention, and demonstrated less depression and confusion.

Television/video/virtual reality

The effectiveness of television, in particular, has been debated, in part because of the impact it has on noise levels. Carlisle (2000) found that women in labor preferred television over magazines and other distractions. Minimally, television could be an effective vehicle for inspirational programming, nature imagery, and other clearly supportive distractions. In a literature review on video and VR presentations, Malenbaum et al. (2008) concluded that such interventions can be beneficial for patients experiencing pain.

Regarding video, two studies support the hypothesis that this medium can help reduce perceived pain. Miller, Hickman and Lemasters (1992) used video visual/audio presentations while changing dressings with burn patents. These patients demonstrated reduced ratings of pain quality and intensity, and lowered levels of anxiety. Lee et al. (2004) also used audiovisual distractions with colonoscopy patients. These patients requested fewer analgesics and reported less pain than individuals who saw videos without music or had no distraction at all. (See Music section above.)

The use of virtual reality (VR) is a more recent development in healthcare settings. Hoffman, Patterson and Corrougher (2000) studied the impact of virtual reality distraction during the treatment of adult burn patients. The VR experience resulted in reduced pain and time spent thinking about pain. Those patients who reported feeling most immersed in the experience had the most significant decrease in pain and stress. VR has also been used with pediatric oncology patients (Wolitzsky et al., 2005). Children experienced an interactive zoo scene while undergoing a port access procedure and showed significant reductions in pain and pulse rate, both before and after.

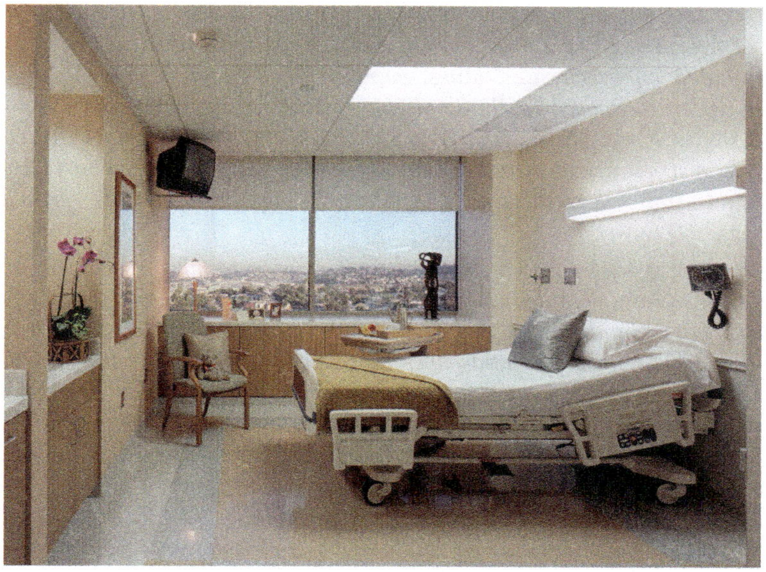

Figure 6.13: *Sculpture, plants, framed art, and television provide multiple venues for positive distraction*
Location: USC University Hospital (patient room): Los Angeles, CA Architect: Lee, Burkhart, Liu
Photo credit: ©Benny Chan/Fotoworks

Conclusions and design implications

Art

Appropriate art is another potential positive distraction and should be incorporated in the design programs for healthcare facilities. Ulrich (1999) makes the following suggestions regarding art selection:

- avoid selecting artwork that is ambiguous in content
- avoid selecting artwork that is abstract in content
- consider selecting artwork that is positive in content and representational in style
- consider selecting artwork that incorporates nature images
- remember that the art preferences of designers may differ significantly from the preferences of laypersons.

Visual art: an evidence-based approach

Upali Nanda, Ph.D., Assoc.AIA

Art has a growing presence in healthcare environments. A significant body of literature argues for the impact of appropriate art on health and satisfaction outcomes (Hathorn and Nanda, 2008). Research shows that art, with nature content, can reduce stress, anxiety and perception of pain, in acute care healthcare patients (for a comprehensive overview of the literature see Ulrich and Gilpin, 2003; Nanda, Eisen and Baladandayuthapani, 2008). In a study with ICU patients, Ulrich, Lunde and Elltinge (1991) compared the recovery of heart surgery patients exposed to six different art conditions: nature art, one dominated by water and trees with a high depth of field, the other a forest scene; abstract art with rectilinear and curvilinear forms equally dominated by greens and blues; a blank screen; and a control of no art. Findings showed that patients exposed to the landscape picture with water and trees experienced less anxiety and less intense pain compared with the other five conditions. By contrast, patients exposed to the abstract art with rectilinear, straight-edged forms, demonstrated worsened outcomes, and had strong negative reactions necessitating the immediate removal of the picture (Ulrich, 2009).

Because of the strong body of research, it is possible today to take an evidence-based approach to art in healthcare settings. Guidelines for evidence-based art have been proposed by Hathorn and Ulrich (2001), Ulrich and Gilpin (2003), and Ulrich (2009) to include: waterscapes (showing calm and non-turbulent water), landscapes (with visual depth, depicting warmer seasons, verdant vegetation, low hills and mountains, and positive cultural artifacts), flowers and gardens (showing healthy and fresh flowers that are familiar, and garden scenes with open foreground) and figurative art (depicting people at leisure in places with prominent nature elements, emotionally positive expressions, friendly and nurturing relationships, and generational and cultural diversity). Authors suggest that characteristics that should be avoided are ambiguity, emotionally negative or provocative content, surreal qualities, restricted depth or claustrophobic features, and closely spaced edges or forms that are optically unstable.

Ulrich (2009) shares two theories that support the research findings discussed above: a) The Evolutionary Theory or Biophilia Theory that holds that millions of years of evolution have left humans to be partly hardwired, or genetically prone, to respond positively to nature settings that fostered well-being and survival for early humans; b) The Emotional Congruence Theory—the notion that our emotional states bias our perception of environmental stimuli in ways that are congruent or match our feelings. This implies that ambiguous art, or art that is open to interpretation, may be interpreted negatively under high stress situations such as critical care.

It should be mentioned that while the research on the impact art can have on patients' healthcare experience is compelling, very little research focuses on the impact of art on different patient populations and different hospital settings. For example, there is research to show that pediatric patients' art preferences (for both style and content) vary by developmental stage (Coad and Coad, 2008; Nanda et al., 2007). There is also evidence that realistic and representational content is preferred over pure abstract (Eisen et al., 2008; Hathorn and Nanda, 2007). Research with long-term care patients shows preference for a social component, in addition to nature features (Nanda and Eisen, 2008).

Hathorn (1998) suggests three aspects of art need to be taken into consideration for healing environments: 1) location of artwork (considering where the artwork is going to be located, and sightlines); 2) needs of special patient populations (evaluating the unique needs of the kind of patients who will view the artwork—for example, images of water that are considered relaxing could be excruciatingly inappropriate for radiology areas where many procedures require a full bladder); 3) the role of demographics in the healing environment (considering the ethnic, gender, and age makeup of the patient population). In critical care settings such considerations are particularly important as patients may be unable to communicate their discomfort. Logistical constraints such as infection control and lack of wall space to install art must also be considered. Further research on art with respect to preferences and health outcomes is warranted within the specific setting of critical care units, across different patient populations, before determinations on appropriate artwork can be made. The existing guidelines, however, serve as a valid start point to undertake an art initiative that can create a better environment for critical care patients and staff.

Upali Nanda is VP, Director of Research at American Art Resources.

References

Hathorn, K., Nanda, U., 2008. A Guide to Evidence-based Art. *Cent. Health Des.* Retrieved Feb 2, 2009, from <http://healthdesign.org/advocacy/adgroups/escouncil.php/>

Nanda, U., Eisen, S., 2008. Art Preferences of Long-term Care Residents with Different Ethnicities. Poster presented at Society of Arts for Healthcare, Philadelphia Apr 16–19.

Nanda, U., Eisen, S., Baladandayuthapani, V., 2008. Undertaking an art survey to compare patient versus student art preferences. Environment and Behavior 40 (2), 269–301.

Nanda, U., Brown, L., Chanaud, C. & Hathorn, K. (2007). Research on Art for Pediatric Patients. Paper presented at Healthcare Facilities Symposium and Exposition. Oct 2–4, Chicago.

Ulrich, R.S., Lunden, O., et al., 1993. Effects of Exposure to Nature and Abstract Pictures on Patients Recovering from Heart Surgery. Thirty-third meeting of the society of psychophysiological research, Rottach-Egern, Germany.

Ulrich, R.S., Gilpin, L., 2003. Healing Arts: Nutrition for the Soul. In: Frampton, S.B., Gilpin, L., Charmel, P.A. (Eds.) Putting Patients First: Designing and Practicing Patient-Centered Care. John Wiley & Sons, San Francisco, CA, pp. 117–146.

Ulrich, R.S., 2009. Healing Arts: Nutrition for the Soul. In: Frampton, S.B., Gilpin, L., Charmel, P.A. (Eds.) Putting Patients First: Designing and Practicing Patient-Centered Care. John Wiley & Sons, San Francisco, CA, pp. 117–146.

Nature

Research suggests that nature is a positive distraction which may reduce stress and, as a result, promote the healing process. Several authors have addressed the physical implications of research which has been conducted on providing access to nature in healthcare environments. Some of their conclusions are as follows:

- exterior environments should provide a contrast to interior environments (Cooper Marcus & Barnes, 1995)
- gardens should take into consideration patients' reduced mobility and extreme sensitivity to microclimate (Cooper Marcus & Barnes, 1995)
- gardens should provide extra security to compensate for heightened feelings of vulnerability (Cooper Marcus & Barnes, 1995)
- gardens should provide sensory stimuli that draw attention to the outdoors (Cooper Marcus & Barnes, 1995)

- gardens should facilitate psychological and physical "journeys" to help patients shift their perspective (Cooper Marcus & Barnes, 1995)
- gardens should provide spaces that include opportunities for social interaction as well as seclusion (Cooper Marcus & Barnes, 1995)
- patient rooms in general medical units should have a space for plants and a window view (Burnett & Hamilton, 1992)
- patient rooms should have window seats (Burnett & Hamilton, 1992)
- designers should consider adding a greenhouse to patient rooms in general medical units (Burnett & Hamilton, 1992)
- designers should consider adding balconies to patient rooms (in general medical units) so that patients can move their beds outside (Burnett & Hamilton, 1992)
- designers should provide views of nature from patient rooms (Ulrich, 1984)
- designers should provide patient-room windows that are large enough and at the right level to be seen from the patient's location in the room (Verderber, 1986).

Music

Although there has been some inconsistency in establishing a significant relationship between music and physiological responses in an ICU, several studies have been conducted that support the hypothesis that music promotes healing (McCaffrey, 2008). In any case, there is no evidence to suggest that music is detrimental to the health of patients.

There are three possible reasons why music may have a positive impact:

1. The structure of the music itself elicits a psychoneuroimmunological response.
2. The music serves as a distraction in the same way a visitor, a television, or a view of nature might distract one from anxiety.
3. The music serves as white noise to absorb unpleasant and threatening sounds. For example, a study by Williamson (1992) found that the sound of the ocean fostered sleep.

Designers, however, should proceed with caution, as the lack of substantive studies addressing the clinical benefits of music has been noted (Richards et al., 2007). Many of the studies involving music have focused on cardiac care patients, whose requirements may differ from other ICU patients. To deal with this potential problem, when music is available it is important that the patient be given the choice of whether to hear it or not. In addition to taking into account the patient's diagnosis and preferences, this choice will provide the patient with an additional source of control—an important psychological factor in healthcare settings.

Regarding the introduction of music in an ICU, the following guidelines should be considered:

- *Control*: Access to music or white noise should be provided in each patient room. The patient should have the ability to control the amount of time the music is on as well as the music selections. Ideally, the music system should allow families to bring music to the unit for the patient.

- *Supervision*: Sound levels should not interfere with the staff's ability to identify alarm sources.
- *Staff spaces*: Staff may also benefit from music, which could be available in lounge areas and selected workspaces. A headphone system, linked into the emergency call system, might allow for individualized "decompression" in staff lounge areas.

Television/video/virtual reality

Access to entertainment and visual/audio distractions should be an integral part of patient care, particularly where pain management is an objective.

6.4 Sunlight

Light, and more particularly sunlight, have been found to have beneficial impacts on medical and behavioral patients. Post surgical patients who were placed in a room with sunlight requested less pain medication than those in dimmer rooms (Walch et al., 2005). Beauchemin and Hays (1998) found that patients in rooms with high levels of sunlight had significantly shorter stays than those who did not, and both sunlight and electrical light may have a positive impact on mood in healthy and depressed subjects (Beauchemin & Hays, 1996; Partonen & Lonnqvist, 2000; Yamada et al., 1995). With regard to depression, Golden (2005) conducted a meta-analysis of studies and concluded that light therapy had the same effect size as pharmacotherapy trials.

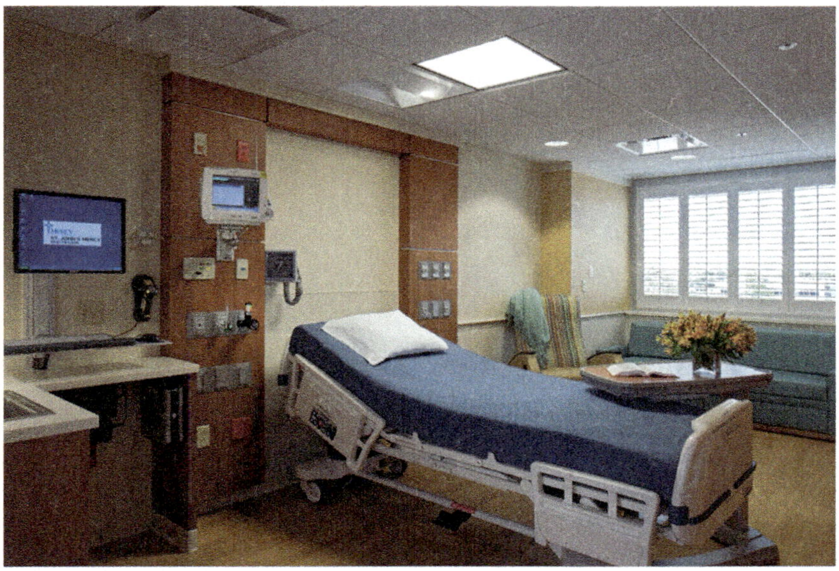

Figure 6.14: *The introduction of natural light, and non-institutional-looking control of that light, may positively impact patient satisfaction*
Location: St. John's Mercy Medical Center, Heart Hospital: St. Louis, MO
Architect: Christner, Inc.
Photo credit: Debbie Franke, Photographer

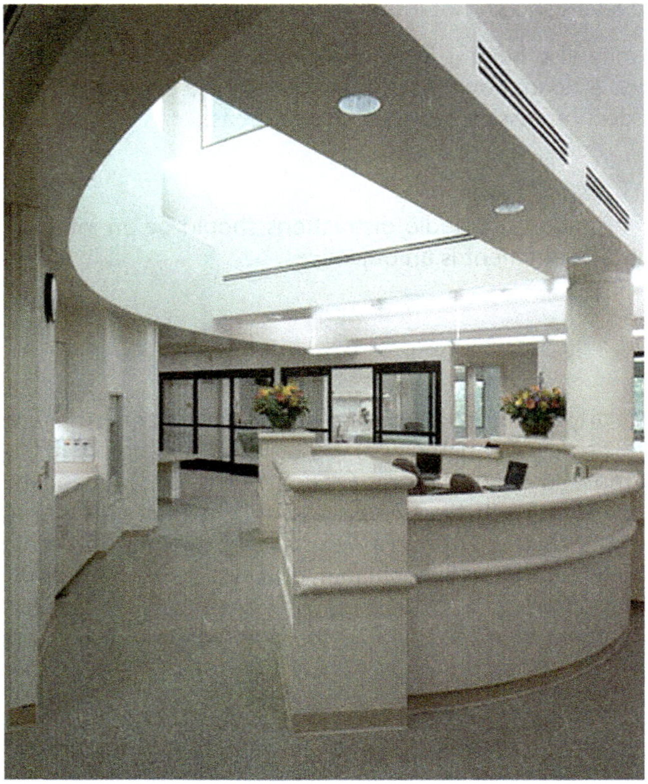

Figure 6.15: *Skylights introduce natural light where windows are not close enough to provide it*
Location: Saddleback Memorial Medical Center—Meiklejohn Critical Care Pavilion: Laguna Hills, CA
Architect: TAYLOR & Associates Architects with Questar Construction
Photo credit: Assassi Productions, photography

Healing by design in critical care

Jennifer Aliber, AIA, ACHA, LEED AP

Angela Watson, AIA, LEED AP

The transformation of critical care facility design is a corollary to the impact of evidence-based healthcare on patient care and treatment. Design of acute and critical care space supports the core focuses of critical care today: quality care, patient safety, and a sense of humanity. In the past decade, three factors have been central drivers of critical care design: treatment of the whole patient; the enhanced delivery of direct patient care by nursing staff; and the role of the family in the critical care environment.

One of the first Pebble Projects, Bronson Methodist Hospital in Kalamazoo, Michigan, included many elements now central to the evidence-based design movement: all single-patient rooms (reducing infection, controlling noise, and increasing patient privacy), locating nursing staff closer to patients (promoting direct care and patient safety), and including gardens, daylight and family spaces as well as intuitive wayfinding. Subsequent projects, including a major specialty hospital within an academic medical center and a community hospital, have incorporated these elements and refined them based on recent evidence and specific requirements.

The emergence of the all single-room nursing unit provides tremendous benefits to patients and their families but at the price of much larger nursing units. Many design challenges today are in fact those of balance between these larger units and the desire to have nursing staff work within a limited area so that the majority of their time may be spent in direct patient care.

At the University of Michigan's Cardiovascular Center, the 24-bed cardiovascular intensive care unit (CVICU) is adjacent to the PACU and ORs, limiting distances for critically ill patients and increasing the ability of anesthesiologists, with offices nearby, to provide care. The CVICU is served by a centralized primary clinician workstation and two flanking sub-stations as well as decentralized workstations between every two patient rooms. A sink near the sliding glass break-away doors promotes handwashing.

These design features should not be considered the exclusive domain of major medical centers. Like the University of Michigan, Concord Hospital, a community hospital in New Hampshire, has decentralized workstations between every two rooms in its 20 single-patient room ICU. As with Michigan, the mirrored arrangement of patient rooms promotes visualization. Corridors terminating in windows introduce natural light into the interior of the unit. Booms in each room accommodate medical equipment, managing space more efficiently and allowing physicians to administer procedures more easily at the patient bedside.

Design has responded as critical care units have come to recognize the valuable role of patients' families in the healing process. Family involvement has been shown to have a demonstrable positive impact, both as a support while patients are in the hospital, and in preparation for caregiving on patients' return home. At the University of Michigan, family space in each room is supplemented with a nearby lounge area, consultation rooms, lockers and kitchenette.

Few changes have been as visually compelling as the integration of light and nature into the healing environment of the critical care unit. Patient beds, long located to face patients away from windows and toward nursing staff, are now situated to give patients access to natural light and views, with the resulting benefit of day/night orientation for conscious critical care patients.

Gardens and access to daylight are central to the design of Concord Hospital's ICU, where a healing garden adjoins the unit. In Michigan, public elevators open onto a multi-storey winter garden, contributing to wayfinding for family members who make their way to the garden level, with its café and resource library, and back to the CVICU. Just as there is a continuum between the ORs, PACU and CVICU, the waiting and lounge areas are also continuous; a family that begins the day in the surgery lounge area simply moves southward along a glass wall and winter garden to the CVICU waiting area.

At Concord Hospital, the impact of design on the quality of critical care is being assessed in a post occupancy evaluation (POE), now underway. Anecdotally, it is captured in the statement made by one of the hospital's senior administrators, who noted that:

A senior surgeon who spends a substantial amount of time in the ICU made it a point to tell me what a difference the new unit has made for both patients and staff. He was used to coming on to the old unit and finding staff stressed and patient care challenging at times because of the environment. Now he goes with confidence that the care our sickest patients are receiving is being provided in a much more positive and uplifting environment and that the staff is much more relaxed and positive about their work. He attributes this significant improvement in care and functionality to the design of the unit.

Jennifer Aliber AIA, ACHA, LEED AP and Angela Watson AIA, LEED AP are principals in the Boston architecture firm of Shepley Bulfinch, Richardson & Abbott, and leaders in the firm's healthcare practice.

Conclusions and design implications

The provision of sunlight, while controlling for glare and solar gain, is recommended. During the winter months, additional electrical lighting should be provided.

6.5 Noise

Noise is a significant problem in ICUs and may play a critical role in intensive care unit psychosis (Hansell, 1984). Multiple studies, beginning in the 1970s, have documented that ICUs have inordinately high noise levels, which are stressful to patients and staff. As with other inpatients, hearing loss is common among ICU patients. Sources include trauma, medications, infections, vascular and hematologic disorders, autoimmune diseases, and environmental noise (Halpern et al., 1999). Seniors are particularly likely to develop hearing loss (Halpern et al., 1999).

In order to interpret the research on noise levels, it is useful to know the definitions of relevant terminology. Three expressions are frequently used: dB(A), L_{eq}, and L_{alm}. DB(A) is the range of frequencies, measured in decibels, that is audible by the average person. L_{eq} refers to the steady sound level that is the energy equivalent of the varying sound over a given period, and L_{alm} incorporates the impact of impulse noise and is usually 5 dB higher than L_{eq} (Meyer-Falcke et al., 1994). The effect of increasing decibel levels is more significant than might be imagined. Hargest (1978) notes that if a piece of equipment generates 60 dB and a second piece of equipment that also generates 60 dB is added to the environment, the resultant sound level will not be 120 dB. The result is likely to be 62 dB because the sound density rather than the sound level changes. It is also important to be aware that decibel levels increase logarithmically, rather than arithmetically, which is to say that 66 dB is much more than 10% louder than 60 dB.

Noise standards

There are several organizations that set standards for noise levels in hospitals. The International Noise Council recommends 45 dB during the day, 40 dB during the evening, and 20 dB at night (Bentley, Murphy & Dudley, 1977). The World Health Organization (WHO) recommends that noise levels do not exceed 40 dB(A) (Tsiou et al., 1998). The Swiss Association of Engineers and Architects recommends 40 dB(A) for peak noise and 30 dB(A) for background noise, and the Environmental Protection Agency recommends an average of 35 dB(A) (Walder et al., 2000). Individual researchers have made their own recommendations regarding noise levels. For example, Bovenzi and Collareta (1984) proposed that the maximum level at night be 20–35 dB(A) and 30–45 dB(A) during the day. Summarizing this literature, it would be safe to assume that a 30–40 dB(A) range is appropriate during the day, and 20–30 dB(A) is recommended during the evening. The following EPA chart (1974) provides typical sound level information for various activities. These levels help provide a comparison for the studies discussed next.

ICU noise levels

Hundreds of studies have documented noise levels in inpatient facilities. ICUs, however, have been found to be among the worst transgressors in creating an offensive acoustical environment. Although contemporary configurations more typically involve single-patient rooms, in 1977 when Bentley, Murphy, and Dudley compared noise levels in a hospital ward, a cubicle off the ward, and an intensive care unit, they found that noise levels were highest and most annoying in the intensive care unit. Average daytime levels in the ICU were 53 dB(A) during the day and 47 dB(A) at night. Bentley et al. (1977) noted that these sound levels were the equivalent of the noise levels in heavy traffic, and that the surges in noise were particularly unpleasant.

A summary of research on ICU noise levels beginning in 1977 and continuing into 2008 follows. Redding, Hargest, and Minsky (1977) found several noises exceeding 70 dB in ICUs. Equipment contributing to the acoustic environment included physiologic alarms. Bovenzi and Collareta (1984) noted that the most common sources of ICU noise were staff activities, air-conditioning systems, and electromechanical instruments. The noisiest parts of the day were morning and early evening, when levels ranged between 55.3 and 60.9 dB(A).

Data on the relationship between unit size and noise are inconsistent. Hilton's 1985 study on ICU noise suggests that increased unit size might be related to increased noise levels. ICU noise levels in large intensive care units ranged from 48.5 to 68.5 dB(A), and 32.5 to 62.5 in smaller ICUs. Levels associated with equipment exceeded 90 dB(A) on occasion. Buemi et al. (1995), on the other hand, found that weekday averages ranged from 41 to 57.3 dB(A) in a four-patient ICU room and from 38.8 to 65.3 dB(A) in a two-patient ICU room. Noise levels in a six-bed ICU in Athens, Greece, were found to range from 60.3 to 67.4 dB(A) (Tsiou et al., 1998).

While the results of most studies indicate dB(A) ranges of between 45 and 60 dB(A), Meyer-Falcke et al. (1994) found that the L_{alm} in their ICU setting was never below 60 dB(A), and maximum peaks were higher than 100 dB(A). Maximum sound levels for equipment ranged from 72.8 to 85.2 dB(A). Balough et al. (1993) encountered some of the highest noise levels in their ICU. For intervals of 20 minutes or more, the noise level fluctuated between 60 and 65 dB(A) and climbed to 70–80 dB(A) for periods of a few minutes. During doctors' rounds, noise levels exceeded 65 dB(A). Meyer et al. (1994) found peak levels in excess of 82 dB, with small decreases at night. Floors in these rooms were finished with marble. While McLaughlin et al. (1996) measured similar background noise levels (L_{eq}) ranging from 57.5 to 61.3 dB(A), they found a high maximum level similar to that of Meyer et al. (1994) of 100.9 dB(A). Akhtar et al. (2000) found average noise levels to be greater than 55 dB(A) throughout a 24-hour period. Ryherd, Persson Waye & Ljungkvist (2008) found noise levels that averaged between 53 and 58 dB, with peaks exceeding 70 dB. Although the data ranges in the literature are broad, it is clear that even in the best cases, noise levels are inappropriately high. Busch-Vishniac et al. (2005) studied noise levels at Johns Hopkins and found unacceptable levels, with minimal, if any, reduction at night.

Noise sources

What are the sources of noise in an ICU? Primary sources of noise identified by Bentley, Murphy & Dudley (1977) and Redding, Hargest, & Minsky (1977) were staff conversations and equipment.

While a high number of hospital staff in a unit results in increased noise levels (Falk & Woods, 1973), unnecessary or overly loud conversations, in and of themselves, may have a harmful effect on patient recovery. The Lomard Effect, which is the tendency of people to raise their voices as ambient sound levels increase, may exacerbate conversation dynamics (Kam, Kam, & Thompson, 1994). In a study involving four intensive care units, Noble (1982) found that the impact of sound generated from machinery, equipment, visitors, and patients was minimal when compared to noise generated by staff communication. Although much of the communication in this study (57–65%) related to patient care, personal communication accounted for 15–16%. Subjective measurements of sound levels suggested that the majority of verbal interactions were found to be loud or moderate.

Noise generated by equipment is often mentioned as being problematic. One of the most significant sources of equipment noise is alarms. There are no default alarm standards (Chambrin, 2001), and alarms may be assigned inappropriate urgency levels (Meredith & Edworthy, 1995), although the setting of alarms is determined by procedures and policies. Lack of consistency among alarms could create a challenging situation for staff. Cropp et al. (1994) exposed healthcare professionals to a tape recording of ICU sounds and found that only 50% of the alarms, and 40% of the non-critical sounds, were accurately identified. False emergency alarms, large numbers of monitors, and noise levels may create confusion among warnings (Meredith & Edworthy, 1995). The location of alarms may also be a factor in generating noise. Russek and Schwartz (1998) found that 91% of subjects who were asked whether they would prefer a traditional decentralized audible alarm system or a centralized audible/visual system preferred a centralized system. Today, most units use annunciators—visual displays—the sounds of which are associated with the alarm triage (Buick, 2008).

Noise levels might be influenced by time of day or day of the week. Christensen (2007) noted that morning noise levels were higher than those in the afternoon and evening. The lowest noise level recorded was 50 dB(A). Additional factors influencing noise are unit configuration and room location. Shepley and Davies (2003) found that circular nursing units had noise levels equivalent to rectangular units, in spite of the fact that the circular units allotted less space per patient. Moore et al. (1998) found that proximity to the nurses' station had an impact on decibel levels. Noise level measurements in the room nearest to the nurses' station were 61.83 dB(A), while measurements in the farthest room were 60.83 dB(A).

Noise reduction

Multiple suggestions have been made concerning how to curtail ICU noise (e.g., Coron, 1994; Dayton, 1994; Suchetka, 1994; Westball, 1994). Kam, Kam, and Thompson (1994) recommend five areas of abatement: modification of the unit's acoustic design, education of staff, good equipment maintenance (squeaky wheels, modulated alarms), noise-conscious patient care activities, and the introduction of white noise. Most studies approach the problem by modifying the larger environment with acoustical materials (such as sound-insulating materials separating the nurses' station from patient areas) or modifying the individual's immediate environment.

Berens and Weigle (1996) examined the effect of ceiling tiles of varying acoustical qualities and equipment cart traffic pattern change (carts entered directly into the storage room vs. traveling in other parts of the unit) on noise abatement and found that the mean decibel level in the ICU decreased significantly from 55 to 53 dB(A). In another study, headphones greatly reduced the subjective perception of noise (Akhtar et al., 2000); however, caregivers preferred not to wear them. Akhtar et al. hypothesized that this reticence may be the result of the interference headphones present when using stethoscopes and other equipment. With regard to the use of "white" noise to promote sleep in patients, Stanchina et al. (2005) found that the change from baseline noise to peak, rather than the peak level itself, determined whether a patient was awakened.

The best way to handle noise, however, is to eliminate the source rather than mollify the impact. Two common interventions to control noise relate to behavioral modification and equipment specification. Regarding behavioral modification, recommendations include shutting doors more quietly, avoiding the banging of garbage can lids, reducing speech levels, and making calls to families rather than having families call in the ICU (Hilton, 1987). This latter step may, however, impede family-centered care.

Moore et al. (1998) examined the impact of behavior education programs and protocol modifications, with discouraging results. The education program, which instituted vibrational pagers and a reduction in loudspeaker announcements, had little impact. Closing patient doors was also ineffective at reducing noise levels in the ICU. Noise levels were higher, as most of the noise emanated from within patient rooms. Other researchers, however, have had greater success using protocol adjustments. Kahn et al. (1998) noted at the outset of their study that 49% of observed sound peaks were associated with television and talking. Subsequent interventions included putting personal pagers on vibration mode, decreasing intercom use, turning down overhead speakers, and controlling visiting hours. Modifications were successful in reducing sound levels during most time periods. Even small gestures have had a significant impact on noise levels in some studies. Researchers in a cardiac ICU reported that by turning down the overhead lights from 2 p.m. to 4 p.m., noise levels decreased 50% because staff tended to be quieter when lights were lowered (Coron, 1994). Lastly, Walder et al. (2000) implemented the following procedures in shared rooms to control noise: careful closing of doors; alarm reductions; limitation of nursing interventions between 11 p.m. and 5 a.m.; conducting conversations with low voices; and no use of phone, intercom, televisions, or radio. These steps resulted in a noise drop from 51.3 to 48.3 dB(A).

Topf's (2000) recommendations regarding policy and behavioral changes include the following:

- orient ventilator bellows (if used) away from the head of the patient's bed
- assign patients to beds located away from nurses' stations
- limit the number of visitors
- monitor sound levels of staff communications
- lower light levels to encourage quiet conversation
- discontinue use of radio and television, or provide the patient with headphones
- turn off unused equipment
- use visual/sign communication in lieu of verbal communication
- modify care protocols so patients hear fewer nighttime sounds
- isolate patients who tend to make loud noises (talking, crying, snoring, groaning)
- oil squeaky equipment
- process night admissions in a separate area
- close patient-room doors
- redirect pedestrian traffic
- keep alarm volumes as low as safely possible

- combine treatments involving equipment
- use rubber-soled shoes
- schedule noisy activities for daytime hours, and
- open supplies away from the bedside.

A second area for potential noise abatement is equipment selection and modification. The noise output of specific pieces of equipment has been examined. High-frequency oscillatory mechanical ventilation was compared to conventional mechanical ventilation (Berens & Weigle, 1995). In addition to measuring noise levels, caretakers rated the noise using a visual scale. Interestingly, twice as much noise was perceived by the staff as was measured on the decibel scale, and the researchers concluded that the oscillatory system was significantly louder. In a study on nebulizers, Berg, Stuttmann, and Doehn (1997) found that a nebulizer could be adapted to reduce the noise level from 70 dB(A) to 55 dB(A).

Impact

The degree to which noise disturbs a person is dependent upon several factors, including one's perception of the meaning of the sound, the location of the sound, age, gender, health status, noise sensitivity, and interference with activities such as sleep (Baker, 1993). Topf (2000) adds other mediating personal variables: personality, culture, outside stresses, preferences, and perception of social support.

Kam, Kam, and Thompson (1994), in summarizing the literature on the physiological effects of noise, note that the hypothalamic-pituitary-adrenal axis is sensitive to noise as low as 65 dB, which results in corticosteroid increases. Increases in urinary measures of adrenaline and noradrenaline have been identified at the 90 dB level. Noise levels higher than 70 dB may result in increased vasoconstriction, heart rate, and blood pressure. Researchers have found that patients who are exposed to noise in recovery rooms require more pain medication (Minckley, 1968). Shertzer and Keck (2001) found that patients who experienced an environment with music and reduced noise reported lower perceived pain than those in the typical noisy environment.

The detrimental impact of noise on sleep is at the crux of the argument in favor of reducing noise in intensive care units. Meyer et al. (1994) found consistent sleep interruptions, in particular in the ICU and respiratory care areas. Sleep is cyclical and involves stages; a night's sleep typically entails four to five cycles of 90 to 120 minutes (Hilton, 1976). When observing ICU sleep patterns, Hilton (1976) concluded that patients had less sleep than usual, and that the sleep stages were not normal; only 50–60% of the total sleep occurred during the night. An analysis of sleep-disturbing factors uncovered various sources: 45.4% of sleep disruptions occurred as a result of assessment, therapeutic procedures, and talking with the patient. The majority of the disturbances involved talking between staff, patient interaction with other patients, and equipment noise. Hilton (1976) noted that six of the nine patients experienced nightmares and other behaviors associated with sleep deprivation. Patients mentioned doors slamming, sudden crashes, ventilator noise, chair movement, footsteps, radio noise, staff conversation, other patients, and discomfort as sources of sleep interference. In a subsequent study, Hilton (1985) investigated patients' perceptions of ICU noise levels and found that their responses ranged from "content" to "highly perturbed." According to patients in a study by Cazoria et al. (2007), aspects of the ICU environment that most bothered them were: communication problems, thirst, lack of sleep, staff discussions at the patient's bedside, noise and light. Sleep disruption is a significant problem in the ICU (Gabor, Cooper & Hanly, 2001).

Researchers have examined the physiological aspects of disrupted sleep. Meyer et al. (1994) suggest that sleep deprivation may impact the respiratory system by decreasing respiratory muscle function and response to CO_2. Westball, (1994) reported that adult men in a CCU had increased anxiety, increased number of awakenings, increased time awake, and shorter sleep stages. Snyder-Halpern (1985) examined startle effect, degree of recovery sleep, and psychological discomfort by observing the sleep behavior of subjects exposed to the noise conditions of a CCU setting. She found significant cardiac rate elevation, which suggests a startle effect, poor recovery sleep based on heart rates, and psychological discomfort based on self-reports. Topf and Davis (1993) also examined the responses of subjects in a laboratory who were exposed to CCU nighttime sounds. Subjects demonstrated poorer REM (rapid eye movement) sleep on 7 of 10 measures. Subjects also reported that they took longer to fall asleep, were awakened more frequently, and slept for a shorter amount of time (Topf, Bookman, & Arand, 1996). In a similarly structured study, subjects were assigned to environments in which they (a) could control noise through a sound conditioner, (b) had no control over noise, or (c) were placed in quiet groups (Topf, 1992). Although the intervention did not have an impact, the results demonstrated that sleep patterns were disrupted.

Noise can have a significant impact on staff as well. Topf and Dillon (1988) found that noise-induced occupational stress was positively related to job burnout and reports of on-the-job headaches. Subjects who reported higher sensitivity to noise were especially susceptible to headaches. Using occupant evaluations in a neurological intensive care unit, Ryherd, Persson Waye & Ljungkvist (2008) found that staff perceived noise to contribute to stress levels.

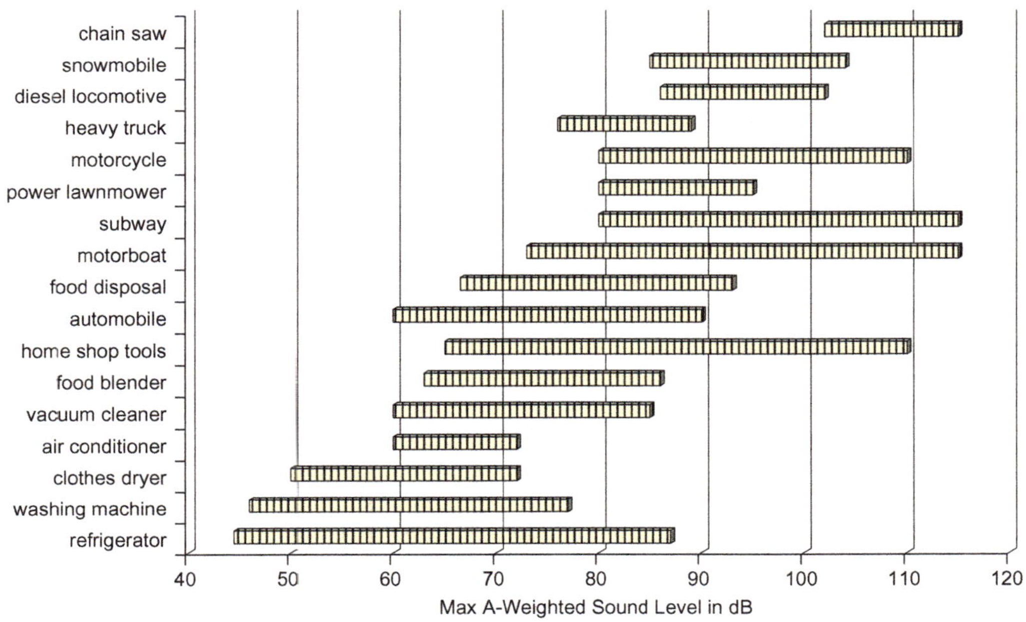

Figure 6.16: *Typical range of common sounds (derived from Environmental Protection Agency, 1974)*

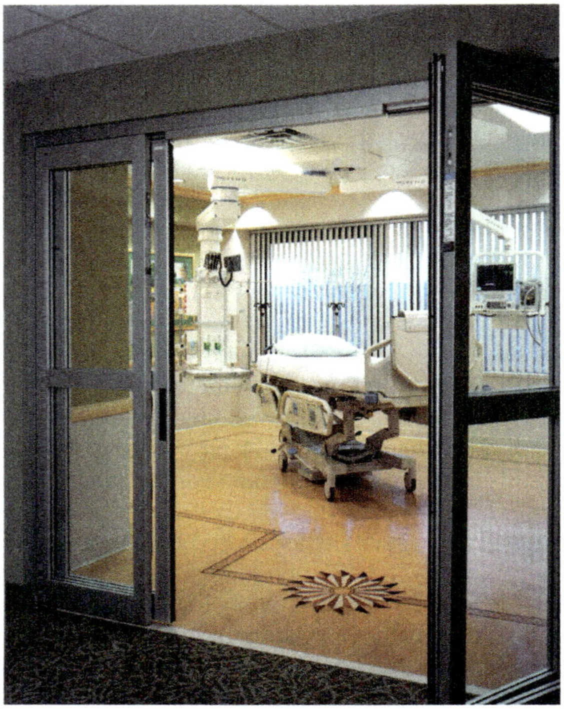

Figure 6.17: *Carpet in non-patient areas helps to reduce sound transmission*
Location: Exempla Lutheran Hospice at Collier Hospice Center, Colorado
Architect: H&L Architecture
Photo credit: Jim Berchert, photographer

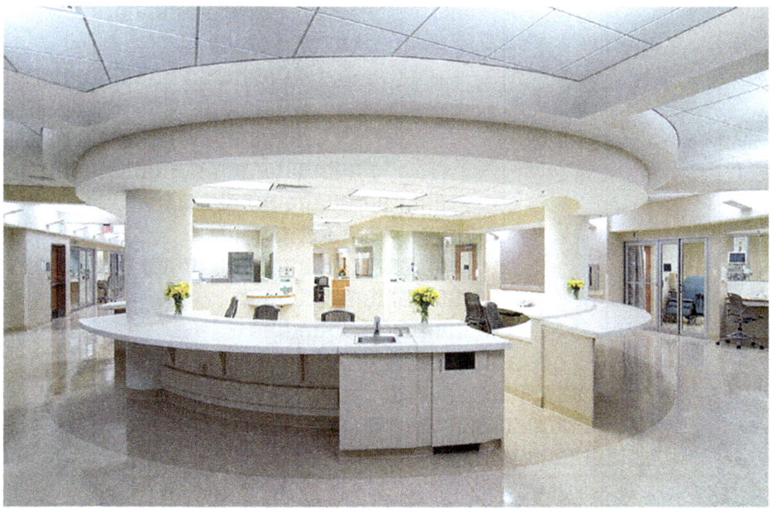

Figure 6.18: *Dropping the ceiling of noise-generating spaces aids in acoustical control*
Location: Cleveland Clinic Health System/Marymount Hospital-ED/ICU Expansion, Cleveland, OH
Architect: Hasenstab Architects
Photo credit: Scott Pease, photographer

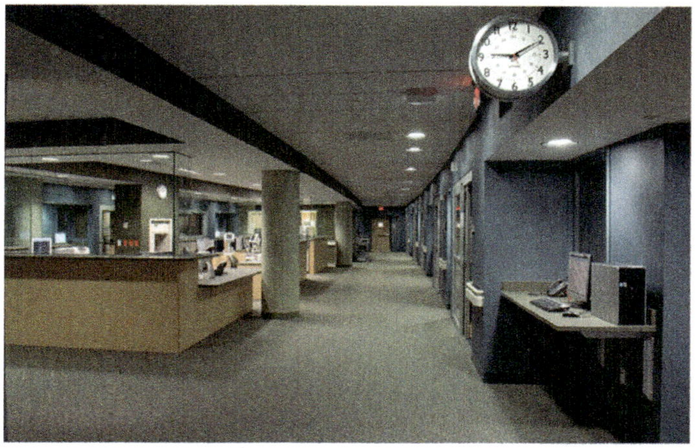

Figure 6.19: *Glass partitions, dropped ceilings and carpeting lower noise levels*
Location: St. Elizabeth Boardman Medical Center
Architect: Strollo Architects and Moody-Nolan
Photo credit: William H. Webb, Infinity Studio, Inc., photographer

Conclusions and design implications

Inappropriately high noise levels impact stress levels and patients' ability to sleep. There are several good articles outlining measures that will reduce noise levels in ICUs. Hargest's (1978) recommendations include the following design interventions:

- eliminate metal drawers, chart holders, and racks
- avoid spring-loaded door hinges on casework
- install baffles at intervals down long corridors
- use glass doors to separate the nurses' station from the patient areas
- install carpet in and around the nurses' station
- lower the ceiling in the nurses' station
- use acoustical tiles on ceilings and walls
- provide dimmer lights (this may encourage quiet behavior)
- install floor finishes that provide acoustical control
- avoid unnecessary thresholds
- use flashing lights instead of bell alarms
- install a flashing light that alerts staff when sound levels have been exceeded.

Topf (2000) also outlines the following complete program of environmental modifications that will reduce noise levels:

- increase unit size
- provide private patient rooms

- install carpet in heavy traffic areas
- install acoustical ceiling and floor tiles
- design a wide hallway between patient rooms and nurses' station
- provide an acoustical barrier around nurses' station
- consider acoustical implications of furnishings in nurses' station
- designate special rooms for staff conversations
- designate special rooms for noisy equipment
- install latch-free doors, when possible
- install rubber stripping in door frames
- install rubber/plastic door latches
- insulate casework in utility rooms
- replace equipment alarms and ringing phones with alphanumeric paging
- provide computers for nurses' notes
- provide plastic covers for charts
- use quiet vacuums and cleaning equipment
- use personal pagers in lieu of overhead paging
- provide headphones for TVs and radios
- specify plastic wheels and rubber bumpers on medicine carts
- specify plastic rails on beds
- provide rubber trash receptacles.

Hilton (1987) also suggests selecting furniture that rolls rather than drags along the ground, and isolating computer printers, and Buick (2008) notes that patient room adjacency to equipment rooms, automatic doors, and exam rooms should be avoided. Regarding patient room proximity to nurses' stations, Buick recommends that a "noisy" space be provided for team reports and rounds. Lastly, and importantly, Snyder-Halpern (1985) suggests that noise levels be evaluated periodically and that patients be interviewed upon discharge to evaluate environmental noise.

6.6 Safety

The issue of providing patient safety is profoundly significant from political, economic, and legal perspectives, and incorporates research topics associated with active living environments, lifespan design research, international/developing country health environment needs, evidence-based design, and practice-based research. Patient safety is *the* design-related healthcare issue of our time, and for the foreseeable future. There are many reasons for this. The Center for Medicaid and Medicare Services (CMS) is implementing "payment by results," a revolutionary reimbursement policy that denies providers payment for bad outcomes related to safety, for instance, all falls, many infections, medical errors, etc. Private insurers are also expected to adopt the CMS/federal policy. This will put huge financial pressure on hospitals and nursing homes to create safer environments.

The detrimental impact of frequent medical errors and unsafe conditions in hospitals was clearly articulated in two publications by the Institute of Medicine (IOM): *To Err is Human* (2000) and *Crossing the Quality Chasm* (2001). The IOM reported that as many as 1 in 343 persons admitted to hospitals die from preventable medical events, and up to 1 in 27 are subject to adverse actions. In response, the IOM articulated several goals to increase quality of care: patient centeredness, effectiveness, efficiency, safety, timeliness, and equitability.

A discussion of the financial implications of emphasizing safety in hospital environments is part and parcel to implementing a program. Clearly, there are capital costs associated with a thorough safe environment initiative. However, in addition to the humanitarian benefits of reducing suffering and mortality rates, there is a business case in support of improved facilities (Ulrich, 1997). Reiling (2004) notes that improved outcomes may result in lower cost per discharge and reduced length of stay, as well as salary saving associated with increased staff efficiency. Research is needed regarding the quantification of the economic benefits.

One of the most widely published experts on this topic, John Reiling, comments that there has been no significant research on the effect of facility design on patient safety (Reiling & Chernos, 2007). While this is true with regard to the analysis of the impact of the accumulated safety interventions of individual hospitals, research which addresses individual components of the environment and their impact on patient safety outcomes is common.

Joseph and Rashid (2007) summarize research on hospital safety by dividing it into three categories: 1) research which has a direct impact on patients, 2) the impact of the environment on staff working conditions, which in turn impacts patient safety, and 3) environmental barriers to safety.

Patient safety

Joseph and Rashid (2007) have reviewed studies, which provide evidence for the following:

- the positive impact of single-bed rooms on the reduction of nosocomial infections
- the negative impact of poor air quality on nosocomial infections
- the negative impact of poor lighting conditions on patient mental health and physiological status
- the negative impact of poor lighting conditions on medication errors, and
- the negative impact of noise on patient sleep and mental health.

Staff ability to deliver safe patient care

Regarding the influence of the environment on staff working conditions, which impact patient safety, Joseph and Rashid (2007) cite studies that suggest that:

- the use of variable acuity rooms results in fewer transfers, medication errors, and falls
- unit layout can reduce walking, and
- noise can increase stress, fatigue and burnout in nurses.

Other research on the impact of the environment on safety

Research which relates to the negative impact of the environment addressed by other authors includes:

- *The environment and staff fatigue*. Studies suggest that fatigue has a negative effect on cognitive performance, mood, alertness, and ability to cope (Onen et al., 2001), which may result in medical errors. While most studies focus on the impact of extended work shifts or sleep deprivation, which are operational issues rather than architectural issues, several organizations and researchers have underlined the negative impact of noise on fatigue (e.g., US EPA, 1978; Buβ & Friesdorf, 2007; Melamed & Bruhis, 1996). Morrison et al. (2002) noted negative physiological stress in nurses exposed to noise levels while conducting care tasks. Apart from the negative impact of noise, Shepley and Davies (2003) found that particular unit configurations can increase walking distance, which may also contribute to fatigue.
- *Negative impact of noise on communication*. Data regarding the negative impact of noise on communication and work tasks is widely available.
- *Inappropriate alarm technology*. Regarding technology, a recent study monitored the use of telemetry and pager systems, and developed a two-way, voice activated hands-free communication technology that resulted in reduced alarm response times from 9.5 minutes to 39 seconds (Gieras & Ebben, 2007).
- *Bariatric patients and falls*. Although it has been reported that the physical environment does not cause falls (Dyer, 2007), studies have shown that standard bed equipment, e.g., bedrails (Boocock, Weyman & McIlroy, 2006) may fail under conditions of extreme weight.

Staff safety

Although the primary focus of the proposed research is on patient safety, studies on the impact of the physical environment on staff safety are available. These studies focus primarily on the ergonomics of the environment (Hignett, 2007; Nelson, Baptiste & Mutz 2007). Safety of staff has been associated with back injury, electricity, pressure changes, violence, radiation, noise, and building-related illness (Behling & Guy, 1993). Kornecki (1994) notes the following events which negatively impact staff: patient falls, cardiac arrest, patient size, the need to transfer physically dependent patients between beds and equipment, and working around the limited confines of hospital beds, bathrooms and equipment.

Gurses and Carayon (2007) asked nurses to identify obstacles which undermined staff ability to focus on patient safety. Although several researchers have reported on the positive impact of the presence of families on patient safety due to their ability to provide additional surveillance (Reiling & Charnos, 2007), the respondents to the Gurses and Carayon study mentioned family tasks as impediments to patient safety.

Conclusions and design implications

"The evidence is overwhelming that current hospital design is not sufficient to prevent medical errors, rates of infection and injuries from falls, and even contributes to slow patient recovery and high nurse turnover" (Barach, 2008, p. 15). Components of safe hospitals might include the following:

- private patient rooms
- same-handed rooms
- adequate patient lifts and bariatric equipment
- noise reduction
- nurse-efficient design
- room configuration and distribution to support clear supervision
- adequate lighting
- communication systems and technology to support charting, and
- ergonometrically appropriate workstations.

References

Coad, J., & Coad, N. (2008). Children and young people's preference of thematic design and colour for their hospital environment. *Journal of Child Healthcare*, 12(1), 33–48.

Eisen, S. (2008). The stress-reducing effects of art in pediatric health care: Art preferences of healthy children and hospitalized children. *Journal of Child Healthcare*, 12(3), 173–190.

Hathorn, K., & Ulrich, R. (2001). The therapeutic art program of Northwestern Memorial Hospital. *Proceedings of the Symposium on Healthcare Design*, Nashville TN (abstract).

Hathorn, K. (1998). Picture of healing. *Proceeds of the Symposium of Healthcare Design*, San Francisco, CA (abstract).

The people 7

There are multiple people who use healthcare environments including patients, families and staff. ICU staff are numerous and include therapists, administrative staff, pharmacists, technicians, and housekeeping staff. The available literature, however, is limited to nurses and physicians. Section 7.1 below discusses patient stress and needs, as well as the phenomenon of ICU psychosis. Sections 7.2 and 7.3 summarize the literature on families and staff, respectively.

7.1 Patient

Patient stress

Of all the participants in the ICU setting, patients are the most vulnerable to stress. Thrust into an unfamiliar environment, deprived of most forms of control, lacking in privacy or personal space—for many patients the trauma of the ICU experience extends long after discharge. Sue Baier has written poignantly about the impact of the ICU experience. Ms. Baier was a victim of Guillain-Barre syndrome, which resulted in her being fully cognizant but completely paralyzed, while in an ICU. Baier's book, *Bed Number Ten* (1986), is an elegant plea to increase awareness of the patient's perspective.

Stress responses originate in the hypothalamus and result in the release of multiple hormones, including adrenocorticotropic hormone, cortisol, antidiuretic hormone, aldosterone, growth hormone, prolactin, testosterone, endorphins, and enkephalins; the release of certain of these hormones has also been associated with a reduction in antibody response (Lusk & Lash, 2005). Externally administered stress hormone levels have also been found to generate traumatic memories in ICU patients (Schelling, 2002).

Lusk and Lash (2005) describe stress as a defense mechanism that normally expresses itself in physical action. According to their theory, the response to primordial stresses, such as potential animal attacks, is physical activity. This activity in and of itself helps mitigate the impact of stress; however, most contemporary stress generators do not require or allow for a physical response. This results in a mismatch between stress and tissue needs (Lusk & Lash, 2005), and the inappropriate internalization of stress.

Lusk and Lash have identified three main categories of ICU stressors: psychological (danger of death, social isolation), treatment-related (artificial ventilation, tubes, painful procedures), and environmental (unfamiliar surroundings, activity and noise, worrisome sights and sensations, sleep deprivation). In addition, stress appears to be higher in patients with small social networks and "low" social status (Fenner & Michels, 2003). Girard et al. (2007) noted frequent occurrence of post traumatic stress disorder in 14% of patients requiring mechanical ventilation. PTSD was most likely to occur in female patients, and patients who were medicated with lorazepam. Symptoms were less common in older patients.

In studies on the impact of stress in the ICU, it is important to separate the portion of the stress that is a result of the patient's health status from that which is a result of the physical design of the ICU itself. In the interest of understanding the contribution of each of these components, Tanimoto et al. (1999) admitted 10 healthy volunteers to an ICU for three days and four nights. Depression was measured prior to and after admission using the Profile of Mood States and the Zung Self-Rating Depression Scales measurement tools. The researchers found that participant fatigue and confusion increased while vigor decreased; however, no physiological effects were found.

Obtaining information directly from ICU patients is difficult; many ICU patients are unconscious or semiconscious. Most studies, therefore, are conducted after the ICU patient has left the unit or with non-patients. Using non-patients to evaluate a patient's stress level may be misleading. Pain and distress may be underestimated by caregivers (Hall-Lord, Larsson, & Steen, 1998). In one study (Novaes et al., 1999), patients, staff, and relatives were asked to complete the Intensive Care Unit Environmental Stressor Scale; all agreed that pain, tubes in the nose and mouth, and inability to sleep were the main stressors. Other stressors that were significant to patients, however, were not high on the lists of staff and families. These included not having control over oneself, not being able to move, and not knowing what would happen next. Although some researchers have found equipment and certain nurse behaviors to be stress producing, Novaes et al. (1999) found that the following experiences were not stressful: seeing equipment hanging over the bed, nurses not introducing themselves, blood pressure measurements, strange machines, and strange smells.

Perez de Ciriza et al. (1996) evaluated the stress levels of post surgical patients using Ballard's Scale of Environmental Stressors in Intensive Care. This tool includes 43 items addressing immobilization, isolation, lack of sleep, space/time disorientation, sensory deprivation, overstimulation, depersonalization, and loss of control. Factors identified by patients as most stressful were associated with the physical environment: tubes in their nose and mouth, difficulty sleeping due to noise, mobility limitations, thirst, and boredom. The attention of nurses was not perceived as a stressor, and patients' overall stress level was relatively low.

Preparation prior to ICU admission may successfully reduce stress levels during the ICU experience. Patients who experienced preparatory sensory information (PSI) regarding the sensations they might experience in an ICU appear to have less stress and a lower frequency of ICU psychosis (Shi et al., 2003).

Conclusions and design implications

Based on the evidence suggesting that the physical environment of the ICU contributes to patient stress, every effort should be made to mitigate negative environmental characteristics. Control of unnecessary noise is a critical factor; see Chapter 5 for design guidelines. Visual isolation from negative sights is also desirable. This can be accomplished through bed location (avoiding views of other patients and equipment, and allowing views of nature and pleasant artwork), among other strategies.

ICU Psychosis

The most comprehensive body of literature regarding the experience of ICU patients addresses a phenomenon known as ICU psychosis or ICU syndrome. Behaviors associated with this syndrome include disorientation and dysfunction. These problems manifest themselves as lack of awareness of one's environment, memory loss, sleep disorders, hallucinations, anger, fear, and depression (Justic, 2000). While some occurrences of delirium may also be specifically associated with a physical life-threatening disorder (Divatia, 2006), most researchers acknowledge the independent impact of the environment as well.

Lipowski (1990) identifies two types of psychoses: hyperactive-hyper alert and hypoactive-hypo alert. In the former case patients are extremely active and agitated; in the latter they are passive but may experience frightening dreams and hallucinations. Elderly patients are at the highest risk of experiencing ICU syndrome (O'Keefe & Lavan, 1996).

While some have argued that the syndrome has not been adequately demonstrated, the anecdotal evidence for its existence is compelling. Almost everyone who has had a family member or friend in an intensive care unit has noted behavioral modifications in their loved one. While dramatic personality changes may be rare, existing traits may become more dominant under the stress of ICU incarceration.

One of the authors experienced this effect in a family member they were visiting in an ICU a few years ago. This individual had a reputation for being concerned about her safety, perhaps more than was warranted, but not so much that it seemed out of the ordinary. Once in the ICU after surgery, however, she demonstrated intense paranoia, imagining that people were lurking outside her window, intending to do her harm. The delusions were evident, but the sources of her delusions were unclear.

The primary causes of delirium, or ICU syndrome, are believed to be physical, psychological, or environmental. Physical causes may be infection, hypoxic conditions, metabolic conditions and medication, chemical intoxication, or withdrawal (Justic, 2000). Psychological sources of ICU syndrome include the reality of an unexpected turn of events, helplessness, humiliation, and changes in body image (Mohta et al., 2003).

Multiple articles have identified the physical environment as a contributor to ICU syndrome (e.g., Gelling, 1999; Lasater & Grisanti, 1975; Mohta et al., 2003). Curtis (1999) notes that the ICU experience may be akin to torture, which involves sensory deprivation. In a literature review by Easton and Mackenzie (1988), the following additional attributes of the physical environment have been implicated in ICU syndrome:

- noise
- constant light levels
- unfamiliar environments
- sensory overload
- dependency
- immobilization.

Immobilization is thought to contribute to ICU syndrome in that it prevents interaction with the physical environment (Easton & Mackenzie, 1998). This notion of the negative impact of a lack of interaction is readily linked to the Prospect and Refuge Theory (Appleton, 1975), which suggests that humans need a balance between new environmental experiences and the ability to insulate themselves from overstimulation. Similarly, the information processing theory of Kaplan and Kaplan (1989) suggests that humans are constantly seeking a balance between understanding and exploration. Information is normally obtained by movement and manipulation. Deprived of this activity, little new learning is achievable—a condition that counters basic human development.

Many of the other negative environmental attributes (e.g., noise, light, sensory overload) lead to sleep deprivation, which in turn may have a critical impact on psychosis. Lack of sleep is very common among ICU patients (Briggs, 1991).

While most authors and researchers believe that the physical environment contributes to ICU syndrome, several argue that it is merely delirium resulting from organic stresses on the nervous system (McGuire et al., 2000). These individuals note that there are few controlled studies demonstrating that environmental changes result in fewer patients with delirium. It is also argued that ICU patients are mostly unaware of their surroundings and therefore unlikely to be impacted by them. However, in a study of recall at two years post discharge, Roberts et al. (2007) found that most patients are aware of their environment. They noted, however that delirious patients had few factual memories.

Conclusions and design implications

The Society of Critical Care Medicine (1995) has established guidelines for designing spaces for patients. "Every effort should be made to provide an environment that minimizes stress to patients and staff" (p. 585). Recommendations are made in support of sensory orientation, including the following:

- natural illumination
- window views
- clock
- calendar
- bulletin board
- pillow speaker connected to radio and television
- elements of visual interest, such as colored walls, graphics, or pictures.

Similarly, Ramsey (1986) recommends creating an orderly environment and reminding the patient of the location, date, and reason for being in an ICU. Weber et al. (1985) suggest placing clocks, calendars, and televisions in the patient room to provide orientation information.

With regard to noise control (see Chapter 6), multiple recommendations have been made such as more conference rooms to eliminate the need for conversations at the patient's bedside, coffee break areas that are acoustically isolated but allow for supervision of patients, better acoustical control, and fewer audible alarms (Hansell, 1984). Another suggestion to reduce noise is to move noise-generating equipment to the foot of the bed (Weber et al., 1985).

The perspective of a patient regarding ICU psychosis is eloquently communicated by Cheryl Misak (2005) in *ICU Psychosis and Patient Autonomy: Some thoughts from the Inside*:

> The experience of madness highlights the fragility of the self. We think of ourselves as being individuated by, or constituted by, a set of memories, beliefs, desires, and priorities. I am whom I am because of my history and a set of memories about and attitudes towards that history and because I have a rather stable, if evolving, set of beliefs, desires, emotional dispositions, and life priorities. Imagining the loss of that relatively stable set of mental states and you have a pretty good picture of what it is like to experience madness. What is most deeply interesting about madness is that it is a disintegration of the self—a profound loss of one's self (p. 427).

Patient perspective

All of the research on the patient perspective has involved post ICU assessments. Most patients have a positive assessment of their experience, regardless of their previous ICU experience or demographic characteristics (Elpern et al., 1992).

Rattray, Johnston, and Wildsmith (2004) developed a questionnaire that focused on the domains of an ICU experience, assessed patient experience, and examined the short- and long-term emotional outcomes of an ICU stay. The domains included awareness of surroundings, frightening experiences, recall of experiences, and satisfaction with care. Patients were surveyed at time of discharge, six months after discharge, and 12 months after discharge. Regarding the physical environment, 58% never knew whether it was day or night, but only 10% thought the unit was too noisy. A relationship was found between recall of frightening experiences and anxiety at discharge, at six months, and at 12 months.

In a similar study (Pennock et al., 1994), surgical intensive care unit patients, who had been discharged within 48 hours, took a 25-item Likert-scale test evaluating the degrees of distressfulness of their experience. The primary stressors were the endotracheal tube and the inability to talk, followed by confusion, sleeplessness, sore throat, and caretaker conversations. With regard to environmental variables, the following items were mildly distressful: noise of other patients, confinement to bed, telephone ringing, noise of alarms, noise of ventilator, lack of bathroom, and loss of privacy.

Swaiss and Badran (2004) interviewed 70 ICU patients one day and five days after discharge. Sixty-eight percent experienced anxiety, sixty percent endotracheal tube discomfort, fifty two percent pain, forty eight percent no tube discomfort, thirty four percent fear, thirty three percent problems communicating, and thirty one percent dreams and hallucinations. Anxiety, fear, dreams, and hallucinations persisted after discharge in six percent of subjects. Bohrer et al. (2002) explored similar issues in German patients. Forty-eight percent complained about restricted mobility, and 29% indicated feelings of helplessness.

Russell (1999) also investigated the perceptions, memories, and experiences of Australian ICU patients using interview and questionnaire techniques. The most significant memory was of the care they received, follow by technological support, relatives visiting, and noise.

In addition to patients' experience *in* the ICU, stress has been associated with their experience just prior to admission as well as after discharge. McKinney and Deeny (2002) used a phenomenological approach to evaluate impressions prior to and after transfer to the ICU. In retrospect, patients perceived both the process of transferring and the extreme nature of the experience in the ICU as problematic. The primary themes associated with the pre transfer experience were acceptance in the ICU, desire for mobility, and relationships with staff. The post transfer themes were mixed, but patients mentioned perceptions of well-being, awareness of differences in the two settings, and the "enormity" of the ICU experience.

In a review of nurse-patient communication, Llenore and Ogle (1999) found that many patients remember events and conversations that occurred when they were in intensive care. The literature suggests, however, that nurse-patient communication is very poor in spite of the competency of the nurses. This is especially puzzling in light of the finding that nurses are very competent in assessing the psychosocial variables in critical care patients (Latour-Perez et al., 1994). In a study by Hafseindottir (1996), it was found that patients on respirators remember their communication experiences clearly and typically describe them as negative. Patients noted that difficulties in communication sometimes led them to giving up on trying to communicate.

Conclusions and design implications

The primary negative spatial experiences expressed by ICU patients are noise, confinement, and loss of privacy. Means of mitigating noise and loss of privacy are discussed in Chapter 5. Confinement might be compensated for via window views and art. Virtual experiences (computer simulations) may help patients psychologically escape from their immediate environment. Although virtual reality has not evolved sufficiently to eliminate the resulting sensations of nausea that occur in some individuals, it is likely that the technology will evolve to make it a viable option in the next several years.

7.2 Family

When Alice, the mother-in-law of one of the authors, was in the open bay Neuro ICU after a head injury suffered in a fall, we found ourselves the unexpected witness to a family tragedy. A young Hispanic man had suffered a severe head injury in an automobile crash. When he was to be taken off life-support, the unit waived the two-person limit to visitors and allowed his entire family to gather at the bedside. In the Hispanic culture of Texas, it is the obligation of every family member to be there as a direct form of social support for the patient and most affected family members. We tried not to watch and intrude as weeping mother, distraught father, brothers, sisters, aunts and cousins gathered around the bed. The cubicle curtain couldn't contain the group of nearly a dozen who tried to keep their voices down and stifle the sounds of their grief. We could not help but violate their privacy, so we slipped away, only to return to our own vigil an hour later. The other bed was empty. If we know strong social support is related to survival from cardiac surgery, what is the likelihood that critical care units should have better accommodations for families who wish to be supportive of a patient, or who wish to say a dignified goodbye?

The case for privacy and dignity for patients and family is less well understood by the clinical staff but has been demonstrated to be a real need (Shepley, Fournier & McDougal, 1998). For many critical care patients the need for observation is no longer one of constant and continuous vigilance. In moments of extreme crisis the fragile psyche is tested to its limits. There are many instances in which an experience would be less traumatic for a patient and/or family if a measure of privacy could be provided. Not all critical care patients are comatose. In totally open units, some patients are exposed to traumatic scenes involving others. Reducing traumatic stress is a positive physiologic outcome that is strongly considered to be associated with the psychology of privacy.

Family members and loved ones have always been visitors to critical care units and ICUs. For much of the past, families have been considered an inconvenience that gets in the way of the intensive care being provided by an expert clinical staff. Some years ago, an ICU nurse commented to one of the authors, "I don't do families!" It was not an uncommon attitude amongst ICU personnel. Families were limited to small numbers of individuals who were permitted to see the patient only in brief, highly controlled blocks of time. When codes were called for crisis intervention, standard procedure was to require family members to leave. Not so today ... at least not in every critical care unit.

Families play roles as advocates for the patient, sometimes making important decisions on behalf of patients unable to communicate. Family members and loved ones of patients provide extra vigilance and frequently play a role summoning assistance or observing and interrupting potential errors. In the case of patients who survive the ICU, these family members will frequently be called upon to deliver care at home, so learning what will need to be done is a potentially important activity before discharge. Finally, in a time of shortages among skilled staff, family members can assist the staff in providing some of the less clinical and routine care.

Family needs

Advocacy for increasing the role of the family in healthcare settings blossomed in the 1990s. Originating from the pediatric healthcare culture, fomented by the now defunct Association for the Care of Children's Health, and currently spearheaded by the Institute for Family-Centered Care, family involvement is now greater than ever in healthcare settings. Many medical staff have turned their energies toward "treating the family", and components of the physical environment are expanding to accommodate the implications of this change in care delivery. Sometimes referred to as familialism (see Chan, 2004), the focus on the family has been associated with specific cultures, although the need to involve the whole family in the care of a single member appears to be universal.

Researchers do not suggest that the participation of families will eliminate family stress. The primary purpose of increased involvement is to mollify the impact of the ICU environment. Understandably, family members are highly stressed by the experience of having a relative in an ICU (Hupcey, 1999). Pérez-San Gregorio et al. (1992) found that more than 50% of family members showed symptoms of depression, while Rukholm et al. (1991) found that family members have high anxiety scores on the Spielberger's State Trait Anxiety Inventory. If the condition of the patient is the result of trauma, stress may be particularly severe (Hopkins, 1994; Leske, 1998). More recently, Paparrigopoulos and colleagues (2006) assessed post traumataic stress, depression, and anxiety in families at intake and discharge, and found high levels of distress throughout the hospitalization of their relatives. Azoulay et al. (2003) recommend that family comprehension and satisfaction should be addressed. Wall et al. (2007) especially emphasize that family members of either dying or surviving ICU patients can benefit from family-centered aspects of care.

Partly due to this stress and partly due to functional and personal requirements, families have many needs in the ICU. While most staff wish to address these needs, studies suggest that staff and families may differ in their perceptions of what might be desired (Blackmore, 1996a,1996b; Forrester et al., 1990; Kleinpell & Powers, 1992; Norris & Grove, 1986). Researchers have uncovered differences regarding the need to be encouraged to cry, have food available, have comfortable waiting rooms, talk about the possibility that the patient may not recover, or have company and a religious advisor (Lynn-McHale & Bellinger, 1988), as well as the need to be integrated into the caregiving team and the need for information (Heyland et al., 2003; Jacono et al., 1990). This misalignment of objectives suggests that more studies must be carried out on the role of the nurse in relationship to the ICU family (Hardicre, 2003). Such studies must take into account the fact that nurses' perceptions of family needs may be influenced by the unit in which they work, their experience in critical care, their education level, and their length of time in nursing (O'Malley et al., 1991).

What is the desired role of the family in ICU settings? Interestingly, Azoulay et al. (2003) found that while more than 88% of caregivers supported family participation in care, only one-third of families wished to directly participate. This is congruent with the findings of Johansson, Fridlund, and Hildingh (2004), who noted that families feel compelled to set their own limits. On the other hand, families express a strong desire to be with their family member. The contradiction can be explained by Engström and Söderberg (2004). These researchers found that families felt it was important to be in the ICU, in spite of the fact that they were afraid to touch their loved one. The primary reason families wish to be at the bedside is to be near the patient and to know that he or she is receiving the best care (Lam & Beaulieu, 2004). This is a very different motivation from wanting to provide medical care. Additionally, adjacency to the bedside and social interactions in the waiting room have been found to inspire hope (Patel, 1996).

A major step in understanding family requirements was the development of an effective assessment tool. The Critical Care Family Needs Inventory (CCFNI) (Molter, 1976) has been used frequently for this purpose (e.g., Blackmore, 1996a; Burr, 1998; Davis-Martin, 1994; Engli & Kirsivali-Farmer, 1993; Forrester et al., 1990; Freichels, 1991; Gournic, 1982; Leske, 1986; Norris & Grove, 1986; Price et al., 1991; Rogers, 1983; Rukholm et al., 1991; Takman & Severinsson, 2006; Warren, 1993; Zazpe et al., 1997) and has been found to be an effective indicator of needs (Bijttebier et al., 2000; Burr, 1998). The CCFNI has been applied in various cultures (e.g., Freitas, Kimura, & Ferreira, 2007; Lee & Lau, 2003). In addition to the CCFNI, other more qualitative methods (such as interviews) have also been effectively employed (Burr, 1998; Coulter, 1989; Thompson et al., 1999).

The issue of family needs has been examined thoroughly. Dracup (1993) notes that at least 22 studies were conducted by 1993 and that "this is the one area of nursing research where replication has been the hallmark" (p. 5). Simpson (1989), Hickey (1990), and Leske (1992b) provide excellent and consistent summaries of the literature on this topic. The five primary categories of needs identified by most researchers are as follows:

- assurance (having questions answered honestly, to be assured that the patient is receiving the best possible care, to feel there is hope)
- proximity (to be called about changes, to receive information every day, to visit frequently)

- information (to know about treatment, to know what is being done to a patient, to talk to the doctor every day)
- comfort (to feel accepted, to have access to telephones, restrooms, and food)
- support (to have explanations of the environment before going into the ICU for the first time, to talk about the possibility of the patient's death, to have friends nearby for support) (Leske, 1992b).

The CCFNI covers a range of needs. The following list summarizes the 45 factors addressed in the inventory, listed in order of preference, as identified by subjects in Gournic's 1982 study. Families need to:

1. talk to the same nurse each day
2. be assured that it is all right to leave the hospital for a while
3. talk about the possibility of the patient dying
4. have questions answered honestly
5. feel there is hope
6. have a telephone near the waiting room
7. have a specific person to call at the hospital when unable to visit
8. have a bathroom near the waiting room
9. have the waiting room be near the patient
10. know how the patient is being treated medically
11. know the prognosis
12. have explanations in understandable terms
13. have comfortable furniture in the waiting room
14. be called at home about changes in the patients' condition
15. receive information about the patient once a day
16. feel that hospital personnel care about the patient
17. have someone be concerned about the relative's health
18. be told about transfer plans while they are being made
19. have explanations about the unit before being admitted
20. know specific facts about the patient's progress
21. know why things are being done for the patient
22. see the patient frequently
23. be assured that the best possible care is being given to the patient
24. have a place in the hospital to be alone

25. know exactly what is being done for the patient
26. have visiting hours start on time
27. talk to the doctor every day
28. know which staff members can be given what types of information
29. have someone help with financial problems
30. be told about chaplain services
31. have visiting hours change for special conditions
32. be alone at times
33. be told about other people who could help with problems
34. help with the patient's physical care
35. be told about someone to help with family problems
36. have a clergy visit
37. have food easily available
38. have friends nearby for support
39. know what kinds of staff are taking care of the patient
40. be encouraged to cry
41. visit at any time
42. have directions as to what to do at the bedside
43. have another person with the relative when visiting
44. talk about negative feelings such as guilt and anger
45. feel accepted by the hospital staff.

In reviewing this list, several items are included that specifically address the physical environment. They are as follows:

- have a telephone near the waiting room
- have a bathroom near the waiting room
- have the waiting room be near the patient
- have comfortable furniture in the waiting room
- see the patient frequently
- have a place in the hospital to be alone
- have food easily available
- visit at any time.

A significant portion of the literature focuses on issues of proximity, as it relates to convenient visiting and access to information. (For information on visiting, see Chapter 9). Regarding visiting, the importance of access to a nearby waiting room with comfortable furniture has been identified as critical (Brickhill, 1995; Halm & Titler, 1990; Lee & Lau, 2003; Raffensberger, 1988; Ramsey & Cathelyn, 2000), and awareness of the importance of waiting rooms has made it a topic of evaluation in several studies (e.g., Fournier, 1995; Lopez-Fagin, 1995; Myhren et al., 2004; Warren, 1993). Myhren et al. (2004) learned that while some families felt comfortable staying in offsite sleeping accommodations, the response was less positive for families of non-survivors. This may be the result of not being able to be with the patient when he or she died. In a study in Sweden, Fridh, Forsberg & Beregbom (2007) found that 40% of patients die without a family member present, and that patients without families were more often located in a shared room.

The need for information has been identified by multiple researchers (e.g., Davis-Martin, 1994; Henneman & Cardin, 1992; Hickey, 1990; Malacrida et al., 1998; Mongiardi, Payman, & Hawthorn, 1987; Price et al., 1991; Spatt et al., 1986; Zazpe et al., 1997). Providing information can be accomplished through private family meetings (Atkinson, Stewart, & Gardner, 1980), family group meetings/support groups (Daly et al., 1994; Halm, 1991; Harvey, Dixon, & Padberg, 1995), or information packets (Daly et al., 1994; Henneman, McKenzie, & Dewa, 1992). The impact of providing information has been measured by several researchers, and the communication of information has been found to reduce anxiety (Mitchell & Courtney, 2004). It may be useful to provide information about the physical environment prior to entering the ICU. Piazza (1983) exposed families to examples of patient care stations, as well as photographs and sounds of the ICU, in advance of admission and found that the intervention resulted in increased comfort levels of families.

The recognition of differences is a core research principle. With this in mind, investigators have examined the potential impact of unit type, stage of illness, and patient type. Regarding unit type, differences in experience have been found based on unit specialty (Foss & Tenholder, 1993; Leske, 1986), while in other studies (e.g., Engli & Kirsivali-Farmer, 1993) similarities have also been noted. Regarding stage of illness, studies have focused on the phases of the family experience, such as the particular needs of families during the early part of their stay (Daley, 1984; Mendonca & Warren, 1998) and the needs of families of patients who are in critical care for extended periods (Davis-Martin, 1994; Freichels, 1991). Additionally, work has been done to examine the needs of families of patients who are dying (Furukawa, 1996; Mendyka, 1993). Related work addresses anticipatory grieving (Breu & Dracup, 1978) as well as bereavement (Granger, George, & Shelly, 1995; Horton, 1995). Regarding patient type, demographic variables such as age and gender have been found to impact perceived requirements (Leske, 1992a). Children, for example, profit by specialized support and education protocols (Baker, Nieswiadomy, & Arnold, 1988; Craft et al. 1993; Lewandowski, 1992). Satisfaction regarding the meeting of needs is also affected by gender and relationship to patient (Johnson et al., 1998).

Many studies have focused on the identification of needs; however, few have focused on the effectiveness of interventions that address needs (Simpson, 1989). In one rare example, Blackmore (1996a) found that, for a specific hospital, the 12 most important needs were met the majority of the time. An existing tool for measuring the degree to which needs are met is the Needs Met Inventory (NMI) (Watson, 1989). Although this tool was not designed to address the appropriateness of the physical environment of the ICU, an expanded version would be an excellent tool for post occupancy evaluations.

Family experience in the intensive care unit

Debra Harris, Ph.D., AAHID

I was 19 years old when, one morning, I received a phone call from my brother—this was an immediate red flag, because the call came at 5 a.m. and he is not a morning person. He told me that our father had suffered three heart attacks and a stroke, and was in the intensive care unit at the hospital near his home. I had only had a few hours sleep because I was a college sophomore and it was Sunday morning, the day after my friends and I had gone to see The Police play for what would be their final concert tour prior to breaking up the band. Needless to say, the sobering news of my dad's health event changed my weekend plans and would impact my immediate future. I managed to get a shower without passing out and ask a friend to contact my professors to tell them that I would not be in class, and then get my dog and myself in the car for the 3-hour drive to the hospital.

Upon arrival to the ICU, I was led to my father's bedside. It is difficult to explain, but probably most have had a similar experience when you see a loved one, in this case my father, tethered to a bed with tubes and monitors and lines and wires—my knees buckled and as I went down, there was a nurse there to catch me.

It is important to note that this was back in the days when enforced visitation hours allowed 15 minutes four times per day to actually spend with your loved one in the ICU. By definition, family members were not invited to participate in the caregiving. The unit, including the patient room and waiting area was cold—sterile with hard finishes and uncomfortable furniture. The waiting room seemed to be a reasonable size but, since time with the patient was so limited, the room was always crowded with family members settling in for the long wait. I guess when I think back on the experience, three things stick out in my mind:

The nursing staff's efforts to provide quality care for the patient and support to the families;
The bonds that are created among strangers based on circumstance; and
The physical environment where it all took place.

The nursing staff was great. Between the events that landed my father in the ICU through the surgery and then recovery, we felt his care was excellent and the willingness of the staff to provide information to keep us apprised of his situation was beneficial. In spite of the "rules" we were able to have other extended members of our "family" come and visit, which I believe was meaningful for my dad. While the nursing team rotated over time, we were always assigned someone to pick up where the other left off and so we developed relationships with our nurses that we grew to count on. In spite of those visitation time restraints, we felt sincerely accepted and included.

Over time, you begin to bond with other visitors in the waiting area. This is kind of a strange phenomenon because the only thing you may have in common is that you are under duress because you have a family member receiving care in the ICU. I remember one particular family that was camped out in the waiting area. With just a few looks and nods of acknowledgement, the seeds of a relationship, however temporary, were sewn.

After the initial fear subsided for my dad's health, my brother and I would try to leave the waiting area to kill the two hours between visitations. I would often bring back coffee or some other treat for the other family who did not seem to want to leave the proximity of the ICU. While we never really knew each other, over time we started to share details and cover for each other if one was out of the range of the nurses and needed to be found. My dad ended up having double by-pass surgery and remaining in the ICU for the first stage of recovery. The other family's loved one was stepped down to a recovery unit before my dad. For all practical purposes that was the full extent of our relationship but now, 25 years later, I still remember each person in that family and what it meant to share that experience through the stress and anxiety; and sharing the news of a positive outcome for our patients.

The hospital where my dad was treated did not have the family-centered care design attributes that we expect today. There was a cafeteria, but it was in the basement and was not a place where you wanted to eat or spend any time. When we were waiting on visitation times, we would go to the restaurant located on a pad site in the parking area of the hospital. It was within walking distance and provided a welcome diversion, food and as much coffee as you could drink.

The waiting area was filled with adequate but uncomfortable seating— it certainly did not welcome families to be there for the long haul. The chairs were arranged around the perimeter of the room. These chairs had fabric-covered padded seats and back on a metal frame. There were no other options for seating, or arrangements for groupings of seating. It would have been nice to have some options. There were older people there as well as children, who may have had more difficulty in finding a comfortable place to wait. I think that we (the families) adjust our expectations to resolve the reality of the circumstance. However, families waiting to see their loved one should be provided with comfortable places to wait, and with accommodations for children.

There were two doors aside from the entry. One led to a restroom and the other to the patient unit. Every time that door opened, everyone would look up expectantly to see if there was news about their family member. There was no designated space for privacy—either to cry, or to meet with a doctor (this was before HIPAA laws were in place). I think our expectation of privacy was different. We knew there was no private place and that others within hearing range were there for similar circumstances, so our expectation of privacy was limited to knowing that others were going to hear part of the comments from the doctor or other member of the ICU team.

Another limitation to our experience was the lack of access to information. There was no library that I was aware of at the hospital. So to learn about my father's health event, heart disease and the options for treatment, I had to leave the hospital and go find sources of information for myself. I think it is important to provide such access in close proximity to the waiting area because I had to choose—do I go learn so that I can be prepared to make informed decisions or do I stay close by in case something happens and I need to be here?

In reviewing my recollections about that experience I have to say that I believed the medical and nursing care that my father received and the support given to my family was excellent. There was confidence in the waiting room—those other families with temporary bonds all received the same level of care which provided a sense of hope for all of us in the waiting room. The limitations of the unit—lack of comfortable seating, access to information, decent food, telephones, no expectation of privacy—are all issues that have been addressed through recommendations for family-centered care and the physical support through design. However, it is the combination of the symbiotic relationship between the care team, the families and the environment that provides support for families in the ICU. One might compensate for the other overall, but creating an environment that supports the caregiver, and through comfort and access respects the family, is the benefit of family-centered care.

Debra Harris is President and CEO at RAD Consultants.

Conclusions and design implications

Because of the potential disparity between medical staff perceptions of family needs and the family's perception of those needs, the programming process should include interactions with family members. Interpolating the results of family needs research on reassurance, proximity, information, and support; the following elements are suggested regarding the physical environment.

Reassurance

The majority of the needs regarding reassurance relate to interactions with the staff. Designers need to provide opportunities for these interactions at the bedside, in the waiting room, and in family conference spaces. A well-designed physical environment can also provide assurance by communicating that the hospital cares enough to make it aesthetically pleasing.

Proximity

Two issues associated with appropriate proximities are visiting (Chapter 7) and telephone/computer communication. Means of contacting family members at home as well as in the waiting room should be incorporated into designers' infrastructural plans.

Information

Architectural programs should include libraries adjacent to family waiting areas, as well as computers to support Internet access and accessible pamphlet storage.

Comfort

Almost all of the family needs items in this category relate to the physical environment. Families have asked to have telephones and bathrooms near the waiting room, to have good food available in the hospital, and to have comfortable furniture in the waiting room. Families have also indicated a need to have furniture/partition arrangements in waiting rooms that allow for both interaction with other families and isolation of the family group, as desired (Fournier, 1995).

Support

Families have requested that staff explain the ICU environment prior to entry. To meet this request, hospitals might install a model of a patient room in a family counseling room. Additionally, family members frequently ask for space in which to be alone. Private family spaces should be available near the waiting room, acoustically separated but with some visibility for emergencies.

While the needs of family are sometimes perceived as burdensome to staff (Levy, 2007), most facilities embrace an environment that supports family-centered care.

Family stress

Stress has been defined in an earlier chapter as the result of an individual's sense that the situation in which they find themselves exceeds their capacity to cope with it. The human component of interpreting a given situation accounts for differences between individuals and their perceptions of a stressful situation. For example, if one has successfully dealt with a problem in the past, that individual's sense of surviving a specific future situation may be greater than someone who has not previously done so.

Some stress is overcome by habituation. In studies of primates, it has been found that repeated and scheduled exposure to shock is more manageable than intermittent yet less frequent exposure. Human research shows that the majority of heart attacks occur on Mondays after a weekend break (Witte et al., 2005). Alternatively, multiple stress experiences, without the opportunity to recover between bouts, can undermine an individual's resources. The key seems to be the duration of the recovery period, which is to say that the pattern of negative health outcomes after a break is dependent upon the duration of that break.

How does this relate to family stress in an ICU? It is likely that families who have been dealing with the health issues of a patient over a period of time are better prepared than those who suddenly find a parent, sibling, or child in an unpredicted life-threatening situation. The role of habituation is evident. Halm et al. (1993) found the stress level of families to be highest upon admission to the ICU, tapering off after the sixth day. The main implication of these findings, however, is that each family and family member will be different in their ability to cope with the ICU experience; architects and medical staff, therefore, must take this into account in their design and medical treatment.

Ærd and Harder (2007) note that family members are both vulnerable and resourceful, but struggle to find a place and determine how to act in an ICU. Researchers have confirmed that families of patients in ICUs experience high levels of stress (e.g., Chartier & Coutu-Wakulczyk, 1989; Jones et al., 2004; Kleiber et al., 1994; Rukholm, Bailey, & Coutu-Wakulczyk, 1992; Rukholm et al., 1991). There are various sources of stress for families with relatives in an ICU. In addition to fear regarding the potential death of the patient, there is anxiety regarding shifts of responsibility, changes in familial roles, and disorientation from the suddenness of the event (Hudak, Gallo, & Morton, 1998). In a study by Paparrigopoulos et al. (2006) women and individuals with high trait anxiety were noted to be at increased risk for high stress. Additionally, the development of post traumatic stress symptoms was associated with early anxiety responses.

Behavioral manifestations of the resultant stress are clearly documented. Family members report fear, worry, and exhaustion (Kleiber et al., 1994); lack of communication among one another; the need to protect children from stress-producing information; vulnerability; disruption of routines; changes in relationships; and role conflict (Titler, Cohen, & Craft, 1991). Family coping strategies may only be slightly effective in dealing with the ICU experience (Twibell, 1998). Family members sleep and eat less, and use drugs and alcohol more (Halm et al., 1993).

Several studies address the impact of stress-reducing interventions. Chavez and Faber (1987) measured blood pressure, heart rate, and subjective stress scales of families who participated in an education-orientation program in comparison to a control group. After a subsequent visit, the families who participated in the intervention had lower heart rates than those who did not. Support group interventions (Halm, 1990) and daily patient-status phone calls (Johnson & Frank, 1995) have also been found to reduce state anxiety. Less significant positive results have been found in families after discharge (Jones et al., 2004).

Incongruencies have been found between staff and family perceptions of the ICU experience (Titler, Cohen, & Craft, 1991). An excellent way to consolidate differing perceptions is to survey the opinions of individuals who have experienced the ICU both as staff and as patient or family member. One such individual, a nurse, who also had the experience of having a family member in an ICU, suggests that interventions should be scheduled in phases: while the family is in the waiting room, after the first visit, or before discharge (Massura, 1982).

Conclusions and design implications

Insufficient attention has been paid to measuring stress in family satisfaction surveys (Latour, 2007). However, families of patients experience high levels of stress that can only be mitigated by providing the infrastructure to support communication, reduce disruption to routine, and support educational programs. Designers can respond to these needs by locating the waiting room adjacent to the ICU, providing adequate numbers of telephones (some of which support privacy), incorporating space for amenities that support routine (such as computers, showers and childcare facilities), and providing libraries and written-information centers.

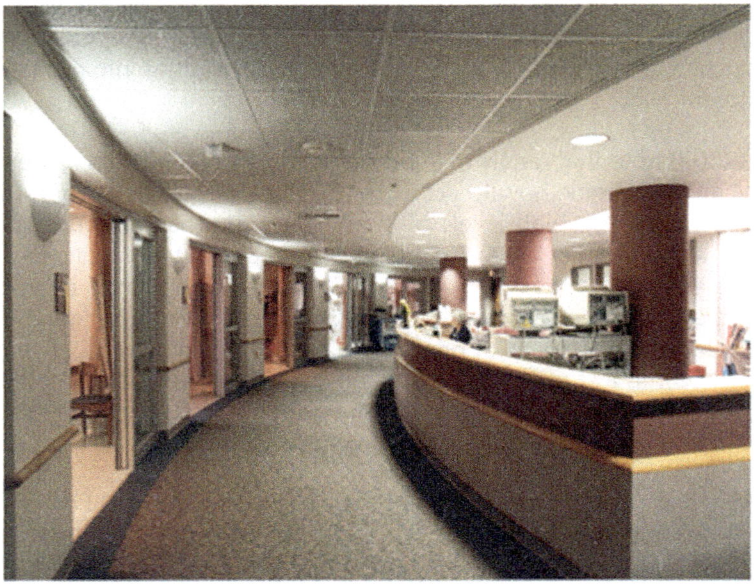

Figure 7.1: *Proximity to staff may serve to reduce patient stress*
Location: Fayette Memorial Hospital: Connersville, IN
Architects: ARTEKNA
Photo credit: William Montgomery, WM Photographic Services

7.3 Nurses and physicians

Patterns of caring

Florence Nightingale is often quoted in the context of idealized care models. The extent of her fame is astonishing. She is probably more widely referenced by the lay public than any single physician or architect. Perhaps this recognition is because she represents quality patient care, which is more lauded than scientific or architectural accomplishments.

Quality patient care is the primary objective of medical staff. Nurses, in particular, may conceive of themselves as nurturers and promoters of life. In this context, nursing staff must define their care styles to meet the objectives of intensive care settings. Because the potential for death plays a significant role in an ICU, patterns of caring must specifically address the dying process. Due to individual differences among nurses, the resulting care patterns range from traditional models to alternative models. This section briefly describes a variety of approaches that designers should be aware of to support diverse care delivery models.

The 1993 American Association of Critical Care Nurses conference on fostering human critical care (Harvey et al., 1993) provides an excellent summary of patient, family, and staff issues regarding care. The conference addressed the need for patients and family to participate in the decision-making process, and the importance of humane care that meets "the patient's personal basic needs in a consistent manner" (Harvey et al., 1993, p. 488). Human care, as discussed in the conference, seeks the integration of caring practices and the technical critical care environment by combining the patient's physiological needs with those pertaining to the "emotional, spiritual, and social well-being" (ibid). Collaboration among the patient, family, and healthcare team forms the foundation of humane care, which fosters an "atmosphere where information is exchanged openly" (Harvey et al., 1993, p. 491). Bearing this in mind, the environment needs to provide the caregiver with tools and resources to facilitate the provision of humane critical care. A collaborative practice diminishes dissension or distrust amongst caregivers and depends on "mutual respect and open communication" (ibid, p. 494). Furthermore, a healthy system is vigilant about the care of the caregivers themselves, promoting their "physical, psychological, and spiritual well-being" (ibid).

Caring behaviors

Four basic caring behaviors are: communication, advocacy, reciprocity, and empathy (Caine, 1991). When asked about the meaning of caring, nurses described the following themes (Ray, 1987):

- maturation (caring is growth)
- technological achievement (caring is technology, technical competence)
- transpersonal caring (caring as touch, attachment, bonding, allaying the person's inner fears, making the patient feel safe, compassion, comfort)
- communication (caring is talking to patients and families, keeping the family informed, collegiality, support from each other, establishing rapport)
- judgment/ethics (caring is understanding the appearance of patient suffering; trust among patients, families, nurses, and physicians; correct decisions; the conflict of values based on differing cultures or personalities; choice for patients and families; economics).

One care technique is called focusing. Focusing is "empathizing concern for the critically ill person and his/her family amid the high technology of the intensive care unit" (Walters, 1994, p. 23). Nurse subjects in Walters's study identified the following three foci: focusing on the patient through personalizing the illness experience, giving the patient an identity, and focusing on relatives. Another caring approach involves Crisis Theory. Wooley (1990), recognizing that the sudden illness of a family member can be perceived as a crisis by the patient's family, recommends that nurses respond to the family's needs using a specific intervention process: assessment and planning, and evaluation and resolution.

Research identifies factors that support caring and factors that undermine caring. Nurses, responding to a questionnaire, identified four factors associated with caring in an ICU: support from colleagues, the impact of role models, interactions with patients and their families, and economic and bureaucratic forces (Barr & Bush, 1998). Positive feelings were primarily focused on the first three. Economic and bureaucratic changes resulted in negative feelings. Chesla and Stannard (1997) used a phenomenological approach to evaluate interviews with nurses and observations of nurse activity. (Phenomenologists describe experiences as they present themselves to consciousness, without a framework of theory or scientific deduction.) Impediments to caring include distancing—separating the family from the patient, distancing oneself from the patient, characterizing family behavior as pathological, and dealing with parts of a patient's circumstances rather than taking a systematic approach. Another potential impediment to care is patient isolation. Evans et al. (2003) found that care interactions were limited with patients in isolation as compared with patients in wards. "Barrier-based isolation precautions are associated with reduced contact time, less frequent patient visits, and a high degree of non-compliance" (Evans et al., 2003, p. 187).

Alternative therapies

Alternative therapies are now commonly employed by caregivers. These techniques, also referred to as complementary therapies, include massage, relaxation activities, music, aromatherapy, touch, modifications of the physical environment (noise and light), and alternative sedatives (e.g., valerian and melatonin) (Richards et al., 2003). Research on the impact of alternative care approaches is limited. Dunn, Sleep, and Collett (1995) evaluated the use of aromatherapy, massage, and rest in an ICU. There were no changes in physiological stress measures as a result of the therapies; however, those who received aromatherapy reported lower anxiety. Meditation and goal setting have been used to support patients, and these activities have been successful in reducing stress. Specifically, in case studies on critical care environments Tiernan (1994) found that imagery was successful in inducing relaxation.

Therapeutic touch is another alternative therapy. Steckel and King (1996) define therapeutic touch as a nursing intervention in which the practitioner uses touch to smooth "electromagnetic energy fields" in the human body (Steckel & King, 1996). Therapeutic touch has been used to stabilize and calm patients, and to reduce pain (Steckel & King, 1996). Although this technique is controversial, most healthcare practitioners will encourage any effort that might have beneficial effects and is non-invasive (Steckel & King, 1996). Dossey (1993) points out that the approach must be endorsed by management before it can be effectively applied in a unit.

Related to alternative therapies is the notion of "holistic nursing". Dossey describes holistic nursing as "the simultaneous recognition and integration of body-mind-spirit unity in nursing practice" (Villaire, 1993, p. 106). A holistic framework should address physiological and psychological adaptation, social interaction, spirituality, growth and development, family processes, and culture/ethnicity (Hudak, Gallo, & Morton, 1998). Spirituality (Pettigrew, 1990; Wagner & Higdon, 1996; Wise, 1998) and culture (Arsenault, 1997; Krumberger, 1996; Wise, 1998) are integral to activities in an ICU. Holistic techniques may include the use of imagery, relaxation, and music therapy.

Death of a patient

The possibility of death is one of the most demanding realities of work in an ICU. In addition to responding to the dying process of the patient, the caregiver must address the grieving process of the relatives. "The challenge of caring for the dying patient in the critical care unit is often compounded by the needs of the family and significant others" (Jastremski, 1998, p. 1150). Strategies employed by nurses to support families include being present, supporting, sharing experiences, involving the family, interpreting the process and activities, and advocating (Andrew, 1998). Andrew points out that the nurse operates in several capacities during this period—as a person, practitioner, and nurse colleague. The complexity of the nurse's role is compounded by the need to support all patients in the context of their cultural attitudes toward the dying process. For a summary of research on culture and dying, see the series on Culture and the End of Life in the *Journal of Hospice and Palliative Nursing* (e.g., Bhungalia & Kemp, 2002; Dinh, Kemp, & Rasbridge, 2000; Kemp, 2000; Kemp, 2001; Kemp & Rasbridge, 2001; Keovilay, Rasbridge, & Kemp, 2000).

Palliative care is a central aspect of nursing in an ICU, and it has been argued that it should be integrated into standard intensive care practices (Nelson & Meier, 1999). The principles of palliative care include the following: communication with the family and the patient, teamwork, focused attention on symptom management, and bereavement follow-up (Levetown, 1998). An analysis of the behavior of nurses who are caring for dying patients in the ICU indicates five categories of activities that must be addressed by each nurse: 1) responding during the death scene, 2) responding to family anger, 3) responding to colleagues, 4) providing comfort, and 5) demonstrating personal growth (Degner, Gow, & Thompson, 1991; McClement & Degner, 1995). Not included on this list is the issue of adequate communication, which has been identified by researchers as problematic. In a survey of family members of patients who had died, most respondents were not fully satisfied with the information received (Malacrida et al., 1998).

Conclusions and design implications

Caring behaviors

Different theories of caring may influence the physical layout of an ICU. Three factors were mentioned in the literature review: personalization, identity, and family. The environment can support a nurse's effort to personalize the ICU experience by enhancing contact opportunities (easier supervision). ICU environments that allow for patient personalization will help endow patients with a history to which medical staff will be able to relate. Large patient rooms and family waiting spaces will serve as environments for nurses to meet with families. The design team and the medical staff should be queried regarding their philosophical approaches.

Alternative therapies

Alternative therapies have specific environmental requirements. Among them are access to music and the potential for acoustical isolation (perhaps through headsets), control of lighting to create relaxation ambience, acoustical and visual privacy to support touch therapies, and aroma isolation to allow the use of aromatherapy.

Death of a patient

When the patient has reached the stage of palliative care, the environment should allow that individual to withdraw from the technological intensity of the environment. A quiet environment, access to nature, and access to family are essential. Shortly after the death of a patient, staff may want to have a support group session. Space adjacent to the unit should be provided for such a session. Private grieving spaces for families should also be provided. Group rooms and grieving rooms require natural light or views to nature to help reduce stress.

Nurse and physician stress

As with families, nurses and physicians are likely to experience stress when there is a lack of fit between the coping skills of individuals and the circumstances in which they find themselves. Regarding the challenge presented by the physical environment, a specific construct has been developed—Environmental Competence/Press Theory (Lawton & Nahemow, 1973; see

Figure 7.2). According to this theory, when the competence level of an individual is inappropriately matched to the challenge presented by the environment, the individual will be negatively affected and will have difficulty adapting to the environment.

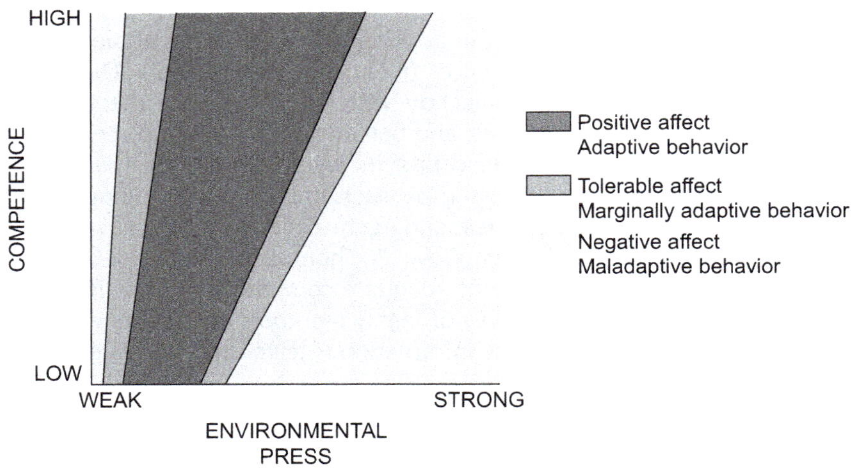

Figure 7.2: *Environmental Competence/Press Theory (Lawton & Nahemow, 1973)*

Effort-reward imbalance and overcommitment can also cause work stress. Buddeberg-Fischer et al. (2008) introduced these factors as threats for mental and physical health as well as life satisfaction.

Lazarus (1993) classifies coping responses in two main categories: problem-focused coping—in which the individual tries to remove the source of discomfort, and emotion-focused coping—in which the individual tries to reinterpret or neglect the source of stress. Chang et al. (2006) provided evidence that emotion-focused coping will deteriorate health. Chang et al. (2007) found that sympathy with co-workers and patients is a variant of problem-focused coping, which is more helpful and less harmful than emotion-focused coping.

Stress has a significant impact on all participants in the healthcare environment; while staff may appear to be less affected, there is significant research to suggest that the medical professions are among the most challenging. In light of the current shortage of nurses, nurse burnout is an area of concern for most hospitals. Burnout is a complex phenomenon and is directly associated with stress[1].

ICU nurses may be particularly susceptible to stress (Patrick, 1979). In a recent study, Mealer et al. (2006) found a higher incidence of post traumatic stress syndrome in ICU nurses. Other studies provide evidence that may contradict this finding. Goodfellow et al. (1997) noted that ICU staff were more stressed than other populations regarding aspects of their jobs relating to career achievement and organizational design. However, the ICU assignment itself was not found to be a significant measure of negative outcomes—personal relationships at work were major factors. However, in healthcare, an intense workload and job tension can play a more significant

[1]A literature review provided by Piemme (1982) outlines the physical, cognitive, psychological, and behavioral changes associated with burnout.

role than positive social environment and organizational justice (Virtanen et al., 2008). Yet other studies suggest that CCU nurses are less anxious than medical and surgical nurses (Johnson, 1979; Maloney, 1982).

Regardless of whether ICU nurses are more stressed that other nurses, it is clear that the job is challenging. The sources of stress for nurses are multiple and include the following:

- inadequate unit management (Adomat & Killingworth, 1994; Bailey, Steffen, & Grout, 1980; Fornes et al., 1994)
- inappropriate and too few staff (Bailey, Steffen, & Grout, 1980; Caldwell & Weiner, 1981; Fornes et al., 1994; Steenkamp & van der Merwe, 1998)
- low salaries (Steenkamp & van der Merwe, 1998)
- interpersonal relationships (Bailey, Steffen, & Grout, 1980; Caldwell & Weiner, 1981; White & Tonkin, 1991)
- emotional reactions to patient conditions (Caldwell & Weiner, 1981; Sawatzky, 1996; White & Tonkin, 1991)
- the need to support families (Caldwell & Weiner, 1981)
- feelings of insecurity regarding clinical responsibilities (Caldwell & Weiner, 1981; Ehrenfeld, 1991)
- difficulty relating theory to the practical sphere (White & Tonkin, 1991)
- unavailability of physicians (Ehrenfeld, 1991; Spoth & Konewko, 1987)
- lack of communication with physicians (Ehrenfeld, 1991)
- little free time (Fornes et al., 1994)
- frequent rotation of shifts, patient assignments, and units, which drains their emotional energy (Millar, 1989)
- too many interruptions (Spoth & Konewko, 1987)
- slow results from the laboratory or pharmacy (Spoth & Konewko, 1987).

With specific regard to the physical environment, researchers have identified other factors that negatively impact staff. These include the following: inappropriate access to equipment, inadequate storage space, poor design and function of biomedical equipment (Gibbons, Geller, & Glatz, 1998), poor equipment, inadequate work space, noise, poor general work environment, lack of supplies, too many people, and inappropriate lighting (Bailey, Steffen, & Grout, 1980).

The literature on ICU physician stress is more limited, although it is clear that doctors experience intense challenges in the medical environment. Unchecked stress is known to result in depression. Coomber et al. (2002) found that one-third of ICU physicians were distressed, one-tenth were depressed, and 3% experienced suicidal thoughts. This research suggested a higher than normal incidence of drug and alcohol abuse among physicians. The highest stressor was allocating beds when the unit was full, because sufficient capacity to provide care may be critical to patient survival. In another study examining the stress levels of physicians in ICUs (Eisendrath, Link, & Matthay, 1986), physicians rated the stress in the ICU as less than that in the non-ICU rotation.

Of the stressors that were reported, the most frequent were the poor prognosis or death of a patient and the physical setting. One explanation for this data is that ICU medical professionals are a self-selected group of individuals who enjoy the challenge of the ICU environment and are not readily vulnerable to stress. Along these lines, Mohl et al. (1982) suggest that stress may relate more to social factors than to primary job assignment. However, the self-reported data on this topic may be misleading. Physiological measures (high cortisol levels) of physician and nurse stress have been found that were independent of subjective stress perception (Fischer et al., 2000).

As there are several studies that focus on ICU physician stress, it is useful to look at data on other physician groups. Ramirez and Graham (1996) examined gastroenterologists, surgeons, radiologists, and oncologists in the United Kingdom and found that 27% experienced psychiatric morbidity (depression, lack of sleep, loss of confidence), with no differences among the specializations. Four categories of stress were identified: work overload and its impact on personal life, poor management and lack of resources, patient suffering, and management assignments. These stress sources are similar to the categories identified by Agius et al. (1996) for Scottish NHS consultants: demands on time, organizational constraints, and clinical responsibilities. Lack of personal confidence was also a stress factor. Firth-Cozens (1998) discovered 22 stressors that correlated with depression; the primary sources of stress were relationships with senior doctors and patients, making mistakes, and conflicts between professional and personal life. In this physician group, 17% were identified as being depressed, 5% frequently contemplated suicide, and 17% reported using alcohol to cope. Other studies involving suicide ideations by physicians range from 5% (Blenkin et al., 1995) to twice that amount (Caplan, 1994). Comparing these studies that suggest that 5–10% of non-ICU physicians experience psychiatric morbidity to Goodfellow et al.'s study that found that 27% of ICU physicians experience psychiatric difficulties suggests that ICU physicians have higher stress levels than other physicians.

Although the evidence regarding sleep and stress in physicians is unclear, lack of sleep may result in impaired job performance. The ICU environment has been criticized for working conditions that increase risk for errors, provider burnout, and negative impact on patients (Dochin & Seagull, 2002), and sleep deprivation is common among ICU staff. In a study by Rosen, Bellini, and Shea (2004), 64% of house staff reported sleep deprivation. Subjects in this study indicated that it was possible that they dozed while making charting notes, reading medical charts and labs, and writing orders.

The cognitive skills required for clinical decision-making include the ability to make an accurate diagnosis and recommend appropriate care for a patient. Weiner et al. (2007) developed a methodology to evaluate physician performance, and argue that it can improve the quality of medical decision-making.

Conclusions and design implications

The stresses experienced by nurses and physicians can be compounded by physical environments that do not support care objectives. Appropriately located and adequately sized storage areas are essential. Links to pharmacy and laboratory should be facilitated. Space for staff gatherings and access to "decompression" spaces (gardens, lounges) are needed. Most importantly for adequate patient care and the minimizing of staff stress levels, a sufficient number of beds must be provided.

Multiple researchers suggest that support groups be used to help nurses with coping (Caldwell & Weiner, 1981; Cassem & Hackett, 1975; Hay & Oken,1972; Spencer, 1994). The space for these group discussions should be located near or on the unit.

Nurse and physician perceptions and satisfaction

Because of the recent growth in family-centered care, a discussion of nurse attitudes and satisfaction in the ICU is dominated by their interaction with the family. Another important issue, however, is the unique psychological and sociological environment of the ICU. Less information is available regarding physician attitudes, although it is clear that the ICU environment is challenging for them as well, in particular with regard to working with families and making decisions regarding admission to the unit.

Nursing and families

Nursing theories tend to be of two kinds: those that focus on the patient as client and the nurse-client relationship, and those that view nursing from an interactional perspective that includes families (Forchuk & Dorsay, 1995). Behaviors that support family-centered care include providing critical support during crises, presenting a positive professional image, making arrangements regarding the amount and frequency of information to be shared, collaborative goal setting, promoting the perception of caring, assuring proficiency, acquainting families with system support, and helping families to set realistic expectations (Long & Greeneich, 1994). As might be expected, Murphy et al. (1992) found that nurses who rated high on a measure of empathy had a greater ability to assess family needs.

As previously discussed, nurses' perceptions of family needs are impacted by the unit in which they work, their experience in critical care, their education level, and the length of time they've worked in nursing (O'Malley et al., 1991). Several behaviors have been found to impede family-centered care: separating the family from the patient (Chesla & Stannard, 1997), separating oneself from or depersonalizing the patient and family (Chesla & Stannard, 1997; Hupcey, 1998), characterizing the family as pathological (Chesla & Stannard, 1997), maintaining a strictly efficient attitude (Hupcey, 1998), displaying a lack of trust in the family (Hupcey, 1998), and looking at things from the perspective of the individual needs of a single patient instead of the patient as a member of a family system (Chesla & Stannard, 1997). Many nurses believe that families should play a supportive rather than a participatory role in the care of patients (Hickey & Lewandowski, 1988), and this attitude may also impede nurses' ability to address family needs.

Although most related research focuses on the impact of staff on families, families also have a psychological impact on staff and can influence interactions between themselves and staff members. Although the onus is on medical staff to share information, the family may also have characteristics that affect the process. According to Dunkel and Eisendrath (1983), interaction with the family can have positive and negative implications. On the positive side, information provided by families can help the nurses make care decisions. This results in mutual trust and encourages personalization of the patient. Additionally, when nurses participate in the bereavement process with families, the nurses are more likely to achieve emotional closure. On the negative side, Dunkel and Eisendrath (1983) suggest that staff may be uncomfortable with unrealistic caregiving goals, may fear family discomfort when painful procedures are being conducted, may have feelings of inadequacy when compared to other nurses, and may experience feelings of loss when a patient dies. In spite of the availability of research on family needs, Hickey and Lewandowski (1988) found that more than 75% of nurses who became involved with families felt they did not have the knowledge to meet family requirements.

Social and psychological environment

Social and individual psychological factors play a significant role in the experience of nurses and physicians. For example, Topf (1988) found that individuals with hardy personalities are less impacted by stress associated with noise. Regarding social structure, the ICU is characterized by a complex set of relationships between members of the medical staff. The relationships between these members have been compared to a family structure in which gender and hierarchy increase the complexity of the social environment (Eisendrath & Dunkel, 1979). The relationship of gender to job assignment as well as competition between individuals who do not work in intimate teams (typically young physicians) may create conflicts.

Advantageous personality traits of individuals working in an ICU include attention to detail, and the need to care and be cared for. Attention to detail is a critical part of the cognitive style of staff who work in an ICU, because errors will have significant negative impacts on patients (Eisendrath & Dunkel, 1979). The inability to meet the high performance expectations that are associated with the detail-oriented personality type may damage self-esteem (Eisendrath & Dunkel, 1979). Eisendrath and Dunkel also suggest that staff who work in ICUs may be attempting to deliver a level of care that they may have wished for but lacked in their early lives. In other words, staff may be attempting to deal with people in ways in which they've never had experience.

There are two other complications nurses and physicians in an ICU face: being subject to the heightened dependency of patients whose demands are insatiable, and confronting the loss of a patient. The death of a patient can result in guilt or depression (Eisendrath & Dunkel , 1979).

Nurse and physician satisfaction

Strong indicators of nurse satisfaction have been associated with good management relationships and an active role in patient care (Darvas & Hawkins, 2002; McNeese-Smith, 1997). Higher levels of collaboration with physicians also increase nurse satisfaction (Baggs & Ryan, 1990), although this phenomenon is more important for nurses than for physicians (Baggs et al., 1997).

Song et al. (1997) compared job satisfaction and turnover in a nurse-managed special care unit relative to a traditional ICU, and found the nurse-managed unit to have higher nurse satisfaction levels and lower absenteeism. Lu, While and Barribal (2007) made a comparison between organizational commitment and job turnover in a hospital in China, and found that high levels of commitment do not reduce the frequency of job turnover, which may be significantly impacted by culture.

Management is a critical factor; it is important to remember, therefore, that changes in the design of ICUs will inevitably result in organizational restructuring, which is likely to result in nursing absenteeism and attrition (Wynne, 2004). A useful summary of the broad body of literature that addresses nurse job satisfaction more generally is provided by Lu, While, and Barriball (2005).

A small body of research is available on physician satisfaction. This research may be particularly important, as it has been found that physicians who are satisfied with their work environment tend to have patients who are more satisfied (Haas et al., 2002). Konrad et al. (1999) have identified several facets and three global qualities that define physician satisfaction. The facets include:

- autonomy
- relationships with colleagues, patients, and staff

- personal time
- intrinsic value of the work
- sense of community
- pay
- administrative duties, and
- resources.

Job, specialty, and career may also impact satisfaction. The resulting document, the Physician Worklife Survey, has been used in subsequent studies to examine physician satisfaction. Wetterneck et al. (2002) noted that general internists are less satisfied than subspecialists and family physicians. Pediatric generalists expressed greater satisfaction than pediatric subspecialists or internists (Shugerman et al., 2001). Differences have also been found between males and females. McMurray et al. (2000) found women to have higher satisfaction with subspecialties but less satisfaction with autonomy, community relationships, pay, and resources. Mean income was $22 000 less than for men, and burnout was more likely for women.

Studies employing other tools have found the following:

- Challenges to both autonomy and the ability to manage patient interactions, as well as the need to provide high quality care, are more strongly associated with satisfaction than with income (Landon, Reschovsky, & Blumenthal, 2003).
- There is conflicting evidence regarding the impact of HMOs and managed care on physician satisfaction (e. g., Bates et al., 1998; Murray et al., 2001; Nixon & Jaramillo, 2003).
- Burnout has been associated with low satisfaction in relationships, professional esteem, and intellectual stimulation (Ramirez & Graham, 1996).

Multiple other medical staff are involved in the success of an ICU. In addition to physicians and nurses, ICU staff includes physiotherapists, radiographers, clerks, pharmacists, dietitians, respiratory therapists, and laboratory specialists. While few studies exist regarding the needs of these individuals, accommodations must be made for their presence in the unit. The majority of these staff members are only on the unit temporarily, but they still need a place to work. Such a space could be shared by other staff who visit the unit, and should be located near the additional ICU staff work locations.

Other non-medical staff also participate in unit activities, such as clerks, maintenance and housekeeping staff, and food-delivery personnel. These individuals play an important role in the smooth operation of the unit and are often encumbered by lack of storage space to support their job objectives.

Conclusions and design implications

The ICU environment is both exhilarating and challenging for staff. Two of the primary challenges are working with families and managing the complex psychological and social environment.

Nursing and families

The physical environment can facilitate interactions with families by incorporating sufficient space and clearly designated territories. If families have adequate space at the patient bedside, they can "stand clear" of medical activities that take place there. The nurses' station lacks territorial definition and creates a zone of discomfort between staff and patient. If staff require separation from distraction, dedicated spaces should be provided to accommodate this need.

Social and psychological environment

Two types of spaces may support healthy social interactions on the unit: spaces where all medical staff come together to relax, and spaces where staff can go to be alone. Group lounges (rather than special lounges for individuals at different levels of the hierarchy) may work in some cultures. Both group and individual spaces should provide natural light or access to nature to create a stress-free physical environment.

Activities and behavior

8

Multiple activities take place on an ICU, but three have been written about extensively: responses and preferences regarding visiting, issues regarding communication, and the impact of technology.

8.1 Visiting

The majority of authors who address the issue of visiting the ICU give broad support to this family activity (e.g., Davies, 1986; Dracup & Bryan-Brown, 1992; Hamner, 1990; Kleinpell, 2008; Lilly, 2008; Molter, 1994; Sosnowski & Ustik, 1994), even with regard to managed visits by children (Shonkwiler, 1985). Unrestricted visiting has been determined to be a top ten need of families (Lee, 2007).

Researchers report that visits are beneficial to patients, but require customized protocols or contracts, depending on the patient and family needs (Marfell & Garcia, 1995; Moseley & Jones, 1991). Dracup and Bryan-Brown (1992) reinforce the notion that families should have access to their loved ones, and point out that excellent information is available regarding family visit needs. They remind us, however, that in spite of the best of intentions, nurses may not have sufficient time to evaluate family functioning and offer education and emotional support.

Studies on visiting

Studies on visiting in ICUs fall into two categories: statistical surveys and preference studies. Results of the latter show that patient preferences for length of visit vary depending on age. They also noted that an understanding of needs varies depending on whose perspective is offered—patients, families, or medical staff.

Statistical surveys

Statistical surveys typically focus on the existence and duration of visiting at hospitals with ICUs. In a survey of multiple hospitals, Stockdale and Hughes (1988) found that 26.9% of units had no set limits on the number of visits per day. Biley, Millar and Wilson (1992) found that 60% of the 107 units surveyed in the U.K. professed to have open visiting, although only 19% actually did. In a study of visitors in Swedish hospitals, 25% had no visitors at all. Those individuals were older and lived alone, which suggests a greater need for social support (Eriksson & Bergbom, 2007).

Preference studies

Multiple studies of patient preference suggest that patients and visitors prefer opportunities for extended visiting (e.g., Abbott et al., 2001; Brannon, Brady, & Gailey, 1990; Marfell & Garcia,

1995; Quinio et al., 2002). Although designers often think of ICUs as supporting one type of patient, the diverse population served may affect visitation needs and preferences. Simpson (1991) found that when a patient's illness was more serious, more visits were desired, and that more SICU patients preferred open visiting than CCU patients. In a subsequent study, Simpson (1993) found that middle-aged and senior patients were more inclined than younger patients to request a limit on the number of visits (2–3 per day), although older patients wanted longer visits.

Studies of ICU patients' physiological responses to visiting have also been examined. These studies suggest that visiting has either a positive or a negligible impact on physiologic measures. Hepworth, Hendrickson and Lopez (1994) found that family visitation was associated with decreased intracranial pressure. In another study, the post visit heart rate of patients with unrestricted visiting decreased significantly relative to patients with restricted visiting (Schulte et al., 1993). Contrary to this evidence, Kleman et al. (1993) examined heart rate, blood pressure, and oxygen saturation, and found that mean physiologic responses did not vary prior to, during, or after visitation. Fumagalli et al. (2006) found that increased visiting hours did not impact septic conditions in spite of higher environmental microbial contamination. The authors suggest that liberalized ICU hours might mitigate cardiovascular complications, through the improved hormonal profile and reduction of anxiety. Eriksson and Bergbom (2007) compared the health outcomes of patients who had no visitors to those who had visitors and found no significant differences. They did note, however, that older patients had fewer visitors.

In order to ascertain whether general social interactions were responsible for physiological changes that were recorded, Simpson and Shaver (1990) compared patients' cardiovascular responses when they were visited by both non-family members (interviewers) and family members. These researchers found that the lowest systolic and diastolic blood pressure values were recorded during the family visit.

A significant issue regarding the development of visit protocols is the role of the patient in the process. Lazure and Baun (1995) found that patient control of visits resulted in increased sleep. Environmental psychologists have identified control as a critical issue for patients, and increased control of the environment is associated with reduced stress. A more in-depth discussion of control strategies can be found in Lazure (1997).

Families

Halm and Titler (1990) found that staff assessment of family needs was not identical to family assessment of their own needs. Recognizing this, several studies have been conducted to obtain preference information directly from family members. Studies confirm that families value visitation in the ICU (e.g., Garrouste-Orgeas et al., 2008; Henneman & Cardin, 1992; Henneman, McKenzie, & Dewa, 1992). In fact, units with the most liberal visiting policies were rated the most highly by patients and visitors (Stockdale & Hughs, 1988). The need for visiting may be greater in ICUs than in other inpatient units. Foss and Tenholder (1993) compared family needs in an ICU and in a general inpatient unit, and determined that the need for visiting hour flexibility in the ICU was more significant. Stillwell (1984) used the Molter Needs Inventory (see Chapter 6) and found that families wanted to visit patients frequently and at will; they also wanted to be oriented before they entered the unit. They expressed no need for a companion and typically were not concerned about their personal privacy. Researchers have found that families would rather negotiate with the caregiver for visiting time than comply with set hours (Brannon, Brady, & Gailey, 1990), but they were willing to accept fewer visiting hours when this reduction resulted in better patient care (Foss & Tenholder, 1993). Stillwell suggests that seeing the patient frequently helps the visitor to avoid inappropriate feelings of denial, and to understand the severity of the illness.

Child visits in the ICU are also given support in the literature. Nicholson et al. (1993) measured anxiety in children before and after a counseling intervention. Children in the facilitated group had fewer post visit negative behaviors and emotional changes. Knuttson and Bergbom (2007) surveyed the reasons raised by physicians and nurses regarding restricting visits to an ICU. Those reasons included severity of patient illness, frightening environment, infection risks, and noise generated by their presences. Nurses were more inclined to support visits by young children. The individuals who brought a child to visit a family member in an ICU felt that providing information before, during, and after a visit was extremely important (Knutsson, 2007).

Staff

Staff generally support family visits in the ICU. Marfell and Garcia (1995) found that 100% of staff supported allowing spouses and parents in the ICU. Ninety-six percent felt that it was appropriate to have the child present, and almost 80% supported having other family members and friends. However, attitudes toward visitation may be strongly influenced by culture. In a study of 531 Flemish ICU nurses, most thought open visiting undermined nursing care and caused nurses to spend more time providing information to families (Berti, 2007). A research project in France, on the other hand, had results similar to U.S. studies. Garrouste-Orgeas et al. (2008) found that neither physicians nor nursing staff found visitation to be disruptive to patient care, and only moderately uncomfortable for staff.

Studies of nurses' perceptions of the impact of visiting on families vary in their conclusions. Hopping, Sickbert and Ruth (1992) found that the shift a nurse is working, and the nurse's background, influenced his or her perception of the visit. In one study (Simpson, 1996), nurses concurred that liberalized visits had a positive effect on patients' emotional state; however, they believed that the impact of the visit was more positive for the family than for the patient or for unit activities. Nurses who were included in a study by Kirchoff et al. (1993) agreed that visitors had a positive psychological impact on patients, although they were not convinced that the positive impact was physical as well. Contrary to Simpson, respondents in the Kirchoff et al., 1993 study felt that the visit was exhausting for families and disruptive to nursing care.

Regardless of their opinions about open visiting, Marfell and Garcia's (1995) subjects felt that nurses only have a moderate amount of control over the visitation process. These nurses approved of liberalized visiting but would like to have more control, perhaps by using visiting contracts. Simon et al. (1997) noted that the following factors influence nurses' decisions about visiting: patient rest requirements, nurse workload, open versus restricted policies, and the potential beneficial effect of the visit.

Patient- and family-centered ICU design

Susan B. Frampton, Ph.D.

One of the most stressful events that individuals and their families can go through is an admission to a hospital intensive care unit (ICU). It is a time often frought with fear and uncertainty for all involved. It is a time when patients and members of their social support system most need and want to be together. Ironically, the ICU environment generally has the greatest restrictions to family access/presence, and often has extremely limited space to accommodate the patient's family and friends. In a commentary published in JAMA (Berwick & Kotaga, 2004), it was noted that "restricting visiting in ICUs is neither caring, compassionate, nor necessary." There is no compelling evidence to support restrictions on family visitation in the critical care setting; in fact, what evidence does exist supports the benefits of family presence in this environment. The literature points to the ability of families to soothe the patient and provide orientation in a very disorienting space, and to provide assistance to staff by monitoring their loved one's condition, alerting staff to any changes in status (Marfell & Garcia, 1995; Krapohl, 1995).

In an analysis of extensive focus group data collected on patient perspectives on ICU care, several cases were identified in which patients believed a visiting family member saved their life (Frampton et al., 2008). In one such case, a physician who had spent several weeks in his hospital's ICU following a stroke recalled one night when he began to choke and turn blue at a time when no staff were close by. His wife, who had fought with the ICU staff to be allowed to stay at his bedside, ran screaming out into the corridor to alert staff. He firmly believed he would have died if his wife had not been with him.

Architects and designers working with hospitals to plan construction or renovation of ICU space can make a significant contribution to a patient- and family-centered care experience. By developing an environment that supports excellent, efficient and safe clinical care, and welcomes the patient's family by providing adequate space and facilities, design teams can address key concerns of staff members trying to deliver the best care in a high stress environment.

An excellent example of a truly patient- and family-centered ICU design is found at Griffin Hospital in Derby, Connecticut. Griffin is a 160-bed community hospital that practices the Planetree philosophy of patient-centered care. When they had an opportunity to redesign their ICU in the early 1990s, they decided to build it around their philosophy, with patients and families foremost in mind. Their existing ICU was built in 1950, with one 12-bed room, no privacy and no storage. The beds were lined up along the walls opposite each other, with the nursing station in the middle of the room. It was dark, noisy, and cluttered. Visiting in this environment was the traditional approach of 10 minutes every hour between 11 a.m. and 7 p.m. This policy is still in place in hospitals across the country that often cite inadequate space as a primary reason for this restriction. The family waiting area was a small, cramped room located on a different floor.

They moved to an innovative, 14-bed, horseshoe-shaped unit with a wraparound corridor called the family corridor, which visitors use to enter each patient room through a family door. A wall phone hangs outside the family entrance doors, so that visitors can call to check should the door be locked for privacy reasons. Most often, patients prefer to have these doors open to the family corridor. Four spacious family lounges are available along the corridor, complete with couches, chairs and televisions, refreshment stations, and bathrooms with shower facilities. The interior of the horseshoe is the clinical area with nursing stations that look into the glass, break-away doors on the "staff side" of each patient room. Artwork adorns the walls, a large water feature bubbles in a glassed-in space viewable by staff and visitors, and ample storage exists in the clinical area.

Several small private rooms for consultations between staff and family, or clergy and grieving families, are accessible along the family corridor.

Once the new ICU was opened, the hospital was able to move to unrestricted visitation, welcoming families 24 hours a day, seven days a week. Contrary to concerns that this might result in gluts of visitors negatively impacting the patient's condition, unlimited access has helped to space visitors throughout the day and evening, and contributes to a quieter, calmer atmosphere. Creating a truly healing environment, including the ICU, has resulted in Griffin Hospital achieving some of the highest patient and staff satisfaction evaluations in the country.

Susan Frampton is President of the Planetree Institute.

References

Berwick, D., Kotaga, M., 2004. Commentary: restricted visiting hours in ICUs: time to change. JAMA 292 (6), 736–737.

Frampton, S.B., Guastello, S., Brady C., et al. 2008. *Patient Centered Care Improvement Guide*. www.planetree.org.

Krapohl, G.L., 1995. Visiting hours in the adult intensive care unit. Dimension. Crit. Care Nurs. 14 (5), 245.

Marfell, J.A., Garcia, J.S., 1995. Contracted visiting hours in the coronary care unit. Nurs. Clin. N. Am. 30 (1), 87–96.

Conclusions and design implications

Visiting policy

Many facilities claim to practice open visiting but do not. Visiting protocols should be explored by the architectural programming team by observing actual practice, and examining written policies. If visiting is truly open, proximity to waiting areas may not be as urgent. However, in these cases room size must increase, security infrastructure must be enhanced, and, because entrances will become more active, they should be visually and acoustically separated from private patient rooms.

Patient needs

Patients appear to benefit from visiting, particularly if they are given some control over the frequency and duration of visits. The amount of visiting may vary depending on the patient population. ICUs that accommodate sicker patients, SICUs, and ICUs with younger patients may require more space for visitation, as the demand may be greater.

Family needs

Families prefer open access to visiting. If families are visiting for long periods, they will require space in the patient room for sitting, resting and possibly sleeping. Clear wayfinding to the unit is also important.

Staff needs

Staff typically approve of visiting, but units may have protocols requiring visiting contracts. A desirable component of ICU design is a place to meet with the family and develop a visiting contract. These activities could take place in a meeting room in the unit or in a consultation room in the waiting area. The patient room should be large enough to allow family members to stand clear during patient-caregiver interactions.

8.2 Communication

"Communication is nursing's finest skill…" (Hall, 1997, p. 104). Clear communication between nurses and other medical staff is essential to meeting the medical needs of patients. Sensitive communication between patients and their families can significantly impact stress levels and perceived satisfaction (Madigan, Donaghue, & Carpenter, 1999).

Literature on communication focuses on two arenas: interaction between staff (e.g., Boyle & Kochinda, 2004; Proctor et al., 2003) and staff interaction with patients and families. The following section focuses on the latter category.

Communication with patients

Difficulty in communication was the most bothersome factor mentioned by patients who had been in an ICU (Cazoria et al., 2007). Factors influencing successful communication between staff and patients are: the presence of family members, an adequate level of patient consciousness, and the provision of a high level of physical care (Baker & Melby, 1996). Circumstances that inhibit communication include the inability of a patient to initiate a conversation, staff's lack of experience in an ICU, and fear on the part of nurses that intimate conversations will put them emotionally at risk (Turnock, 1991).

In an intensive care unit setting, the communication skills of most patients are compromised due to medication, paralysis, intubation (Hagland, 1995), noise, pain, and sleep deprivation (Helton, 1980). Patients' auditory ability is also often reduced. Researchers have found a prevalence of hearing impairments in the ICU patient population (Hamill-Ruth et al., 1998). Because of these reasons and others, nurses spend approximately 5% of their time verbally communicating with non-responsive patients, providing reassurance or informing them about procedures (Baker & Melby, 1996).

Much of the literature on communication with patients focuses on interactions during the respirator treatment period (e.g., Salyer & Stuart, 1985). Ventilator patients tend to remember their communication experiences clearly, and they are typically negative (Hafsteindottir, 1996). These patients report difficulty breathing and fear of choking, as well as hallucinations and confusion (Hafsteindottir, 1996). Because of their intimidating circumstances and their inability to speak, finding means of communication may be even more critical than with other patient populations. This lack of ability to communicate is also stressful for nurses. Inability to communicate with a ventilated patient may result in feelings of incompetence, despair, or stress (Bergbom-Engberg & Haljamaë, 1993).

Apart from lack of communication, some of the most stress-inducing experiences a patient can have include inappropriate communications that undermine their feelings of security (Noble, 1979). One form of communication advocated in the ICU is touch. In a review of related literature, Verity (1996) identifies three kinds of touch: comforting touch, task touch, and affectionate touch. Non-verbal communication (body language, facial expression) is also important (Vincent, 1997). A study by Estabrooks (1989) notes three ways in which touch is used: to communicate caring, to accomplish a task, and to protect. The use of touch for caring and to accomplish a task is readily understood. Interestingly, Adomat and Kilingworth (1994) found that there was no relationship between the frequency of touch type employed and a patient's diagnosis. The use of caring touch, however, was positively related to the number of years he or she has been a nurse.

Communication with families

Because most ICU patients are unconscious, communication interaction typically shifts to the family (Azoulay & Pochard, 2003). Regarding communication with families, Azoulay et al. (2000) found that, in 54% of the cases reviewed, families of ICU patients experience inadequate communication with physicians regarding diagnosis, prognosis, and treatment. Speaking with the family prior to surgery and as soon thereafter as possible, providing orientation to the ICU, and attempting to maintain the same caregivers are recommended to support communication (Oyarzun, 1996).

Confusion about whose responsibility it is to share information (physician or nurse) can be a barrier to communication. Other factors undermining this important activity are the perception that speaking with relatives may seem like a low-order activity (Scullion, 1994), and staff's lack of time (Vincent, 1997). Regarding lack of time, researchers have found that structured communication programs may reduce the number of spontaneous phone calls made by the family to the ICU, and may maintain family satisfaction (Medland & Ferrans, 1998). Liaison programs can also enhance communication with families (Madigan, Donaghue, & Carpenter, 1999). Unfortunately, in some cases the family may also have characteristics that interfere with communication. These characteristics include an inability to understand, age, nonnative language, and employment status (Azoulay et al., 2000).

The primary outcome of communication is information. Information has been identified as one of the primary needs of families. Informational support consists of anticipatory guidance, explanations of terminology, frequent status updates, comfort information (visiting schedules, food services, chaplain and social worker resources), and encouragement (Gaw-Ens, 1994). Adequate communication is among the most significant determinants of satisfaction for families of patients who are dying in the ICU (Heyland, 2003).

Conclusions and design implications

Communication is an essential aspect of providing care in an ICU. As in other settings, the physical environment can support or impede this activity.

Communication with patients

Aspects of the environment that will support communication with patients include control of noise and the reduction of other sensory stimulation that may inhibit sleep.

Communication with families

Clinician-family communication is critical to family satisfaction in the ICU. The availability of appropriate settings for speaking with family members will support communication. Family consultation rooms near the waiting area are commonly used for this purpose, although sometimes medical personnel will have discussions in the waiting room to avoid the intimidating circumstance of having a specialized meeting space. Many conversations take place after medical staff, patient, and family have had an encounter in the patient's room. Some of these conversations should not be held in the room (so as not to frighten or disturb the patient), and the corridor lacks privacy. Special rooms or alcoves directly in the unit are recommended.

8.3 Impact of technology

"The hospital of the future will be a concentration of extraordinary technologies" (Coye, 2007, p. 9). From a layperson's perspective, the primary characteristic of the intensive care unit is the technology it brings to bear on the healing of patients. The ICU is intended to represent state-of-the-art science, the purpose of which is to cure the most ill of the ill. Advances such as wireless networks for patient records and mobile X-ray picture archiving may free staff to spend more time with patients (Thomson, 2008), and to improve patient outcomes (Krizner, 2008).

One of the effects of this relatively new health environment typology, however, is potential dehumanization (Dean, 1998), and caregivers recognize the philosophical conflict that this dichotomy generates. Specifically, Hudson (1993) identifies two aspects of the nursing process—curing (technological/physical) and caring (empathetic)—and suggests an effort be made to incorporate both. Interestingly, however, nurses who perceived the ICU situation as "complex physiologic care" requiring medical and technological procedures tended to view the family as an impediment (Chesla, 1996).

The primary differences between ICUs and other units is the layout and openness that permits increased supervision, as well as the increase in use of technology. The focus of the following section is a review of the effectiveness of technology.

The effectiveness of ICU care as opposed to home care and regular-unit care has been examined by researchers. Although most agree that ICU care is lifesaving in the majority of cases, there have been challenges to the position that it is the best alternative for all patients. Shortly after ICUs became established, initial studies brought broad support for the decreases in morbidity associated with patients using these units. However, these studies were challenged regarding their methodological integrity (Siegel, 1987). Subsequent research (e.g., Mather et al., 1976) suggested that myocardial infarction patients actually had improved outcomes when they returned home, in comparison to those patients assigned to a CCU. More recent comparisons of a traditional ICU and a special care unit (SCU) for chronically critically ill patients demonstrate that the high-technology ICU did not result in better outcomes (Douglas et al., 1996; Rudy et al., 1995). The need for intensive treatment for heart patients can be reduced by stratifying the patients by risk and placing intermediate-risk patients in intermediate coronary care units.

Means of assessing the cost-effectiveness of emerging therapies in the ICU have been proposed by Chalfin (1999), who reminds us of the "moral imperative to ensure that allocation proceeds according to areas and problems of greatest need and chance for highest potential benefit" (p. 270). Cost is linked to effectiveness. Ahrens (1998) recommends that in order for technology to be effective it must: 1) be clinically proven to be effective, 2) be addressed in a technician education program, and 3) involve incentives that will affect use patterns.

Regarding the reactions of patients and their families, technology can create fear and anxiety, immobilization, and depersonalization (Halm & Alpen, 1993). Equipment often overcrowds the patient's space, is noisy, results in sensory overload and deprivation of normal environmental sounds, and creates sleep deprivation due to monitoring. Stanton (1991) notes that the technology in an intensive therapy unit (ITU) may result in anxiety, sensory deprivation, and sleep disturbance, and will often, as in the case of intubation, interfere with communication. Respirator-treated patients, in particular, found that the inability to communicate resulted in anxiety, pain, and lack of sleep (Bergbom-Engberg & Haljamae, 1989). Stroud (1997) reminds us, on the other hand, that staff can increase family members' confidence by demonstrating competence with technology.

Technology can be intimidating for staff as well. Kjerulff et al. (1992) define technology anxiety as fears associated with working with medical equipment. In their study, nurses who were more intimidated tended to have lower scores on care planning and scored lower in adaptability. Mann (1992) identifies the following potential limitations of increased technology for caregivers: 1) nurse roles must become more complex, and a focus on technology may result in reduced personal contact; 2) unfamiliar equipment may be frightening; and 3) technology may intimidate the nurse into focusing on or disregarding the equipment. Lastly, Mann suggests that the use of high-tech equipment may result in increased autonomy and therefore increased liability for the nurse.

The majority of researchers praise the power of technological advancements, but they strongly recommend that its limitations be recognized. "Preserving humanity and maintaining normalization must continue to be paramount in delivering nursing care" (Mann, 1992, p. 59). Russek and Schwartz (1998) advocate the integration of "mind-body values" and technology.

Conclusions and design implications

Is it possible that the dominance of technology in an ICU "silences the subtle attempts of ill people," "muffles the whispers of death," and "compromises the competence of caregivers" as suggested by Almerud et al. (2007, p. 157)? Although there is evidence that the ICU may not be the most appropriate treatment mode for all critically ill patients, these environments are life-saving for many. The dominance of technology in these settings, however, can be mitigated by designers. Distracting patients' attention from the equipment to outdoor views, art, or music is helpful. Enclosure of equipment in casework when not in use has been an effective technique in single-room maternity care. Surfaces in the ICU must be highly maintainable, however; a single wall that is in view of and away from the patient bed and that is dedicated to a visual softening of the environment would be helpful. Medical staff should also have views free of technology and machinery.

Part Four: Path to a Bright Future

The purpose of Part Four of this book is to summarize research issues which must be addressed when seeking to uncover evidence to be used in the design of critical care units (Chapter 9), and to provide a brief summary of the most salient trends in the future on intensive care unit design (Chapter 10).

Research issues 9

The process of writing this book has involved a vigorous journey through references provided by multiple data engines and libraries. While the search has frequently strayed from traditional design literature by traversing medical, engineering, sociology, and psychology journals, its objective has not changed; the purpose of this book is to identify research that can be applied to the design of intensive care unit settings.

Many healthcare design professionals have expressed the need for quality research in health design (Marberry, 1996), although there is a lack of clarity regarding the definition of design research and how to identify superior studies. Additionally, there is a lack of consensus concerning which type of research should receive priority. The following chapter addresses these issues.

9.1 Definition of design research

Design research is the exploration of the relationship between physical and virtual/representational environments and psychological, behavioral, physiological, and mechanical responses. Examples of each of these constructs of the world of design research are provided in Figure 9.1.

Evidence-based design, or knowledge-based design, suggests the application of design research. These terms refer to the integration of design research into actual projects. Studies that address a direct relationship between the physical environment and outcomes can be defined as primary design research. Studies whose outcomes indirectly suggest spatial implications can be referred to as correlate design research. An example of correlate design research would be a study whose outcome suggests that social interaction between nurses results in higher nurse satisfaction and retention. Although the purpose of this study would probably not be to investigate the environmental implications of such interaction, the results suggest that spaces such as lounges must be provided to support these activities.

Regrettably, there are misconceptions among practitioners regarding the definition of research. In a survey of 134 healthcare architects, Dr. Kim (2001) found discrepancies between the academic definition and the widely held perspectives of practitioners. More than 88% of practitioners defined site visits as research, followed by 82% who identified post occupancy evaluations (POEs) as research. Also designated as research were behavioral observation (79%), questionnaires (77%), interviews (77%), literature reviews (66%), feasibility studies (55%), programming (51%), and schematic design (39%) (Kim, 2001).

From an academic's perspective, only post occupancy evaluations, observation, questionnaires, interviews, and programming would potentially involve research, and only under certain

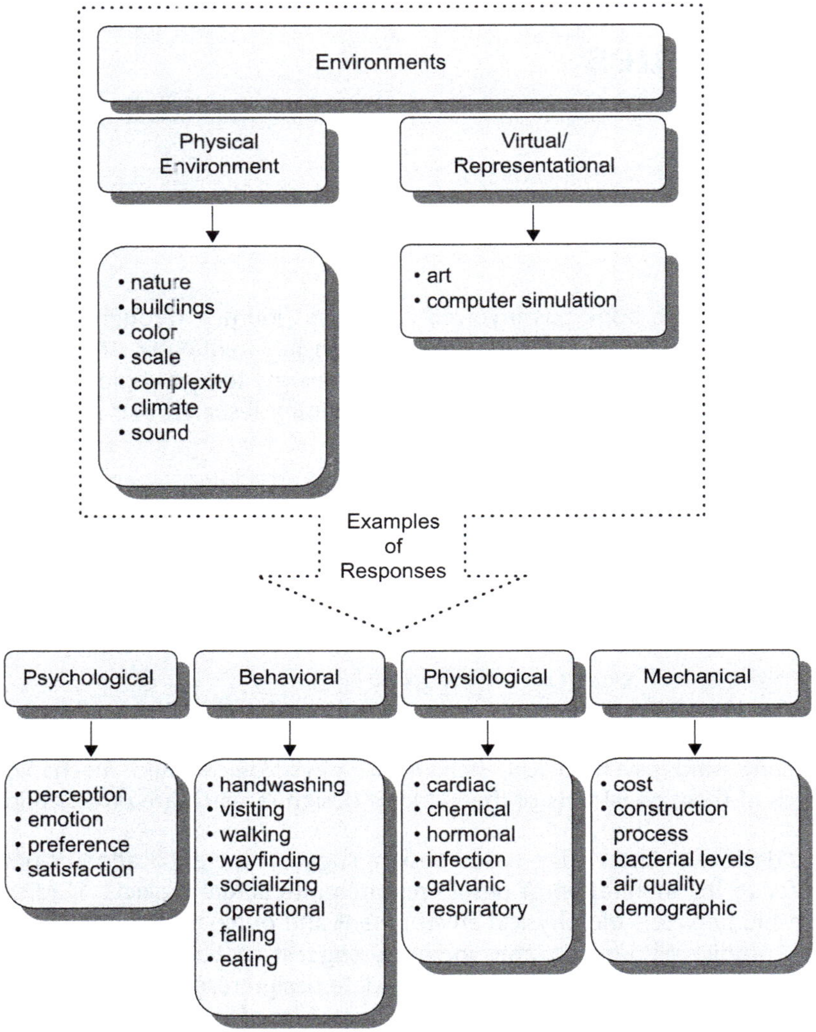

Figure 9.1: *Categories of environments and examples of responses*

conditions[1]. For example, post occupancy evaluations would only qualify if the methods they employed were rigorous and objective, and if they entailed the examination of hypotheses. In the case of a POE, a hypothesis might serve to provide a structure for studying whether the specific intentions of designers were met. In the case of programming, hypotheses regarding nurse preferences might be explored, such as structure interviews regarding nurse preference for a centralized communication center.

[1]Programming may involve observation, questionnaires, and interviews, but rarely to a degree that would meet the rigors of "hard science".

Evidence-based design and evidence-based medicine

Ray Pentecost III, PHD, AIA, ACHA

Embracing an evidence-based approach to healthcare facility design that draws its inspiration from an evidence-based approach to medicine is a gesture of enormous symbolic significance, and one which predictably invites comparisons between the two. First, invoking the claim of "evidence" inevitably begs the question of quality. How strong is the evidence? How credibly was the evidence gathered, and how reliably was it interpreted? Stories of doubt and frustration abound in the world of evidence-based medicine where researchers, convinced of the merit in their findings, nevertheless encountered challenge after challenge from their peers. The assault of legitimate rival hypotheses to otherwise apparently worthy research conclusions can leave researchers fatigued and frustrated, but the industry is better for it. Design practitioners relying on the work of those who have studied the facility-impacting research and drawn design-influencing conclusions therefrom would be well served to respectfully, maybe even cautiously, consider the source and quality of the research underlying the resulting design principles. Second, researchers learn quickly that, notwithstanding the merits and potentially far-reaching impact of their work, their conclusions are also firmly bound by limitations. In the domain of medical research it is common for the proper use of a new drug to require numerous disclaimers and exceptions that define those populations for whom this drug or that discovery is inappropriate. Again, it simply must be so for an evidence-based approach to design. The contents in this book that speak eloquently to the proper design of critical care units may, or may not, be applicable to the design of other kinds of healthcare facilities for different patient populations. The possibility of the external validity of any researcher's conclusions beyond the initial study must be as conscientiously contemplated as the original research itself, and may, in many cases, suggest a roadmap of additional research that needs to be done to explore the applicability of findings in one study to the participants in another. Of course, to be true to the comparison between evidence-based medicine and design, the two aforementioned points inescapably call into focus a third point, which is that everyone using this book to enrich their practice should, in fact, become a practitioner researcher. It happens in medicine when physicians share their experiences in recommending new medications for patients, and it should be happening to a greater degree in design. Whether by the direct use of an evidence-based design guideline from this book (attempted replication of known results), or by the use of the evidence to shape a new design direction (attempted innovation and discovery of new design-impacting evidence), practitioners naturally position themselves to make their own contribution to the world of research-influenced design – if only they will. Their experiences are vitally important in the natural research cycle of both further validating current evidence and discovering new findings. Unless practitioners are willing to take up the mantle of being healthcare design practitioner researchers who share their results, the profession may never know how fully the use of evidence in design could reshape the healthcare design experience.

Ray Pentecost is Vice-President, Director of Healthcare Architecture at CLARK NEXSEN.

The lack of mutual understanding regarding the meaning of research is a significant limitation to the promotion of design research. Currently, most research is conducted by members of academic institutions or by specialized consultants. Because of this, the gap between practitioner and scientist continues to be problematic.

9.2 Other barriers to knowledge-based design

Another impediment to research is obtaining funding to support potential studies (Shepley, 1996a). A handful of organizations, in particular the Center for Health Design (CHD), the Coalition for Health Environments Research (CHER) (now combined with CHD), and the Academy of Architecture for Health (AAH), have made an effort to promote research through the provision of grants. Additionally, highly qualified academic teams have been successful in acquiring support from universities and national organizations, such as Texas A&M University, Georgia Institute of Technology, the National Science Foundation, and the Robert Wood Johnson Foundation. Although funding for health design research is generally limited to individuals with advanced academic credentials, opportunities may be available within professional practice.

Unfortunately, there are a limited number of grants available, and office practice has not traditionally lent itself to billing clients for research activities. In order to be compensated for this activity, designers should suggest the potential inclusion of a research phase when they are conducting interviews and proposal processes. By recommending that research be included in the service package while in the proposal/interview and negotiation phases, designers might be able to be compensated for research-related tasks. There are additional benefits to promoting research. From a marketing perspective, a firm's ability to offer such services should set them apart from other design firms and facilitate the acquisition of new projects (Shepley, 1996b). Reports from the "trenches" have been varied regarding the success of this technique. However, it is the authors' belief that persistence will pay off—design research is a notion that is just coming of age and is likely to be highly marketable in the near future.

Another problem is the absence of in-house expertise in design firms (Shepley, 1996a). Although an increasing number of architecture schools are incorporating research skills in their curricula, this training is still uncommon. If a continuing education program is in place, however, specialization in a specific area could be obtained after graduation. Courses in questionnaire and interview methodology can be accessed from many major educational institutions, and, with the increase in distance learning opportunities, interested individuals could obtain such knowledge remotely. Several institutions, including Texas A&M University, are planning certificate courses that will help practitioners understand design research. If, however, a firm is not able to invest in continuing education, an alternative option would be to collaborate with research faculty and graduate students at nearby universities (Shepley, 1996b).

Apart from financial/logistical difficulties, there are other impediments to promoting research in practice. One problem is maintaining objectivity. Most in-house studies are conducted by staff, who are currently participating in or have previously participated in the building project under consideration. When a study is done in-house—even when the need for objectivity is recognized—experimenter bias may be introduced into the construction of the evaluation tools and the interpretation of the results. For example, in the construction of a questionnaire for a post occupancy evaluation, the number of questions is virtually infinite. In the process of selecting the questions, the in-house researcher may limit the topics in such a way as to skew the outcomes. Participation of an outside party, therefore, is highly desirable.

Another barrier to the growth of the discipline of design research is the lack of alignment between the approaches of researchers and designers (Shepley, 1996a). Rouse (1985) has identified three differing perspectives separating scientists and practitioners: 1) the goal of university research is to understand the problem, while the goal of industry is the "incremental improvement of particular situations"; 2) researchers tend to scale down problems (possibly beyond their applicability), while practitioners may utilize methods that are scaled up (possibly beyond their reliability); and 3) the university tends to emphasize individual accomplishment, whereas industry focuses on organizational teamwork. These contrasting perspectives are not irreconcilable, but they may frequently result in a research product that is unappreciated by the group that was not involved. An adverse outcome of these individual approaches is that the work of researchers and designers is published in journals not typically accessed by both. This problem is evident when perusing the library of a typical firm. The journals normally include *Architectural Record, Landscape Architecture,* and *Modern Healthcare,* all of which rarely publish research. Researchers, on the other hand, are publishing in *Environment & Behavior, Environmental Psychology,* or the *Journal of Architectural & Planning Research.* A new journal has recently been created, *Health Environments Research and Design,* which offers additional publishing opportunities. Hopefully all these journals will find their way to the bookshelves of both healthcare architects and researchers.

Perhaps the most significant obstacle to conducting research in private practice is the reluctance of firms to allow their projects to be scrutinized (Shepley, 1996a). This is particularly true for post occupancy evaluations in which even the best buildings are likely to have significant faults. Neither the designers nor the building owners want "bad publicity" about their buildings. Unfortunately, if these individuals request permission to review the results of the study prior to publication, they might request omissions of negative outcomes, thereby creating compromises in the study. Conversely, when collaboration is not permitted, the designer and owner are likely to feel alienated from the research process. There are two ways to address this problem. One is to keep the results confidential, and the other is to publish the results without identifying the name of the institution involved. The obvious shortcoming of keeping the results in-house is that other designers and researchers cannot benefit from the studies. Keeping the study site anonymous is helpful, but anonymity is difficult to achieve if drawings and photographs are incorporated in the document.

The only way to circumvent the problem of research outcome "paranoia" is to change our culture as architects and designers. If self-evaluation were commonplace, the results of these studies would be less likely to stigmatize the building product.

A final impediment to the integration of research into design projects is difficulty sifting through the literature and determining which studies are of highest quality. Even if a practitioner fully embraces the power of applied research, distilling the significant literature is challenging. The following section provides some guidelines for identifying quality design research.

9.3 Quality standards for design research

For those who are not acquainted with design research, it is useful to have criteria by which to judge the available literature. The following seven criteria, referred to as the SUPPORT system (Shepley, 2005), are useful when reviewing studies.

***S**ubstantive methodology.* Does the project describe a credible methodology? There is a common misperception that a study must be quantitative to be credible. Qualitative studies will be highly respected by the academic community if they are carried out in an orderly manner using a previously explored methodological process. A good example is naturalistic inquiry (Lincoln & Guba, 1985). This qualitative method, which was developed by statisticians, involves a structured analysis of naturally acquired data using auditing, member checking, and case reporting techniques.

Uncovers new knowledge. Does the study provide new knowledge? Is it a rehashing of old ideas, or does it draw new conclusions? A literature review does not provide new knowledge unless it draws original conclusions through a synthesis of the articles that are reviewed.

Peer-reviewed or refereed. Has the article describing the research been published in a peer-reviewed or refereed journal? A peer-reviewed journal is one in which the manuscripts are evaluated by reviewers who are experts in the research topic of the article. A refereed article is one that is reviewed by individuals who are not on the editorial board. Information regarding whether a journal is peer-reviewed is contained in the author's guidelines in the hard copy or website of the journal in which the article appears. Lists of peer-reviewed journals are also available in reference books, such as *Ulrich's Periodicals Directory* (Bowker Staff, 2003) (also online) and *Magazines for Libraries* (Laguardia, Katz, & Katz, 2003).

Problem or hypothesis. Does the research described in the article outline the specific problem or hypothesis that it addresses? As in design, the intentions of the researcher need to be clearly articulated at the outset of the manuscript. For example, a good hypothesis might be, "patients who are able to adjust patient-room light levels will have greater feelings of control than patients who cannot." If the discussion of the topic meanders without clarifying the objectives, then the study is likely to be insubstantial.

Objective researchers. Has the study been conducted by objective researchers? Is there a possibility that the design of the study or a description of the outcomes is influenced by the individual who has generated the study?

Repeatable methodology. Is the methodology clearly articulated? Is it descriptive enough so that it could be repeated by future researchers? When conducting a study, part of what can be learned by others is how to conduct subsequent experiments. It is important, therefore, to make research techniques accessible to others.

Triangulated outcomes. This term refers to using multiple methodologies or studies to obtain information on a single study question. For example, if researchers were interested in understanding the impact of a healing garden, they might make behavioral observations, conduct interviews, and distribute questionnaires. A common form of triangulation occurs when researchers use qualitative and quantitative approaches for the same problem. Another form of triangulation is comparing the outcomes of different studies about the same topic.

9.4 Directions for future research

According to the architects and designers in Kim's study (Kim, 2009), at the macro level the two areas most in need of research were trends in healthcare needs (based on demography and disease type), and healthcare systems and financing. Applying these findings to ICU settings, it would seem that the field needs data regarding both the demographic and diagnosis characteristics of ICU patients of the future as well as information on reimbursement and financial issues. Interestingly, these two research needs would influence the building program more than the essence of the design.

On the micro scale, functional requirements, health outcomes issues, technology issues, and user/patient issues were mentioned most frequently in Kim's study (2001). Studies on functional requirements might involve behavior mapping of the relationships among ICU spaces. Health outcome issues are at the core of most academic research and could include an expansion of existing studies on the role of nature and art to non-adult populations. Technology issues are critical, and many medical staff suggest these issues will be the driving force in future design of ICUs. Technology manufacturers should address the noise, efficiency, and space implications of their products. Lastly, user/patient issues are a significant factor in a market that is influenced by client satisfaction, and studies regarding the impact of environment on behavior will be critical to future design projects.

What research is currently available, and what directions should it take? A partial answer to the question regarding current status is provided by researchers at The Johns Hopkins Program for Medical Technology and Practice Assessment. Rubin, Owens, and Golden (1998) examined 78761 articles in search of those that were based on sound methodology, and suggested a correlation between patient outcomes and the physical environment. Only 84 studies successfully met their criteria. Table 9.1 is a summary of the 10 studies relating to adult intensive care.

The following become apparent after reviewing the studies in ICU design research described above. Firstly, two major topics have dominated the field—music and noise. These studies have been motivated by two commonly agreed upon hypotheses: a) music helps soothe patients and therefore may positively impact health outcomes; and b) noise can cause anxiety, interferes with sleep, and negatively affects outcomes. Secondly, most studies are very specific in terms of the environmental component that they address; they are of limited use to designers. For example, while we know that options for music are desirable, apart from providing the infrastructure and proper acoustics, there is very little known about additional requirements for the patient room.

Subsequent to this literature review, Shepley and Quan (2003) conducted an analysis for the period between 1998 and 2002. Examining 2000 titles, an additional 35 were selected for inclusion, three of which were applicable to adult ICU design. The increase in appropriate studies over the Johns Hopkins study was likely due to the availability of better search systems in 2002 combined with an increased interest in the field. Even more recently, Ulrich, Zimring Quan, et al. (2004) conducted an expanded review, incorporating the results of a broader range of disciplines, which identified more than 400 studies that would be useful to designers. The document summarizes evidence indicating hospital design can promote healing and addresses the impact of design on patient falls, hospital-acquired infections, medical errors, and noise levels.

What direction should research take in the future? Rather than trying to randomly identify specific research topics, it might be better to develop theories around which research projects might be focused. Perhaps more grounded theories are needed. Grounded Theory, which is most frequently associated with the work of Barney G. Glaser, is a method of comparative analysis, the purpose of which is to generate theory (Glaser, 1978; Glaser & Strauss, 1967). The utility of this approach is particularly appropriate in investigations of new problems or to gain a fresh perspective on an old problem (Stern, 1995). Glaser was quick to recognize the importance of this approach in healthcare settings; some of his earliest work was conducted with dying patients (Freiherr von Manteuffel, 1998). With the exception of a few research areas, such as the relationship between nature and stress and studies involving noise and music, there is very little theoretical structure around which studies can be generated. This book proposes, therefore, that

Table 9.1 *Studies of effects of healthcare environments on patient outcomes (Rubin, Owens, & Golden, 1998)*

Citation	*Environmental Variables*	*Subjects*	*Outcome Variables*	*Results*
Baker, C. F. (1992). Discomfort to environmental noise: Heart rate response to SICU patients. *Crit Care Nurs Q,* **15**(2), 75–90.	Noise level and type of noise	SICU patients after surgery	Heart rate (HR)	HR higher with non-talking noise than with ambient noise
Baker, C. F et al. (1993). The effect of environmental sound and communication on CCU patients' heart rate and blood pressure. *Res Nurs Health,* **16**, 415–421.	Noise level and type of noise	CCU patients	Heart rate and blood pressure	Higher heart rate during conversation in room
Davis-Rollans, C. & Cunningham, S. G. (1987). Physiologic responses of coronary care patients to selected music. *Heart & Lung,* **16**(4), 370–378.	Three music pieces	CCU patients	Heart rate, emotional state, respiratory rhythm	No physiological differences; patients happier with music
Gast, P. & Baker, C. (1989). The CCU patient: Anxiety and annoyance to noise. *Crit Care Nurs Q,* **12**(3), 39–54.	Noisy vs. non-noisy hour	CCU patients	Anxiety, annoyance	No differences
Guzzetta, C. E. (1989). Effects of relaxation and music therapy on patients in a coronary care unit with presumptive acute myocardial infarction. *Heart & Lung,* **18**, 609–616.	Music	CCU patients	Apical heart rate, peripheral temperatures	Music + relaxation resulted in a rise in temperature
Hilton, B. A. (1985). Noise in acute patient care areas. *Res in Nurs & Health,* **8**, 283–291.	Noise level	ICU and other wards	Self-reported sleep and satisfaction	ICUs had high sound levels; ICU patients reported lack of sleep/rest
Humphreys, H., Johnson, E. M, & Warnock, D. W (1991). An outbreak of aspergillosis in a general ITU. *J Hospital Infection,* **18**(3), 167–177.	ICU	ICU (ITU) patients	Aspergillosis infection	Less infection after construction with false ceilings and artificial ventilation system

(*Continued*)

Table 9.1 (Continued)

Citation	*Environmental Variables*	*Subjects*	*Outcome Variables*	*Results*
Peolsi, P. et al. (1996). Effects of heat and moisture exchangers on minute ventilation, ventilatory drive, and work of breathing during pressure-support ventilation in acute respiratory failure. *Crit Care Med*, **24**(7), 1184–1188.	Hot water humidifier and heat/moisture exchanger	ICU patients	Ventilation, static pressure, ventilatory drive, work of breathing	Exchanger increased ventilation, static pressure, ventilatory drive, and work of breathing
Shirani, K. Z. et al. (1986). Effects of environment on infection in burn patients. *Arch Surg*, **121**, 31–36.	Ward and private enclosure; ICUs	Burn patients	Infection and mortality	Patients in private enclosures had fewer infections; ICUs had lower mortality rates
Zimmerman, L. M. et al. (1988). Effects of music on patient anxiety in coronary care units. *Heart & Lung*, **17**, 560–566.	Music, white noise, and control group	Myocardial CCU patients	Anxiety, blood pressure, heart rate, digital skin temperature	No differences

in addition to the quantitative studies that are taking place, scientists and designers should consider embracing a more qualitative approach to health design research.

Research has typically been portrayed as a dry and dull subject and has rarely been thought to be the realm of architects and designers. In actuality, it is an opportunity for creative enrichment of the design experience. For healthcare architects who are eager to provide the highest quality facilities to their clients, research is a critical part of their service.

Design and performance 10

The design of any space, along with its equipment and furnishings, can serve as an enabler of high performance or as a barrier to effective operations. Durham and Hayward have written about hospital design strategies for operational restructuring (1996). Clearly, a goal of better designs would be to enable better performance. The question that must be asked is how can we know that performance is better? And further, what design interventions will bring about improved performance?

Evidence-based designers and their critical care clients need to develop measures of performance that will allow comparisons; especially pre and post design implementation comparisons.

10.1 Measures of organizational performance in healthcare

Determining whether critical care unit designs have an effect on organizational performance requires an understanding of organizational effectiveness in the healthcare setting. The national Baldrige awards, established by the United States Congress and awarded by the President, are a highly visible recognition for organizational excellence (National Institute of Standards and Technology, 2002). The Baldrige National Quality Program (BNQP) reviews healthcare organizations for the purpose of establishing national benchmarks and challenging them to improve performance.

One healthcare organization that won the Malcolm Baldrige National Quality Award is the 21-hospital SSM Health Care system based in St. Louis. The system has used the Baldrige model for evaluating its performance for seven years (Modern Healthcare, 2002). Bronson Methodist Hospital in Kalamazoo was honored with the Baldrige Award in 2005 (Knapp, 2006; Thompson 2006). There have been additional healthcare recipients: North Mississippi Medical Center in 2006, Sharp Health Care and Mercy Health System in 2007, and Colorado's Poudre Valley Health System in 2008 (Baldridge National Quality Program, 2008). The Baldrige criteria serve three roles for organizations seeking performance improvement: to facilitate the sharing of best practices, to serve as a tool for understanding and managing performance, and especially "to improve organizational performance practices, capabilities, and results" (Baldridge National Quality Program, 2002, p. 1).

The Baldrige program uses six categories for results to evaluate organizational performance in healthcare:

1. Healthare outcomes
2. Patient- and other customer-focused outcomes
3. Financial and market outcomes

4. Workforce-focused outcomes
5. Process effectiveness outcomes
6. Leadership outcomes (Baldridge National Quality Program, 2008, p. 3).

These Baldrige criteria for organizational effectiveness can be lumped within the categories of economic, clinical, or consumer and staff perspectives. These categories correspond to the material published by the Joint Commission on Accreditation of Healthcare Organizations (Joint Commision on Accreditatior of Healthcare Organizations, 1994, 2004). In their textbook on hospital administration, Shortell and Kaluzny (2000) use financial, clinical, and human resources as their three labels for these same performance categories. Measures of organizational effectiveness can be used to examine the impact of a facility design at a hospital. The following sections broadly review these categories.

10.2 Economic performance in healthcare

Samuel Levey, Ph.D., a professor of health management and policy, reports that "the national health bill has skyrocketed to well over $1 trillion, or 14% of the nation's gross domestic product, in contrast to $42 billion in 1965, the watershed year that witnessed the passage of Medicare and Medicaid" (Shortell & Kaluzny, 2000, p. xii). Today's healthcare environment is attuned to performance and improvement as the rising cost of healthcare places pressure on managers to economize (Coile, 1998, 2002, 2003; Morrison, 2000; Parmenter, 2001). Healthcare costs are now rising again "with little prospect of meaningful control" (Morrison, 2000, p. 52).

Factors that influence economic effectiveness for hospital patient units include recruitment and retention of staff during times of labor shortage, job design, quality of the work experience, the efficiency of the work process, the leverage of work-saving technologies, and the cost of supply inventory (Coile, 2002).

Economic and financial measures

A question for this book's readers is what measures do healthcare executives and members of your governance structure consider important indicators of performance? What indicators related to critical care services are important to them? There is certainly a relationship between some financial measures and the design of the facility.

One category of measures falls in the area of revenue, margin, operating expense, and capital debt. Management may be concerned about revenue per patient and the cost of providing care. Many of the factors contributing to these measures fall out of the critical care unit's control, but some clearly are affected by staffing efficiency, distribution models for pharmaceuticals and supplies, available technology, and so forth.

Capital cost versus operating cost

One of the most important realities for designers and their clients is the need to recognize the difference between capital cost and operating cost. Standard accounting procedures put the cost of acquiring facilities and equipment into capital costs, which may be financed by operating surplus, cash reserves, or debt. The day-to-day operation of the hospital comes from a completely different category of funds—the operating budget. What is important for designers and their clients to understand is that management and governance groups have strong incentives to contain and reduce capital cost and associated debt. This incentive is so strong that many projects deliberately avoid an investment in construction that is clearly known to offer dramatic potential savings in future operating costs.

Some enlightened organizations, and some with large cash reserves, are prepared to invest capital to reap savings in operations. Organizations which do not, or cannot, are certainly able to see the argument for future benefit, but until the standard accounting rules are changed, the leadership will be held accountable to this counter-productive model. The implication of this reality is that designers must work as much as possible to produce efficient and effective designs for the same cost as a standard budget.

The product of design is firmly in the realm of capital cost. The outcomes of performance are clearly in the realm of operating cost. Measuring the relationship between the two will lead to better understanding of when an investment in design will pay off with a desired performance outcome.

Operational efficiency

The relationship between operational efficiency and facility design should be self-evident. The efficiency of patient flow, ready access to equipment and supplies, ability for staff to rapidly perform their tasks, the convenient arrangement of related spaces, and appropriate environmental factors such as lighting, noise control, and thermal comfort are all potentially impacted by the design of the unit. Flexible design of rooms and equipment has been described as a means to achieve streamlined care processes (Gallant & Lanning, 2001). Among the many measures that might be used to track operational efficiency are:

- average length of stay (ALOS)
- departmental throughput
- equipment & systems utilization
- energy consumption & efficiency
- workdays lost to illness or absence.

What outcome measures do nurses feel are important to represent an accurate view of staffing efficiency? How do these measures then relate to the design of the space in which the staff perform their work? Some designs are more suited to efficient delivery of care than others.

The relationship of staffing efficiency to facility design can be quantified with a variety of measures, such as:

- number of assigned staff per occupied patient bed
- nursing hours per adjusted patient day

- number of minutes of hands-on caregiving per patient per shift
- travel distance & location of supplies or equipment
- location of communication & information technologies
- availability of labor saving technologies.

What outcome measures associated with systems efficiency can be related to facility design? There is a relationship between design of your critical care unit and the efficiency of the information systems, materials management and supply system, pharmacy model, food service system, and conveyance systems like pneumatic tubes, cart lifts, and dumbwaiters.

It should be clear that any attempt to improve operational efficiency can involve system redesign, facility design, and redesign of the work itself. Work redesign is a powerful way to address performance issues (Hackman & Oldham, 1980). Numerous authors have proposed methods for assessment of the work and redesign of healthcare roles and tasks to improve outcomes (Beckman & Simms, 1992; Tonges, 1993; Hanson & Sayers, 1995; Kelly, 1995; Coulter, 1997; Larson, 1997). Design of the work and design of the facilities in which it will be performed should occur together for maximum coordination.

10.3 Clinical effectiveness

Two additional aspects of healthcare organizational effectiveness are clinical outcomes and patient safety. Examining the impact of facility design on clinical outcomes and safety can contribute to the understanding of organizational performance and effectiveness. The Institute of Medicine issued a widely circulated report on medical safety entitled *To Err is Human* (1999), which concluded that large numbers of patients are harmed as a result of medical errors. Two studies when extrapolated to the population of over 33 million United States hospital admissions in 1997 "imply that at least 44,000 and perhaps as many as 98,000 Americans die in hospitals as a result of medical errors" (Kohn, Corrigan, & Donaldson, 2000, p. 26). The Institute of Medicine followed its first report with a second and final report that "focuses more broadly on how the health care delivery system can be designed to innovate and improve care" (Institute of Medicine, 2001, p. ix).

These Institute of Medicine quality reports influenced many in the field to address clinical improvement, or to redouble their efforts. Organizations that responded in this manner include individual hospitals and systems along with non-provider organizations such as the Institute for Healthcare Improvement (IHI), the Leapfrog Group, Agency for Healthcare Research & Quality (AHRQ), and the Center for Health Design. Measures for clinical effectiveness, therefore, can include medical errors and medication errors.

One organization devoted to higher standards for patient safety is the Institute for Healthcare Improvement (Wysocki, 2002). It plays a major role in developing and demonstrating effective strategies for improving healthcare. Its work primarily concerns process improvement and rapid-cycle pilot projects. Much of the work done by the Institute for Healthcare Improvement and the hospitals or systems it works with is based on Langley et al.'s (1996) Plan, Do, Study, Act model for improvement. One hundred fifty-five hospitals enrolled in improvement collaboratives attended a conference held by the Healthcare Improvement Institute in February 2003 to discuss study methods and to report on their results (http://www.ihi.org).

A 37-site IHI project focused on critical care units documented drops in pneumonia, reductions in complications, shorter patient stays, and cost reductions of as much as 30% after data had been gathered, small-scale rapid-cycle changes had been piloted, and successful pilots were expanded to full units (Wysocki, 2002). This suggests that other measures of clinical effectiveness and safety could include rates of hospital-acquired or nosocomial infections, re-admission rates, and average length of stay.

Role of facilities design and quality improvement

Roger Resar, M.D.

The relationship of facilities design and the quality improvement capabilities of an organization deserve discussion. The methodologies of lean or six sigma have their proponents, but when all is said and done a process needs to be designed, or improved, and then subsequently reliable. In my role as a consultant to teams attempting to design reliable processes for intensive care units, I have had a chance to observe the effects of facilities design on the ability to execute quality improvement strategies. Two concepts regarding the relationship between facilities design and quality improvement are pertinent:

- *Current Design Needs: Those facility designs that might aid in the execution and implementation of current suggested improvement strategies.*
- *Future Design Needs: Those facility designs that would permit the intensive care unit to more easily design and test new strategies related to future unknown needs.*

Current Design Needs

The application of quality improvement principles in the daily work of the intensive care unit has been dramatically demonstrated by a precipitous drop in ventilator associated pneumonia rates, or by the increased teamwork and communication seen in the use of multidisciplinary rounds. Both of these processes are enhanced by the utilization of the basic facility design concepts of unit size and shape.

One of the components of the ventilator bundle is to reliably elevate the head of the bed for ventilated patients. The use of visual cues to assure head of bed elevation is obviously much easier and generally more reliable when a circular open environment exists, as opposed to when a rectangular or loss of line of sight design is present.

Veteran intensives skilled at the use of multidisciplinary rounds have generally limited these teamwork exchanges of vital information to about 45 minutes. Rounds taking longer usually are not sustained due to the time constraints on most of the participants. A unit of 12–16 units is the ideal size to achieve rounding in the time interval. Large units create a volume of patients too great to make those multidisciplinary in an efficient and useful manner. The trade-off of larger units with possible efficiencies of scale must hence be measured against the known benefits of effective use of the multidisciplinary rounds on daily goals and length of stay in the intensive care unit.

The design specifications of size and shape can have an influence on the functionality of the rapid response team. The team commonly uses intensive care resources. A unit design that allows a sudden dispersal of unit staff to respond to a deteriorating patient needs to take advantage of the ability of the remaining staff to cover those patients already in the unit. Here, considerations of size and visual observation of those patients currently in the unit become very important design concepts. A unit of fewer than 10 beds may not have the ability to provide coverage, while a unit larger than 16 beds will commonly lose visual advantages.

Future design needs

The future obviously is a time period commonly understood to contain all events that have yet to occur. It is truly thought provoking to consider how facility designs could enhance future improvement efforts, or, put another way, how the surety of change could be accounted for in the original design. To truly foster the concept that changing facility designs will be needed, the current facility design must be flexible enough to anticipate the need for improvement, and then create the ability to test ideas and execute the changes.

Two additions to current design come into play. The first is an initial design that allows for a change in physical layout of the unit or of the patient rooms. This would include the ability to easily rearrange the linkages of the patient rooms to the outside environment, such as plumbing, gas lines, vacuum, electrical and communication needs. This would allow new equipment, processes and care teams to quickly change the functionality of the room based on new ideas. The second would be having at least one room in which patient care would regularly occur, but which would be set up for simulation activities. These simulations would involve testing ideas that would involve new equipment and patient care processes. The room itself would be designed to be very observable and have movable plumbing, gas lines, vacuum, electrical and communication connections allowing easy changes.

With a design strategy for the facilities of the intensive care unit to both have the initial design conform to the structures, needs to be implemented with high reliability. The known current improvement strategies combined with an attempt to be flexible for future needs is a powerful partnership between structure and the improvement capability of those within it.

Roger Resar is Senior IHI Fellow at the Institute for Healthcare Improvement.

Clinical and quality measures

There is a growing body of credible research that links clinical outcomes to design of facilities (Ulrich et al., 2004; Ulrich et al., 2008). An important question for the next generation of researchers is what clinical outcome measures do critical care physicians, nurses, managers, and healthcare professionals consider important indicators of best practice? And further, what measures associated with clinical outcomes can be related to facility design? Examples of relevant measures might include the following:

- reductions in length of stay (ALOS)
- reductions in re-admission rate
- reductions in non-surgical infection rates
- reductions in medication error or near misses
- reductions in patient falls and staff injuries.

It is possible for outcomes to be related to specialized initiatives. These initiatives could be based on delivery of care and treatment protocols, or upon the structure of the organizational delivery model.

- Outcomes Associated with Evidence-Based Clinical Pathways
  - Facility Design in Support of Best Practice Clinical Pathways
- Improved Outcomes in Specialty Centers
  - Design to Support a Center of Excellence
  - Facility Design in Support of Clinical Specialties.

One of the single most important issues is the relationship of patient safety to facility design. Safety has become the highest priority at many institutions. There are aspects of patient safety in which the design of the physical environment plays a part. Each critical care unit should be asking what issues are most important to the safety of their patients and staff.

In the case of nosocomial or hospital-acquired infections (HAI), the question is which facility elements have an impact. An important area is the level of compliance with the Centers for Disease Control (CDC) guidelines for the washing of hands. Studies have shown that the physical location of sinks and alcohol gel dispensers has an impact on hand-hygiene compliance. A study currently in press by Xiaobo Quan, while completing his doctoral work at Texas A&M University, compared compliance with CDC guidelines in three settings: an open bay ICU with scattered sinks and gel dispensers, older private rooms with relatively inconvenient locations for sinks and gel dispensers, and a new unit described as "well-designed" that featured sinks and gel dispensers immediately accessible to the entrance of every private patient room. The results showed an increase in compliance in the private rooms, and a dramatic improvement of 70% in compliance from the open bay to the well-designed room. The conclusion of Quan's study (2005) is that properly located hand-hygiene elements make a greater difference in compliance than educational programs, and result in sustained performance as opposed to the temporary improvements associated with staff education campaigns.

An area for further study is selection of materials for surfaces that could harbor vectors. This includes horizontal work surfaces like counter tops, walls and wall coverings, flooring materials, ceiling materials, and materials found in furnishings. The issue for these various surfaces is the ability to clean, the tendency to harbor moisture, and antimicrobial characteristics or treatments.

A study conducted on behalf of the Coalition for Health Environments Research (CHER) for the Facilities Guidelines Institute (FGI) has concluded that there is strong evidence that multi-bed patient rooms are a safety risk for patients (Chaudhury, Mahmood, & Valente, 2005). This data has influenced the consensus body revising the 2006 edition of the *Guidelines for Design & Construction of Hospitals and Health Care Facilities* to mandate all private rooms in new construction (American Institute of Architects, 2006).

Articles have appeared suggesting that high reliability organizations like the aircraft or the nuclear industries may have lessons for healthcare (Hudson, 2003; Gaba, 2004). Several institutions have designed facilities in which all patient rooms are precisely identical, or single-handed rather than mirrored back to back (Reiling et al., 2003). Examples include the Saperstein Critical Care Tower at Cedars-Sinai in Los Angeles. It is too early to tell whether single-handed room designs will be correlated with reductions in error or reduced adjusted mortality. Studies to support or refute the hypothesis are eagerly awaited by many in the field.

Burrington (1999) performed a study on the safety aspects of bedpan cleaning. She found numerous citations indicating the dangers inherent with carrying, spilling, spraying, and flushing bedpans and their contents. Of particular concern are the pathogen-laden aerosols associated with the typical cleaning process. This raises the question of whether a sealed maceration process involving paper-based containers for bodily fluids and human waste would reduce infection transmission, and be safer for the staff.

The airborne transmission of pathogens and infectious agents has become increasingly important as the world has been exposed to potential epidemics and pandemics in the post SARS era. An important performance question for critical care in the future is whether a modest number of isolation rooms will be sufficient. The M.D. Anderson Cancer Center in Houston has built a patient tower that features 100% HEPA-filtered air, and they are convinced it is very important for their immuno-compromised patients (McKahan & Hamilton, 2006).

Another question: which facility elements have an impact on medication errors? While computer verification of medication administration records (MAR) and positive patient identification with bar coding has improved results, drug preparation and administration tasks are subject to human factors such as distraction, fatigue, and confusion. In addition to designing for technological interventions, design elements such as effective task lighting, refreshing air movement, sound control, resilient flooring, and the absence of distracting overhead paging can all contribute to reductions in medication errors.

Which measurable outcomes associated with patient safety can be addressed in whole, or in part, by a facility design intervention? The same characteristics that impact performance in medication preparation may be associated with other types of error. Can the staff hear verbal communication from the team, or nearby alarms? Does the writing surface and lighting support error-free recording? Does the signage or bar code system enhance positive patient identification?

In addition to errors, another important category would be falls. Most if not all critical care units experience some level of patient falls (Hairon, 2007). How many are preventable through improved design? Ann Hendrich, a Robert Wood Johnson Fellow, has done much pioneering work in this area (Hendrich et al., 1995; Morse 1997; Hendrich, Bender, & Nyhuis, 2003; Hendrich, 2006). The size of the patient toilet doorway may be a major issue as many falls appear to occur when the assisting staff member is "peeled off" by the narrow opening. Other designs, such as St. Joseph's in West Bend, Wisconsin (Reiling, 2005), have dramatically reduced the distance to the toilet and built a handrail that extends over the entire route from bed to toilet. A question for a researcher might be: what facility elements have an impact on falls associated with critical care stays?

Other clinical and quality issues exist, and when described can be examined for a relationship to the environment in which they occur. An example might be the overall mortality statistics associated with a hospital's critical care service. When adjusted for acuity and other factors, did a change in facilities correlate with a significant change in mortality? Some issues may be described as related to safety rather than clinical quality, as in the example of failure to rescue data. Each organization will likely have slightly different categories for data, along with unique ways to bundle and study the data, while the larger field would be best served by consistency in methodology and reporting.

10.4 Role of design in creating therapeutic environments

Can design contribute to improved clinical and quality outcomes? If the measures listed above can be linked to features of the environment, the environment surely must qualify as a treatment modality. Determining a common definition for a therapeutic environment could be an important research study. No single definition exists today. It seems that a therapeutic environment can only be identified by the collection of evidence indicating which outcomes had been positively influenced. Evidence is required to make a therapeutic claim about the environment's role (Hamilton, 2005b). On the other hand, the often-used term "healing environment" would seem to be an inexact choice of words. While the environment may have a measurable impact on outcomes, it is hard to believe that the environment actually heals. The term has importance in popular use among designers and others who believe the facility plays a powerful role in the healing process (Heuelat, 2003).

It is believed that stress exacerbates every known clinical condition, and actually causes some types of illness (Selye, 1956; Benson, 1975). If this is the case, one positive role that the environment can play is the reduction of stress for patients, families, and staff (Ulrich, 1997).

Some of the obvious ways in which the environment can contribute to reduced stress include: noise reduction, fewer auditory alarms, less or no overhead paging, indirect lighting, elimination of glare, appropriate artwork, the presence of live plants, elimination of antiseptic or chemical odors, as well as views of nature and the outdoors (Ulrich, 1997; Ulrich et al., 2004; Ulrich et al., 2008). In the same way that patients may exhibit elevated blood pressure and stress hormones in the case of "white coat syndrome" (Verdecchia et al., 2002), an overly institutional appearance and associated technology can be a source of stress.

Some have given attention to the role of the diurnal cycle in the critical care unit. Disorientation leading to a condition often described as "ICU psychosis" may include lack of any outside view and a loss of grounding in the day-night cycle (Gelling, 1999; Hewitt, 2002). Windows are required in critical care rooms, but some beds remain in windowless rooms designated for "recovery," or in multi-bed settings removed from a window. Some bed positions simply make it impossible for the patient to experience the window which may be behind their head. There have been suggestions that the critical care patient should not be subjected to a continuous situation of bright lighting suited for careful examination, particularly overhead lighting that is directly into the patient's eyes.

Research in neonatal critical care has shown better results associated with lighting tuned to a diurnal cycle (White, 2004). Could this also be true for adults? At the same time, there is research from the arena of the shift worker that suggests workers perform better in conditions of bright light during night shifts (Knauth & Hornberger, 2003). This might suggest an environment in which the corridor lighting modulates with time of day, patient rooms are darkened for some or most of the night, and staff areas have bright task lighting on the night shift. This is an area suited to important further research.

The availability of natural daylight is an issue for patients and hospital workers. Some suggest that in artificial lighting situations, designers should specify full-spectrum lighting which contains most of the wavelengths found in natural light (Ott, 2000). Fluorescent and incandescent light sources have significantly less of these wavelengths. Natural light contains a certain amount of specular reflection that can be mimicked by quartz light. An interesting hypothesis is the suggestion that patient rooms lit with full-spectrum sources, and supplemented with a bit of quartz lighting for specular reflection, would be closely correlated with improved outcomes. An important potential experiment would be to measure outcomes in patient rooms that would allow comparisons between different light sources.

A newly emerging field called psycho-neuro-immunology includes the study of the environment's influence on the human immune system. Aspects of the environment have an impact on psychology and physiology, and the work of this field is to trace the subsequent impact on the immune system. Success in this area may eventually lead to a clear description of the elusive "healing" environment (Orr, 1989; Horsburgh, 1997; Dilani, 2001).

10.5 Relationship of staff performance to facility design

Staff performance is often described in the language of efficiency or productivity. This implies a certain expected amount of work to be performed within a certain expected amount of time. These words are inadequate to describe the extraordinary variability included in the performance of staff working long hours to care for increasingly sicker patients in the context of shortages of skilled nurses, therapists, and pharmacists. It may be simpler to measure the negative aspects of the performance equation. What then are the elements of the physical environment that contribute to fatigue and error on the part of critical care personnel?

Staff members at the end of a long shift may be fatigued, and in the case of 12-hour shifts, nearly exhausted. These conditions may contribute to error. Aspects of the environment play roles in the process of fatigue. Long hours walking long distances on hard-surface floors can lead to soreness, aches, and fatigue. Lighting conditions, especially glare, can contribute to eye strain, headaches, and fatigue. Absence of daylight and the flicker of fluorescent sources at consistent wavelengths can also contribute to eye strain and headaches. The absence of fresh air and air movement can lend to the fatigue process. Environments that are unusually hot or unusually cold will require additional energy expenditure on the part of working staff.

Common design decisions, such as whether the floor will be hard surface or carpeted; length of travel distance to supplies and equipment; whether the work areas will be lit by daylight, full-spectrum artificial lighting, conventional fluorescent sources, or task-specific lighting; availability of labor saving equipment; installation of patient lifts; and what sort of heating, cooling, and ventilation system will be specified, all have an impact on staff performance.

Staff performance is also impacted by the interaction among team members. There is a need for staff to have an opportunity for healthy socialization, mentorship from experienced colleagues, and development of the norms and behaviors associated with creation of a positive work culture. This can include the conference and report rooms, along with places for education and carrels for skill development, but should also allow for staff toilets, lockers, lounge, coffee, and break settings. Work on a critical care unit can be highly stressful, and there should therefore be some place for retreat, emotional recharge, or meditation.

When the staff is in a retreat or recharge mode, they should be away from the public. A popular contemporary design concept in healthcare is that of "off-stage" space, based on the Disney concept that the guests never see the "cast" except when they are on stage (Lee, 2004). We are never supposed to see Mickey relaxing on a cigarette break. In a critical care setting, this translates to providing areas where the staff can decompress and recharge away from the patients or families, and keeping the cart traffic out of the public's view. The critical care unit at Griffin Hospital in Derby, Connecticut has an off-stage corridor running through the middle of the unit's support space which keeps carts and supply traffic out of view. They also have a perimeter corridor on the exterior in which family members and visitors circulate, leaving the quiet, carpeted work corridor for staff.

Relationship of staff safety to facility design

A high percentage of healthcare workers, especially nurses, have reported experiencing one or more workplace injuries (Yox, 2004). Fear of injury among healthcare workers is a contributor to workplace stress. This leads to the question: what are the health-related risks associated with staff roles in critical care? They will fall into categories such as injury, infection, chemical exposure, and workplace violence.

What are the most common injuries to critical care staff members, and which are most harmful? Back injury, falls, needle sticks, and repetitive motion injuries are among the most common and potentially harmful (O'Brien-Pallas et al., 2004; Trinkoff, Brady, & Nielsen, 2003). In each case, there is an environmental or design aspect to the problem.

Back injury

Injury prevention through design can include the provision of labor saving equipment such as ceiling-mounted patient lifts to reduce staff back injury (Joseph & Fritz, 2006). The design of efficient layouts to reduce unnecessary walking, carpeted corridors to reduce foot-strike impact of thousands of steps, electrical outlets positioned well above the floor, and storage locations neither too high nor too low are among many other considerations to reduce back injury. Architects are notorious for designing cabinets and shelving at heights off the floor which no normally sized female nurse can reach.

Falls

Design for protection from falls can include simple provision of rails and grab bars at appropriate locations. Interior designers specify rounded corners on counters and cabinets to reduce the chance of injury in the case of a fall. Design to reduce falls may also include oversized toilet doorways to allow staff to better assist patients. Cushioned or carpeted flooring surfaces can make a difference. Slip-resistant surfaces can be designed for hard-surface flooring. Inventors are currently working on high-tech solutions in which the floor senses the impending fall and alters its surface characteristics. It remains to be seen whether these exotic technologies will prove effective and within the purchasing power of healthcare organizations.

Repetitive motion injury

In the case of repetitive motion injury, such as carpal tunnel syndrome or variations of "tennis elbow," the field of ergonomics is most involved in assessment, diagnosis, and redesign. These injuries can be impacted by the height and angle of work surfaces, keyboards, screens, and chair positions. Equipment design and mounting height can be an issue. A properly designed work environment should minimize the risk of repetitive motion injury and ergonomic problems.

Infection risk

Healthcare workers are exposed to infectious organisms. While the adoption of universal precautions is spreading, there are numerous situations in which workers may be inadvertently exposed to infection. The most common methods of transmission of infectious organisms are through contact and airborne means.

Airborne transmission is promulgated by the breath of an infected patient, a cough or sneeze, including those of staff or unit visitors, air movement associated with the changing of dressings and open wounds, the aerosols generated in the process of cleaning a bedpan, air movement associated with opening or closing a door, and the action associated with floor cleaning, among other activities. The standard design interventions for these risks include relatively high levels of ventilation and filtration, along with a designated number of isolation rooms which are on independent air systems.

Engineers refer to the number of "air changes" to indicate the volume of air that enters and is removed from a space. Higher numbers of air changes suggest a higher level of protection from airborne transmission, but no degree of volume entering and being removed guarantees that any specific atom of air or particle suspended within it will be removed.

Filtration is the companion to volume of air supplied to a space. All air supplied to a critical care unit should be filtered (2003). HEPA filtration is 99.9% filtration, which one engineer has likened to blowing air through a brick (Morris, 1998). The Alkek Tower at M.D. Anderson Cancer Center in Houston, in which all critical care units are located, along with a significant portion of the acute beds, has been designed with 100% HEPA-filtration. They are convinced that the high level of filtration provides significantly cleaner air and protects their high percentage of immunosuppressed patients (McKahan & Hamilton, 2006).

As critical care units plan for increased acuity and disastrous epidemic or pandemic situations, concern must be given to the air systems on the unit. This raises the question as to whether a few isolation rooms (in the United States, usually 10% of the unit's total beds) are sufficient in the case of an outbreak of a highly contagious strain of infection, such as the SARS episode in China and Canada, or the prospect of an avian flu pandemic. Concern over biological attack by terrorists is another possible reason to consider higher levels of isolation capacity. Future critical care units may well be designed to have higher proportions of isolation rooms, universal provision of patient isolation, or rooms easily converted to isolation status in a crisis.

Contact transmission appears to be more serious than airborne transmission (Ulrich et al., 2004). The elements of contact transmission include staff and family behaviors, cleaning methods, choice of materials like countertops, cubicle curtains, furnishings, or flooring, retention of moisture on surfaces and materials, and antimicrobial characteristics of the materials used. When designing a critical care unit, one should consider what facility elements can help inhibit the spread of infectious organisms to hospital personnel, and subsequently to other patients.

Outbreaks of resistant infections, such as recent *methycillin resistant staphylococcus aureus* (MRSA) episodes in the United Kingdom, appear to be spread entirely by contact. Multi-bed rooms that are hard to clean between discharges, along with inadvertent contact with beds, equipment, instruments, furniture, records, keyboards, and items like stethoscopes seem to favor the spread. Hand hygiene is considered to be an important protection against such spreading, but even the most scrupulous clinician can end up touching things of which they may be unaware. The lab coat may barely touch the bed rail and go on to touch the outside of the sink in which the hands are being properly scrubbed.

Design to resist contact transmission includes the provision of private rooms, along with convenient locations for gloves, disposable gowns, and masks near the entry to the room. There must be handwashing sinks with properly designed basins and hands-free faucets located in such a way that a staff member cannot enter the room without encountering it. There should always be a gel dispenser for alcohol-based cleaners. Materials in the room should be easily cleanable and the housekeeping staff must be properly trained in the most effective cleaning methods. Surfaces should be designed to shed water and avoid any puddles or pooling. Where possible, the materials should have antimicrobial characteristics. Family and visitors should be made aware of the dangers and given quick instruction on the way to avoid spreading contaminants. Rooms should be properly decontaminated between occupants.

Hazardous materials

A serious problem for healthcare workers is exposure to hazardous and toxic chemicals. These can come from a variety of sources such as medications, materials or substances used in treatment, cleaning solvents, and in some cases the chemicals in building materials used in construction. Poisoning is a continual threat to the healthcare worker. Many have developed allergies to widely used materials such as latex. Design features responding to these concerns include specification of inert materials and substances to avoid the so-called sick building syndrome, and choice of materials that can be cleaned with less toxic chemicals (Atkins, 1996; Yeoman & Paisley, 2005; MAPEI, 2006). Other measures include proper lighting and ventilation where medications and toxic substances are likely to be in use. In the case of hazardous materials, a fume hood may make the best environment for performance of the task. An obvious design feature for protection is the presence of a safety shower to drench an eye or body part that has been exposed.

This important area of concern leads to some interesting questions for future research studies. What are the principal environmental issues associated with staff safety and workplace injury in critical care? What design interventions can have a measurable impact on staff safety and workplace injury in critical care?

Relationship of staff security to facility design

Security is an important issue for staff. Threats to security include the potential for workplace violence and theft. Preservation of the worker's individual identity in the case of computer information and work with medications and the like are important. Similarly, an employee should be secure in the knowledge that personal possessions will remain safe when kept in lockers or drawers on the unit. A critical care worker should be able to work without constant attention to monitor persons on the unit for unauthorized access. Facility design, of course, can assist in accomplishing many of these objectives, but security cannot be an issue for a single unit. Security design and implementation is an issue for the entire organization, and at times for the neighboring community as well.

Reports of workplace violence seem to have increased, especially in the emergency department. Many of those who pass through the emergency department end up in the critical care unit. The critical care worker might face the potential of violence from three sources: patients or persons associated with a patient, other staff members, or individuals associated with their personal lives, such as a spouse.

What environmental factors can help increase staff security on critical care units? Most design interventions for security involve control of the perimeter, increasing observation and surveillance, or the process of "hardening" an important element. A first step is to make sure the critical care unit is a part of an otherwise safe and secure hospital environment. Attention to the critical care perimeter can mean minimizing the number of entrances and exits, securing locked doorways with keypads and other means of controlling authorized access. Increasing observation and surveillance can include designs with broad expanses of glass, view panels in doors, and cameras to monitor waiting rooms, corridors and otherwise unobserved locations. Staff can be surveyed to discover spaces in which they feel least secure, and interventions made to correct perceived problems. In the case of "hardening," sensitive locations such as narcotics cabinets, lockers, and locked drawers can be chosen with better grades of protection from potential thieves.

10.6 Consumer and staff perception of the organization

Consumers pay a larger proportion of their healthcare costs out-of-pocket (Morrison, 2000). These consumers play greater roles in directing their own healthcare and are also demanding higher quality (Morrison, 2000; Coile, 2002). The Leapfrog Group is an example. It is a consumer action group of more than 130 public and private organizations that purchases healthcare through employee insurance programs and reviews hospital quality (Morrissey, 2003). Its work culminated in three quality-based initiatives: computerized physician order entry, evidence-based hospital referral, and the use of intensivist physicians to manage the intensive care unit (http://www.leapfroggroup.org).

Universal adoption of these three Leapfrog initiatives by all non-rural hospitals would serve to prevent more than half a million serious medication errors and save more than 58 000 lives each year (Birkmeyer et al., 2000). The Leapfrog Group believes that making quality indicators public and proposing improvement initiatives will pressure healthcare organizations to improve or face rejection from powerful collective buyers of care (Lovern, 2002).

The typical healthcare consumer has no means of evaluating clinical quality and must rely on the cascade of tangible symbols the hospital presents as a proxy for quality (Berry, 2002). Quality indicators available to consumers include the facility's physical appearance, cleanliness, neatness, and noise, staff courtesy, and other observable indicators of the organization's attitude toward patients and their families.

The popularity of the annual 100 best hospitals issue of *U.S. News and World Report,* annual rankings of hospitals listed by Solucient (Reilly, 2002), and hospital rankings by the American Association of Retired Persons (AARP) further indicate the public's interest in quality of healthcare. Multiple sources of hospital ratings exist, each with websites that report on hospital quality (Scalise, 2001). Hospitals recognized frequently cite the reports in advertising, or on their own websites.

Most hospitals routinely measure patient satisfaction (Press, 2002), either through a national survey firm or through their own survey. Runy (2002) suggests that patient and employee satisfaction are key benchmarks for evaluating organizational performance.

The satisfaction of employees and patients is intertwined. Numerous studies indicate that if an employee is unhappy, it reflects negatively on a patient's perception of care. When patients are satisfied with the care, employees feel a greater sense of accomplishment and are happier in their jobs. Research also shows that a satisfied workforce leads to lower turnover rates, increased productivity, better care and enhanced outcomes (Runy, 2002, p. 58).

Patient satisfaction has also been shown to consistently correlate with staff satisfaction (Press, 2002; Malone, 2002a; www.pressganey.com). Causation between these two has not yet been examined, but knowledge that they are related has implications for organizational effectiveness (Malone, 2002b). An example would be an intervention designed to address staff satisfaction could be expected to influence staff turnover, and also may have a positive impact on patient and family satisfaction.

Patients can articulate their healthcare preferences related to the environment (Picker Institute, 1999). Results indicate that acute care patients readily articulate that they want environments that: (a) are convenient and accessible, (b) are conducive to well-being, (c) are confidential and private, (d) are caring for the family, (e) facilitate connections to the staff, (f) are considerate of people's impairments, (g) are safe and secure, and (h) offer a relationship to nature. These desires expressed by patients seem to be equally relevant to critical care populations. It would be interesting to repeat the study with a critical care population.

Satisfaction measures

Critical care departments and units are continuously interacting with a variety of constituents, including patients, their families, physicians, nurses, clergy, staff members of all types, along with visitors and members of the general public. In every case, the interaction is accompanied by a cascade of physical and environmental clues that suggest how the organization perceives the individual (Berry & Seltman, 2008). The quality of the daily or intermittent interactions leads the individual to form an impression. A number of satisfaction measures may be used to identify how these constituencies feel about the organization.

Patient and family satisfaction

The relationship of patient and family satisfaction to facility design can be fairly direct. If you are initiating a design process, you will want to know what facility issues are important to patients and their families.

One available method to discover patient and family opinion is to refer to the satisfaction survey results. Nearly every hospital uses some standardized instrument to collect regular feedback from patients or their family members. The data from these surveys is highly reliable (Press, 2002), although it lacks many questions related to the environment. Organizations are generally permitted to customize a few of their own questions in addition to the nationally standardized items; this could be a way to gather more precise data on their reaction to your facilities.

An interesting research study might ask what useful information can be found about facility design from Press Ganey and other typical satisfaction surveys. One could ask what information specific to the patient and family experience with critical care would help with an improved understanding of the impact of the physical environment on them. It seems clear that the current standardized surveys are inadequate in their questions about the environment. That raises the question: what type of survey would better answer facility questions?

Focus groups are another way to gather information from those who have experienced your care model and your space. You can collect groups of volunteers who are willing to discuss their experience and impressions and have them answer questions or explore alternate concepts posed by a trained facilitator. This method is recommended if you are approaching the initiation of a design and construction project.

A potential source of useful information about the environment is the collection of complaints from patients or their families. Cataloging complaints is a form of measurement. Some patients and family members who show an interest in working with the hospital, the unit, and the staff to improve conditions may be invited to join patient advisory groups. These advisory groups can be effective in helping the staff learn what the patient and family experience is like. An advisory group can be especially helpful during the design phase of a construction project.

Relationship of staff satisfaction to facility design

Staff or nurse satisfaction is related to the quality of their work experience. The workplace plays a role in the quality of work experience. Does the workplace support the tasks a nurse or staff member needs to perform on a regular basis? Does the physical environment make life easier for the nurse—or make life more difficult? What environmental features of the critical care unit contribute to a positive or negative work experience?

Staff satisfaction surveys are not conducted as frequently as patient and family surveys. This means that every opportunity to gather information is all the more precious. As is the case with patient and family surveys, relatively few questions about the physical environment are asked on the standard staff surveys. Units might be well served to develop their own instrument to discover the physician, nurse, and staff perceptions about the environment in which they spend every working day.

A particularly important aspect of the environment in a time of shortages of skilled staff is the role it plays in recruitment and retention. There are high costs associated with the loss of a qualified staff member and the subsequent recruitment of a replacement (Mattke & Mattorel, 2005; Jones, 2006). Potential employees can be influenced by their observation and impressions of your workplace. A combination of a beautiful new facility and a positive culture caused the new Woodwinds facility in Woodbury, Minnesota to create a waiting list for employment after using the University of Chicago to help them with an instrument to help determine which applicants were best suited to work there. They had many times more applicants than positions in a community that has a persistent shortage of healthcare workers.

In the same way that the environment can impact potential employee perceptions, the workplace can play a role in staff retention. Workers in a pleasant, supportive workplace are more likely to stay on-board.

One method for gathering data about the environment is to track grievances which mention aspects of the unit's design, equipment, and furnishings. Similarly, a standard question set for exit interviews might ask about the role played by the environment. These potentially negative comments could serve as an indicator of areas needing improvement.

An important question for future research might be: what facility issues are perceived to be important by the staff of critical care units? It would be relatively easy to conduct a session with the staff of a unit to provide a little basic information about the role of the environment, allow for a period in which they are encouraged to make personal observations about their interactions with the environment, and then follow up with a survey to discover their opinions about the role of that specific unit's environment.

Physician satisfaction

It seems obvious that there must be a relationship between physician satisfaction and some aspects of facility design. Unfortunately, physician satisfaction is measured less often than patient or staff satisfaction. This is an area where much work might be done to determine how critical care physicians feel about aspects of their working environment.

For physicians to effectively perform their work they need to have the appropriate lighting and access to examine patients, the ability to record their observations and make notes, the ready availability of clinical information and reference materials, and the proper conditions for clear communication with nurses and other members of the interdisciplinary team. Surely many of these issues have a physical design aspect. Physicians may also have an interest in procedure rooms, lounges, call rooms, and spaces in which to consult with families. A potential research question would be to identify what facility issues are important for physicians. Their reactions may be measured in conjunction with subsequent physician satisfaction surveys.

It is plausible to contend that physician satisfaction depends to some degree on the quality of their work experience. It is clear that the workplace plays a role in the quality of work experience. Does the workplace support the tasks a physician or intensivist needs to perform on a regular basis? Does the physical environment make life easier for the physician—or make life more difficult? What environmental features of the critical care unit contribute to a positive or negative work experience?

Physician loyalty, sometimes described as not splitting admissions, or choosing to work at a single hospital, is important to an organization. The measure for this type of loyalty is obvious from its definition. Factors in physician commitment to one institution over another may include reputation or benefits, but will often relate to the degree of physical connection a physician has to the institution. Is the physician housed on the hospital campus, conveniently available to the critical care unit? Is the physician a rent paying tenant, or located at some distance from the hospital? While these questions are somewhat less relevant for the typical intensivist housed on the unit, the degree of other physicians' linkage to the hospital can be described empirically.

10.7 Participation roles in the design process

Some versions of the design process are configured to involve users of the intended facility in the activities associated with creating an approved design. This method, sometimes described as a participatory design process, is intended to allow the design team direct contact with individuals who have specific knowledge of the function, and to build organizational enthusiasm for the project. The goal is to have a better design that meets the needs of the users, and to obtain their "buy-in" for the project.

Some questions in the participatory design process involve selection of representative groups, management of the types of decisions user groups can make, and the range of participants. Will former patients and their families have a role in the design process? Will management set a budget before a wider group is involved? If involved in the design process, will staff find the new space to be efficiently designed? A research study that asks how a participatory design process influences the ultimate facility users might be interesting.

10.8 Measures of community support

It is important to note the level of community support for an organization, such as a hospital or its critical care elements. Some aspects of community support may be influenced by the facility design. How, then, do communities exhibit support for healthcare organizations? There is the willingness of community leadership to serve on boards, or participate in development and fundraising. The level of volunteerism is an indicator, and clearly philanthropy is a tangible declaration of support. The question is what aspects of facility design make a positive contribution to this kind of support?

Another measure of the public and community support can be the reputation of the organization. Reputations and "brand" loyalty can be measured with surveys and focus groups. Press coverage, as in the frequency of mention, the number of lines devoted, and the percentage of positive versus negative editorial comment, can be an indicator, as can be the number of minutes or seconds allotted to televised coverage. Consumer preference is measured every day as patients and their physicians choose one institution over another. Market share is a rapid and constant feedback measure of community support.

Different sources such as management textbooks, the Joint Commission, and the Baldrige criteria all address these types of measures as important to understanding organizational performance. Each uses a slightly different set of labels. Perhaps this entire category ultimately speaks to the issue of *commitment* to the organization from physicians, nurses, staff, patients, families, community leaders, ordinary citizens, philanthropists, and potential collaborating organizations of all kinds.

10.9 Relationship of design to culture

Organizational culture, sometimes called corporate culture, influences organizational performance (Wilkins & Ouchi, 1983). Culture is sometimes casually described as "the way we do things around here." Culture is composed of shared values, prescribed behaviors, policies and procedures, along with the artifacts and symbols of the organization (Schein, 1992). The physical setting of an organization is a tangible artifact, symbolizing the organization's attitude towards its staff and the public. Leonard Berry has said that the environment provides a "torrent of clues" about the organization for the observer (Berry & Seltman, 2008). Facility design clearly plays a role in the culture of healthcare organizations (Hamilton & Orr, 2006; Hamilton, Orr, & Raboin, 2008).

The joint optimization of culture and related facility interventions offers the potential for synergy (Cherns, 1976; Appelbaum, 1997). Culture change is difficult, and attempts to create change often fail as the resilient former culture reasserts itself. When a design intervention accompanies an attempt at culture change, it may be possible to physically restrict the behaviors that are intended to change, and to physically enhance the desired behaviors. Design to enhance the desired culture, and to create barriers for the old behaviors, can support a culture change initiative. The result is a simultaneous set of coordinated interventions to improve the technical and physical healthcare *environment*, along with positive change in the social and cultural aspects of the healthcare *experience*. This means purposeful design of both the physical and social aspects of the organization. One possible outcome is that the design of a critical care unit will be better correlated with the redesigned organization, and can result in measurable performance improvements and medical outcomes.

There are examples of joint efforts to alter the culture and simultaneously redesign the physical environment in healthcare organizations. The Planetree organization had its beginnings in California during the mid-1980s (Gearon, 2002). A significant element of their philosophy is to change hierarchical, physician-centric healthcare delivery to a collaborative, patient- and family-centric model. From the very beginning, the Planetree model depended on a physical change of art, color, carpet, wood trim, furnishings, and room types (Orr, 1992). In addition to the original unit at what was then Pacific Presbyterian Medical Center in San Francisco, other widely described examples include the Mid-Columbia Medical Center in The Dalles, Oregon and Griffin Hospital in Derby, Connecticut (Frampton, Gilpin, & Charmel, 2003).

Hamilton (2003b) performed a study of two hospital designs for a master's thesis in which the unobtrusive data, triangulated by survey and interview results, indicated the success of a joint design project and culture change intervention at Harbor Hospital in Baltimore. The other successful design project for St. Michael Health Center in Texarkana was shown to be supportive of a strong preexisting culture which the new building strengthened.

It will be important to learn more about this important relationship between design and the culture of a critical care unit, or the larger hospital culture. What forms does culture take in healthcare organizations and in critical care units? Which of these cultural forms have a positive influence on performance? Can results of joint culture and facility interventions in critical care be shown to be more effective than either type of independent intervention?

10.10 Measures specific to a proposed design intervention

When a design is intended for only a portion of the organization, such as a partial renovation or the addition of a single new element, one can select performance measures associated with that specific design intervention.

An example might be the renovation of an adjacent space to add a procedure room to the ICU. The design hypothesis would be something like: *The new procedure room will reduce dangerous transfers from the ICU, resulting in fewer crisis interventions and improving mortality among ICU patients requiring procedures.* The hypothesis leads naturally to the development of measures to support or refute the intended purpose of the design. One would record data before the project is complete to set a baseline for crisis interventions associated with transfers out of the unit for procedures, and would collect mortality figures for patients who had procedures while admitted to the ICU. Comparison data would then be collected after the new room had been constructed and put into use.

The resulting analysis of data could show several things, ranging from validation of the concept of reduced travel for ICU patients, through inconclusive results, to a surprising increase in crisis interventions or mortality. The researchers would try to determine whether confounding factors were involved. Did physicians order more procedures for patients because of the new proximity? Was movement on the unit just as much a problem as movement off the unit? What would happen if procedures could be performed in the patient's room without any transfer?

The types of measures used for project-specific situations will vary as widely as the nature and the purpose of the project. The design hypothesis, based on interpretation of credible evidence, could be about clinical outcomes as well as staff efficiency, infection control, patient and family satisfaction, lighting, comfort, HVAC performance, building materials, appearance, technology, and a myriad of other factors. What is important is that the measure be appropriate to support or refute the hypothesis associated with the planned design concept.

10.11 Commitment to improved performance

What is important is to recognize how important continuous improvement is to the evolution of healthcare delivery. Nowhere are measurement and improvement more important than in critical care. There is a strong relationship between the design of critical care environments and their performance. It is hoped that every reader will take away a commitment to explore the ways in which physical design can enhance the important work being done in these intensive care settings.

Conclusion

Those who are designing the critical care units of the future would do well to review what has been done in the past, and to take the opportunity to visit and observe as many other units as possible. Thoughtful assessment of the impact of current trends is another important task for the planner and the user. Then an effort should be made to imagine an ideal future—one that offers the prospect of exceptional care and superior outcomes.

How can the work of the physician and nurse be simplified and made more effective? How can technology improve the diagnostic and therapeutic process for these critically ill patients? How can the endless stream of medications, supplies, and food be made to flow more efficiently? What can be done to involve family and friends in effective social support for critical care patients? What can be done to accommodate families with dignity and genuine concern for their stress? How can redesign of the work process itself contribute to improved performance?

The need is great. The earliest critical care units are now quite obsolete. Reliable predictions suggest that the United States will spend more than $200 billion on hospital construction in the next decade, much of which will be in new or replacement hospitals (Babwin, 2002; Carpenter, 2004, 2008). It is clearly a moment of rare opportunity.

The only way to achieve a better future is to be able first to imagine it. We must learn what we can from the best of today's examples, but make sure *your* design for critical care goes much farther towards an ideal model. Then be sure to document and share your results.

The design of the ICU of the future will be the result of decades of extensive research on the impact of the physical environment on patients, family, and staff. These superlative facilities will represent the ultimate marriage between art and science—they will be characterized by the inherent visual beauty associated with design solutions that address human physical and psychological needs.

In spite of their high quality, these inpatient facilities will be designed to serve as laboratories to collect data in support of the more distant future, as the needs of patients (e.g., culture and diagnosis) and staff (e.g., demographics and training) shift over time. It is the social responsibility of designers to measure the success of each design and disseminate the information so future facilities benefit from the lessons learned. There is no "standing still" in the search for good design solutions.

The future ICU will be more effective than the modified recovery rooms which pioneered the critical care concept. The ICU will have larger rooms with important staff support functions directly at hand, closer to the bedside. The monitoring and hospital information computers will be integrated systems with full connectivity. These rooms and the equipment in them will be served by powerful and flexible utility infrastructures suited to uncomplicated changes.

There is no question that the future ICU will better address the clinical needs of the intensivist-led interdisciplinary team. It will accommodate new types of equipment and advanced technologies specifically designed for critical care use. These resources, in a properly designed environment, will make it possible to achieve improved outcome measures.

The ICU of the future will be efficient and cost effective. The economic implications of evidence-based design will be balanced against cost savings associated with improved patient and staff outcomes. Whether in the United States, Canada, Europe, or in the developing world, if the critical care unit is not economical there will be no incentive to make an investment in better facilities.

Safety precautions will permeate all facets of the unit design. Infection control will be paramount in the development of mechanical systems, selection of materials and cleaning methods, and location of hygiene devices. Patient falls will be curtailed due to enhanced supervision techniques, amenity location, and floor finishes. Staff injuries will be vastly reduced through effective lift devices and improved lighting. Medical errors will be virtually eliminated through communication-enhancing technology, improved lighting, and noise reduction.

The ICU of the future will be a model of green building design. Generous provision of natural daylight will reduce electrical lighting needs, while building materials and furniture finishes which reduce off-gassing will be selected. The physical environment will support recycling protocols with convenient collection points.

We seem to have learned that art and a mildly stimulating environment helps diminish the negative aspects of an institutional character. In the end we have apparently discovered that staff and patients are more threatened by the cubicle curtain, stethoscope, keyboard, and plumbing than by pet therapy animals and house plants. Adding a little comfort, joy, and unconditional enthusiasm will nearly always be welcome.

The new ICU will offer the patients and their family a positive, nurturing environment supportive of the healing process and psychosocial needs. The contribution of the physical environment to ICU psychosis and similar psychological conditions will be profoundly reduced through noise reduction, access to natural light and nature, attention to uplifting décor, and enhanced interaction with families and staff.

In the same way, designers will recognize the important psychosocial needs of the critical care staff and begin to offer a supportive environment for a highly stressed professional team. The ICU of the future will be a better place to work, as well as more supportive of staff efforts to treat serious illness.

In today's climate of nearly continuous change, flexibility in the design of critical care environments is important. Adaptable flexibility can be achieved through decentralized staff support, increased room size, provision of a complete utility infrastructure, multiple computer and data connections, provision for mobile technologies, changeable life support systems, and sophisticated environmental controls. Before flexibility became a "buzz word" for clinicians, managers and their architects, the well-designed unit anticipated zones for future growth, contained shell space for later conversion to an anticipated use, and sometimes was located adjacent to "soft space" that could be relocated at minimal expense. This type of planning provided convertible flexibility. Convertible flexibility can also be achieved through unit configuration, decentralized staff support, increased room size, multiple locations for computer and data connections, preparation for a complete utility infrastructure and routing of antennas for telemetry.

The critical care environment of the future is exceptionally important because of an aging population that will increasingly require acute hospitalizations. The total numbers of ICU cases will increase, with higher levels of acuity, to represent a larger proportion of the total inpatient hospital census. As care is increasingly performed on an outpatient basis, the ICU and the trauma service become the most important components of the future hospital. We can only presume additional change in the future, and that the flexibility to adapt or convert will continue to be prized.

The authors are excited by the potential results of collaborations between enlightened designers and engaged clinicians in the creation of the critical care environments of the future. We wish all of you well in the process of designing yours.

Appendix
An alternative method for human waste disposal in critical care

This is a reprint by permission of Burrington and WHR Architects, the successor to the 501(c)3 Center for Innovation in Health Facilities. In 1999 Burrington was employed by WHR as a nurse with an interior design education. She produced this document in response to questions from participants at the ICU 2010 conference held in College Station, Texas in 1999 (Hamilton, 2000). The original was a white paper which was never widely circulated, and, although it was written a decade ago, it raises important points. It is reprinted in its original form. Infection control experts today question whether contaminated human waste should end up in the sewer system, so there is an interest in devices which can sterilize the waste before it is flushed or macerated. Burrington has since gone on to become a dietician working with obesity research at Baylor College of Medicine.

Abstract

The following study was initiated in response to a question raised during the April 1999 ICU 2010 conference focused on Critical Care Design. The purpose of this article was to evaluate the use of an alternative, closed system for handling and disposal of human waste to hospital critical care environments. This closed waste disposal system consists of recycled, biodegradable molded pulp paper products (bedpans, urinals, commode liners, etc.) that are intended for single use by the patient. A specially designed closed disposal unit macerates the paper receptacles and their contents, then flushes them into the sewage system. Issues concerning infection control, environmental factors, and cost-effectiveness of this type of system are discussed. Information was obtained through literature review and interviews with ICU Nurse Managers and Charge Nurses currently using this type of system. The conclusion is that a closed waste management system could be a favorable alternative to traditional methods of bedpan washing and human waste disposal in the ICU environment. The author, a Registered Nurse with a degree in interior design works for an architectural firm that specializes in healthcare design.

Problems with bedpans in critical care

Infection control, rising costs of medical waste disposal, and concern for the environment are among the myriad of issues facing healthcare providers as well as architects and designers who work closely with them in planning new or renovated healthcare facilities.

One issue to consider is the choice of a human waste/bedpan disposal system. Although the portion of patients in hospitals who require the use of a bedpan is surprisingly low, giving bedpans is still an important and significant part of hospital life and nursing care, especially in critical care areas (Gibson, 1976).

In the event that a private bathroom exists, very few ICU patients are able to walk to the toilet. A survey of nurse/supervisors in 29 cardiac care units indicated that the use of a bedside commode or patient care module (swivette-type toilet) caused significantly less physiological stress to the patient than using a bedpan or ambulating to the toilet (Clipson, 1972). The use of built-in bedside commodes that rotate into a cabinet is common. These, however, are often associated with odors and leakage, potentially leading to contamination and infection transmission. Caregivers using flushable bedside units near the patient to empty soiled bedpans may increase patient exposure to contaminated aerosols and splash (Harvey, 1998). Conventional methods for disposal of human waste, i.e. manual systems of emptying, rinsing, and washing bedpans are not only unpleasant for healthcare professionals but can pose a risk for cross infection to staff and patients. Even automatic bedpan washer disinfectors can be inadequate since the limited heat conductivity of the plastic receptacles most commonly used in hospitals today may make proper disinfection more difficult (Gibson, 1976). Furthermore, healthcare facilities using disposable petroleum-based plastic receptacles pay high disposal fees to collect and haul plastic waste to limited landfill sites.

A closed system alternative

Could a system offering a completely closed disposal method for biodegradable pulp products be a feasible solution to these issues in the ICU environment where patients often require the use of bedpans or bedside commode chairs?

One such closed system, the Vernacare Waste Management Disposal System is a range of biodegradable, molded pulp paper products (all made from 100% recycled newsprint) including bedpans, commode liners, emesis basins, graduates, and bowls. Products are designed for one-time use by the patient and are then placed in a special, closed disposal unit about the size of a dishwasher. A maximum of four utensils can be disposed of in one cycle. The pulp receptacles and their contents are macerated and then discharged into the sewage system. This closed method of waste disposal limits the exposure and spread of fecal bacteria associated with splashes that often occur during manual bedpan washing.

"Paper mache" bedpans (as they were once called) and bedpan macerators have been used in hospitals across Europe for over 35 years. The idea is progressively gaining acceptance in healthcare facilities throughout North America with approximately 600 Vernacare units now operating in the United States and Canada.

According to Timothy Emo, Vernacare Product Manager, Emergency Rooms are currently the most common application for this system in the U.S. ERs generally treat high volumes of patients on a short stay basis, therefore Vernacare addresses the environmental and cost-related concerns associated with disposing such large quantities of single use plastic products. The closed disposal system is more recently seeing increased application in the critical care environment as well, primarily due to the potential infection control advantages that it offers.

Infection control and waste management

Patients in intensive care units represent only 8–15% of hospital admissions, yet suffer a disproportional percentage of nosocomial infections (infections acquired during hospitalization) compared with patients in non-critical care areas.

Although the gastrointestinal tract is one of the less common sites of infection seen in ICU patients, nosocomial diarrheas continue to be an important problem in hospitals and in critical care units in particular.

It has been established that outbreaks and spread of the gram-positive organism, *Clostridium difficile*, cause virtually all cases of infectious nosocomial diarrhea. This organism, a resident of the human colon, does not normally cause disease unless allowed to proliferate. *C. difficile* proliferation in the colon can occur when the normal colonic flora is compromised by the use of antibiotic medications. Antibiotics induce the elaboration of toxins from *C. difficile* in the gastrointestinal tract that produce intestinal inflammation and diarrhea. Widespread use of broad-spectrum antibiotics is common in the treatment of many ICU patients. Other factors involved in the colonization and infection with *C. difficile* include age and underlying illness (Richards & Edwards et al., 1999); (Cunha, 1998).

The exact source from which *C. difficile* gains access to the gastrointestinal tract during outbreak situations is not known, but data suggest that hospital environmental contamination may be a potential source of infection. *C. difficile* spores can survive desiccation for months, and are relatively resistant to conventional disinfectants. Because this organism can lay dormant in its spore form in the environment for extended periods of time, infection control measures are necessary to prevent the spread of *C. difficile* throughout the institution (Mulligan & George et al., 1980). Due to the progressive emergence of antibiotic-resistant organisms within hospitals (Bonten & Weinstein, 1999), even high compliance rates with basic infection control methods may no longer effectively reduce the spread of *C. difficile* and other disease-causing enteric pathogens. The annual cost of treating *C. difficile* can easily exceed $600000 in larger healthcare facilities (Wilcox et al., 1996).

A study performed by Wilson and Frederick at a tertiary referral hospital within the Department of Veteran's Affairs in 1996 looked at the environment around areas where bedpans were manually washed. For study purposes, a plastic bedpan was contaminated with fluorescent marker dye called glo-germ, a substance commonly used by infection control practitioners to evaluate hand-washing techniques. The bedpan was washed manually using the standard technique for this hospital. The room was then observed under a fluorescent woods lamp. Extensive contamination of both the room and personnel was shown with the fluorescent dye. Dye was found on the walls, floor, and shoes of the person who had washed the bedpan. The dye material also continued to be detectable on the bedpan itself.

A second part of the same study used Rodac culture plates to detect colonization of actual *C. difficile* spores in two patient rooms and the sink where bedpans were being washed. The areas tested were found to be heavily contaminated with *C. difficile* spores. The rooms were cleaned with sodium hypochlorite and tested for *C. difficile* again one week later, with similar results. Data concludes that spores were disseminated widely throughout the area and therefore presented a substantial risk for transmission of *C. difficile*-related disease within the hospital. It was noted that the degree of contamination seen could likely be attributed to the method of bedpan washing used Wilson & Frederick (1996). According to Mary Moorefield, Infection Control Practitioner at the Durham North Carolina VA Hospital where this study was conducted, "since the closed waste disposal system was introduced in the older medical-surgical units of the hospital, there has been a decrease in *C. difficile* spread." The older ward-type areas were treating higher-acuity patients with limited toilet facilities and no automatic bedpan washing machine. Durham VA hospital is not using Vernacare in their intensive care units yet due to budgetary limitations. The ICUs had recently been completely renovated, including conversion to all private rooms with toilet areas, prior to installation of the closed disposal system on the patient wards. Ms. Moorefield presented results of the VA study at the 1998 Healthcare Design Symposium.

Bedpan macerators – past and present

As mentioned previously, disposable bedpan systems have been used in hospitals overseas for approximately 35 years. Since their introduction, these systems have always addressed the risks of cross infection by providing patients with a clean, dry waste receptacle for each use. Some primary criticisms of earlier models included flooding after blockage of main drains, production of contaminated aerosols, and frequent breakdowns usually associated with blockage. As in earlier models, the most common cause of blockage continues to be overloading or placement of inappropriate objects into the disposer unit. Repeated training of users is a necessary component in reducing the incidence of blockages even in view of newer, more efficient models.

A disadvantage of the earlier paper-mache bedpans themselves as compared with those made of plastic or steel was their relatively rough surface, which could potentially damage thin or tender skin over pressure points. Manufacturers have responded to such criticisms by improving the design of both the paper products and the disposer machines (Collins, Deverill, Taylor, & Oates, 1980) [11]. For example, the new Vernacare "2000" system has an airtight chamber which eliminates aerosols, and a locking lid to prevent accidental opening during cycle. A foot pedal provides controlled opening of the lid in order to prevent a coarse, sudden action, which could otherwise produce contaminated water spray upon opening. In addition, if a foreign object is accidentally placed inside the disposal unit, it cannot travel beyond the internal hopper, thus reducing costly plumbing and maintenance calls.

A major disadvantage of the system to date is the need for a carrier or support for the pulp bedpan as the paper receptacle alone cannot support the weight of a patient. The support consists of a plastic form that is not disposable, therefore adequate disinfection of this piece is a potential problem. The present need for this type of support appears to be a basic defect of the entire system (Collins, Deverill, Taylor, & Oates, 1980)[11]. Although the support piece may not come in direct contact with the patient, it could become contaminated while sliding in and out of the patient's bed. Once again, frequent education of staff is required to ensure regular and proper cleaning of the support piece. The plastic supports can be sterilized by autoclave and reprocessed for multiple use.

User interviews: pros and cons

Telephone and e-mail interviews were conducted with Nurse Managers and Charge Nurses at 10 facilities (nine in the U.S. and one in Canada) that are currently using the Vernacare System in critical care settings. Nine out of the 10 users interviewed expressed an overall positive opinion of the system. Some miscellaneous comments regarding perceived benefits of the closed disposal system included: no splash-back from bedpan washing; clean, more convenient; time saving; more time for "real" nursing functions; and controls contamination.

Eight of the ICUs surveyed, ranging from seven to 25 beds, have one or two closed disposal units in a centrally located soiled utility area. In these facilities, the system was subsequently added to an already existing ICU. Nurses in these units generally felt that their situations were adequate, however those in the larger ICUs would prefer to have additional disposal units. One user commented that carrying used receptacles through the patient unit to the soiled utility room was a problem.

At the other two facilities surveyed, Washoe Medical Center in Reno, Nevada and University of Iowa Hospital in Iowa City, Iowa, installation of the Vernacare System was a programmed part of the design process from the onset. ICUs in both hospitals were designed to accommodate an approximate ratio of one disposal unit per every two patient rooms. Sandy McIntosh, Nurse Manager of the SICU at the University of Iowa Hospital believes that "the biggest benefit (of the closed disposal system) is the location of the disposal units. Most of our disposal units are shared, one unit between two patient rooms in a separate, closed anteroom and some rooms have their own disposal unit, also in a closed area." When questioned about data to support the waste disposal system from an infection control standpoint, most of the nurses interviewed had no knowledge of available statistics and found it difficult to determine noticeable differences with regard to outbreaks of infectious diarrhea. Susan MacMillin, Infection Control Practitioner at St. Michael's Hospital, Toronto, Ontario, Canada, explains,

> This is difficult. Our *C. difficile* diarrhea rate dropped when the system (Vernacare) was brought into the medical floor. However, at the same time we had also introduced restrictions on *clindamycin* and *cefuroxime* (two antibiotics associated with nosocomial diarrhea) and we do not allow *cefoxitin* use, due to its high risk for causing *C. difficile* diarrhea. Lateral transmission (of *C. difficile*) is always a possibility on a unit where there are commodes and bedpans used. Of note to date, we have never had a *C. difficile* diarrhea outbreak on any floor that already has the closed waste disposal system in place. Outbreaks have occurred on units that do not have the system, but other variables also play a role, as in the case of *clindamycin* use.

MacMillin also commented on the cost-effectiveness of the closed disposal system. "We have two systems that have been in use since 1986 and they are still in operation, so this is cost-effective. If you speak to nurses, they believe it is cost-effective for them. Remember, it's not that fewer nurses will be needed, it's outbreak avoidance and more time to perform nursing functions. If one factors in the nursing labor to clean bedpans after every use, then it (waste disposal system) is cost-effective." Two of the other facilities interviewed had conducted an initial cost analysis upon installation of their Vernacare System. Although specific figures were unavailable, both hospitals reportedly found the system to be more cost-effective than traditional bedpan washing and disposal methods.

According to the ICU nurses interviewed, one of the greatest benefits of this waste disposal system is the convenience or time saving factor. A time and motion study was conducted at Riverview Health Center, a 338-bed long-term care facility in Winnipeg, Manitoba, Canada to determine if the Vernacare System really did save nursing time. Using traditional washing methods, staff required anywhere from 28 to 100 seconds to rinse out a bedpan. The average time was 60 seconds. In contrast, the average time to use the closed disposal system was 16 seconds, with a range of 10 to 33 seconds. Findings suggest that Vernacare was saving nursing time. Calculating the difference between the two methods, the disposal system required an average of 36 seconds less than manual washing. Saving 36 seconds on each bedpan used in this facility in a year translates into 24 967 minutes, or 416 hours, of saved nursing time—time that could be better spent caring for patients[12].

During the interview process, the ICU nurses were asked to describe the noise made by a system disposal unit during its two-minute cycle. Several users compared the sound to a common kitchen garbage disposal. They virtually all agreed that the unit should be placed in a closed area because of the noise factor.

Inquiry was made regarding patients' reactions to the disposable paper products. Nurses generally responded that because they are in an ICU setting, many of their patients are too ill to respond. Those patients that are awake and alert are often initially unsettled by the strange look and feel of the paper products, but they generally become more accepting as they do not have to sit on a cold bedpan.

Some additional comments were noted during the nursing interviews. One nurse suggested that the disposable products are better than plastic from an aesthetic standpoint because the reusable plastic bedpans tend to pick up odors even with regular washing/disinfecting. Another remarked that the disposable bedpans stack/store more easily than the conventional plastic variety. None of the nurses described problems with leakage or crushing of the molded paper receptacles.

The ICU nurses were also asked to explain from their experiences any negative aspects of using the Vernacare System. The most common response was the issue of overflow and/or blockage. This is usually associated with objects other than the manufacturer's disposable products being placed into the disposal unit. Nurses agreed that repeated education of staff is necessary in order to limit the frequency of these incidents. Two users commented that the plastic bedpan supports were often thrown away rather than being sterilized for reuse, thus breaking down the overall cost-effectiveness of the system; similarly, this is an issue of staff education, not necessarily a defect in the system itself. None of the nurses made comments about potential infection control problems relating to use of the plastic supports. Two other IC nurses mentioned that odor in the utility room is sometimes a problem, even when using Bio-Waste, the manufacturer's digestant deodorizing liquid, in the disposal units.

Conclusions

Due to acuity of illness, most critical care patients are confined to the use of a bedpan or bedside commode unit requiring a bedpan. Research has shown that nosocomial infections continue to be a serious problem in critical care areas, and that gross contamination with enteric pathogens can occur while manually washing plastic bedpans or commode chair liners in a sink or patient toilet area. Implementing a closed waste disposal system could reduce the risk of cross infection of *C. difficile* and other virulent organisms like *Vancomycin Resistant Enterococci* (*VRE*) and *Methicillin Resistant Staphylococcus Aureus* (*MRSA*) for the most part; application of a closed waste disposal system in the ICU setting could prove to be a cost-effective way to reduce the exposure and spread of disease-causing bacteria. This type of system could also save precious nursing time. The use of recycled biodegradable pulp products helps to greatly reduce the amount of paper and disposable plastic being sent to landfills.

Most of the negative comments about this disposal system revert back to the issue of necessary staff re-education regarding its proper use.

Nursing staff currently working with closed system macerators in the ICU appear to be pleased with the system as a whole, and are spending less time in the unpleasant and potentially dangerous task of emptying and washing bedpans. Facilities with shared disposal units between two patient rooms especially enjoy the convenience of not carrying soiled bedpans through the nursing unit to a central utility room. The Vernacare company has started to examine the feasibility of a smaller "patient room model" but representatives say they are still some time away from anything concrete.

As a result, designers may wish to consider the closed waste disposal system as an innovative alternative to traditional toileting and waste disposal methods in the critical care environment.

References

Gibson, G.I., August 5, 1976. The bedpan and cross infection. Nurs. Times 72 (31), 1198–2200.

Clipson, C,W., 1972. Wehrer II: Planning for Cardiac Care. The Health Administration Press pp. 138–139.

Harvey, M.A., 1998. Critical care unit bedside design and furnishings: impact on nosocomial infections. Infect. Cont. Hosp. Ep. 19 (8), 597–601.

Richards, M.J., Edwards, J.E., et al., 1999. Nosocomial infections in medical intensive care units in the United States. Crit. Care Med. 27 (5), 887–892.

Cunha, B.A., April 1998. Nosocomial diarrhea. Crit. Care Med. 14 (2), 329–338.

Mulligan, M.E., George, W.I., et al., November 1980. Epidemiological aspects of Clostridium difficile-induced diarrhea and colitis. Am. J. Clin. Nutr. 33 (Suppl. 11), 2533–2538.

Bonten, M.J.M., Weinstein, R.A., 1999. Bird's-eye view of nosocomial infections in medical ICU: Blue bugs, fungi, and device-days. Crit. Care Med. 27 (5), 853–854.

Wilcox., et al., September 1996. Financial burden of hospital-acquired *Clostridium difficile* infection . J. Hosp. Infect. 34 (1), 23–30.

Wilson, K.H., Frederick, J. (1996). Clostridium difficile—*contaminating the environment around a bedpan washing unit in a Veterans Hospital*. Unpublished study.

Collins, B.J., Deverill, C.E., Taylor, L., Oates, K., 1980. A survey of the use and abuse of bedpan macerators. Nurs. Times 76 (9 Suppl. 13), 4–6.

References

Abbott, K., Sago, J., Breen, C., et al., 2001. Families looking back: one year after discussion of withdrawal or withholding of life-sustaining. Crit. Care Med. 29, 197–201.

Administration on Aging, May 31, 1997. Aging into the 21st Century. National Aging Information Center, Bethesda, MD.

Adomat, R., Killingworth, A., 1994. Care of the critically ill patient: the impact of stress on the use of touch in intensive therapy units. J. Adv. Nurs. 19 (5), 912–922.

Ærd, A., Harder, I., 2007. Relatives' experiences in intensive care—finding a place in a world of uncertainty. Intens. Crit. Care Nurs. 23 (3), 170–177.

Agius, R.M., Blenkin, H., Dreary, I.J., et al., 1996. Survey of perceived stress and work demands of consultant doctors. Occup. Environ. Med. 53, 217–224.

AHA Commission on Workforce for Hospitals and Health Systems, 2002. In our Hands: How Hospital Leaders can Build a Thriving Workforce. American Hospital Association, Chicago, IL.

Ahrens, T., 1998. Utilization of intensive care unit technology. New Horiz. 6 (1), 41–51.

Akhtar, S., Weigle, G.M., Cheng, E.Y., et al., 2000. Use of active noise cancellation devices in caregivers in the intensive care unit. Crit. Care Med. 28 (4), 1157–1160.

Allekian, C., 1974. Intrusions of territory and personal space. Psychiatr. Med. 5 (1), 27–39.

Almerud, S., Alapack, R., Fridlund, B., Ekebergh, M., 2007. Of vigilance and invisibility—being a patient in technologically intense environments. Nurs. Crit. Care 12 (3), 151–158.

American Institute of Architects, 2006. Guidelines for Design & Construction of Health Care Facilities. AIA Press, Washington, DC.

Anderson, R., 2000. Pharmacy. In: Hamilton, D.K. (Ed.), ICU 2010: ICU Design for the Future. Center for Innovation in Health Facilities, Houston, pp. 84–90.

Anderson, R., Mackel, D.C., Stoler, B.S., Mallison, G.F., 1982. Carpeting in hospitals: an epidemiological evaluation. J. Clin. Microbiol. 15 (3), 408–415.

Andrew, C.M., 1998. Optimizing the human experience: nursing the families of people who die in intensive care. Intens. Crit. Care Nurs. 14 (2), 59–65.

Appelbaum, S.H., 1997. Socio-technical systems theory: an intervention strategy for organizational development. Manage. Decis. 35 (6), 452–463.

Appleton, J., 1975. The Experience of the Landscape. John Wiley, London.

Arsenault, S., 1997. Assessing the family: the importance of culture. Crit. Care Nurs. 17 (4), 96.

Atkins, E.H., 1996. Sick building syndrome. J. Am. Med. Assoc. 275 (21), 1634–1635.

Atkinson, J.H., Stewart, N., Gardner, D., 1980. The family meeting in critical care settings. J. Traum. 20 (1), 43–46.

Aubin, H., 2005. Superhospital study raises some new questions. Montr. Gaz., July 12, A19.

Azoulay, É., Pochard, F., 2003. Communication with family members of patients dying in the intensive care unit. Curr. Opin. Crit. Care 9, 545–550.

Azoulay, É., Chevret, S., Leleu, G., et al., 2000. Half the families of intensive care unit patients experience inadequate communication with physicians. Crit. Care Med. 28 (8), 3044–3049.

Azoulay, É., Pochard, F., Chevret, S., et al., 2003. Family participation in care to the critically ill: opinions of families and staff. Intensive Care Med. 29, 1498–1504.

Babbie, E., 2002. The Basics of Social Research. Thomson Learning, Belmont, CA.
Babwin, D., 2002. Building boom. Hosp. Health Netw. 76 (3), 48–54.
Baggs, J.G., Ryan, S.A., 1990. ICU nurse-physician collaboration & nursing satisfaction. Nurs. Econ. 8 (6), 386–392.
Baggs, J.G., Schmitt, M.H., Mushlin, A.I., et al., 1997. Nurse-physician collaboration and satisfaction with the decision-making process in three critical care units. Am. J. Crit. Care 6 (5), 393–399.
Baier, S., 1989. Bed Number Ten. Holt, Reinhart & Winston, New York, NY.
Bailey, J.T., Steffen, S.M., Grout, J.W., 1980. The stress audit: identifying the stressors of ICU nursing. J. Nurs. Educ. 19 (6), 15–25.
Bailey, K.D., 1978. Methods of Social Research. Collier-Macmillan, London.
Baker, C., Melby, V., 1996. An investigation into the attitudes and practices of intensive care nurses towards verbal communication with unconscious patients. J. Clin. Nurs. 5 (3), 185–192.
Baker, C.F., 1992. Discomfort to environmental noise: heart rate response to SICU patients. Crit. Care Nurs. Q. 15 (2), 75–90.
Baker, C.F., 1993. Annoyance to ICU noise: a model of patient discomfort. Crit. Care Nurs. Q. 16 (2), 83–90.
Baker, C.F., Nieswiadomy, R.M., Arnold, W.K., 1988. Nursing interventions for children with a parent in the intensive care unit. Heart Lung 17 (4), 441–446.
Baker, C.F., Garvin, C., Kennedy, C., Polivka, B., 1993. The effect of environmental sound and communication on CCU patients' heart rate and blood pressure. Res. Nurs. Health 16, 415–421.
Bakker, R.G., Faoagali, J.L., 1977. The effect of carpet on the number of microbes in the hospital environment. N. Z. Med. J. 85 (581), 88–92.
Baldrige National Quality Program (BNQP), 2002. Health Care Criteria for Performance Excellence. Baldrige National Quality Program, Gaithersburg, MD.
Baldrige National Quality Program (BNQP), 2008. Health Care Criteria for Performance Excellence. Baldrige National Quality Program, Gaithersburg, MD.
Balough, D., Kittinger, E., Benzer, A., Hackl, J.M., 1993. Noise in the ICU. Intens. Care Med. 19 (6), 343–346.
Barach, P., 2008. Strategies to reduce patient harm: understanding the role of design and the built environment. Stud. Health Tech. Inf. 132, 14–22.
Barr, W.J., Bush, H.A., 1998. Four factors of nurse caring in the ICU. Dimens. Crit. Care Nurs. 17 (4), 214–222.
Bates, A.S., Harris, L.E., Tierney, W.M., Wolinsky, F.D., 1998. Dimensions and correlates of physician work satisfaction in a midwestern city. Med. Care 36 (4), 610–617.
Beauchemin, K., Hays, P., 1996. Sunny hospital rooms expedite recovery from severe and refractory depressions. J. Affect. Disord. 40, 49–51.
Beauchemin, K., Hays, P., 1998. Dying in the dark: sunshine, gender, and outcomes in myocardial infarction. J. R. Soc. Med. 91, 49–51.
Beckman, J.S., Simms, L.M., 1992. A Guide to Redesigning Nursing Practice Patterns. Health Administration Press, Ann Arbor, MI.
Behling, D., Guy, J., 1993. Industry profile: healthcare – hazards of the healthcare profession. Occup. Health Saf. 62 (2), 54–58.
Bencko, V., Kapek, J., Vins, O., 2003. Hospital waste treatment and disposal in the general university hospital – current situation and future challenges. Indoor Built Environ. 12, 99–104.
Benson, H., 1975. The Relaxation Response. William Morrow & Company, New York, NY.
Bentley, S., Murphy, F., Dudley, H., 1977. Perceived noise in surgical wards and an intensive care area: an objective analysis. Br. Med. J. 2 (6101), 1503–1506.
Berens, R.J., Weigle, C.G.M., 1995. Noise measurements during high-frequency oscillatory and conventional mechanical ventilation. Clin. Invest. Crit. Care 108 (4), 1026–1029.
Berens, R.J., Weigle, C.G.M., 1996. Cost analysis of ceiling tile replacement for noise abatement. J. Perinatol. 16 (3), 199–201.

Berg, P., Stuttmann, R., Doehn, M., 1997. Larm auf intensivstationen: ein beitrag zur larmreduktion durch modifikation der atemgasbefeuchtung [Noise pollution in intensive care units. Noise reduction by modification of gas humidification]. Der Anaesthesist 46, 856–859.
Bergbom-Engberg, I., Haljamaë, H., 1989. Assessment of patients' experience of discomforts during respiratory therapy. Crit. Care Med. 17 (10), 1068–1071.
Bergbom-Engberg, I., Haljamaë, H., 1993. The communication process with ventilator patients in the ICU as perceived by the nursing staff. Intens. Crit. Care Nurs. 9 (1), 40–47.
Berkman, L., Syme, S., 1979. Social networks, host resistance, and mortality: a nine-year follow up study of Alameda County residents. Am. J. Epidemiol. 109 (2), 186–204.
Berry, L., 2002. Presentation to the Board of the Center for Health Design. San Francisco, August, 2002.
Berry, L., Parker, D., Coile, R., et al., 2004. The business case for better buildings. Front. Health Serv. Manage. 21 (1), 3–24.
Berry, L.L., Seltman, K.D., 2008. Management Lessons from Mayo Clinic: Inside One of the Worlds Most Admired Service Organizations. McGraw-Hill, New York, NY.
Berti, D., 2007. Beliefs and attitudes of intensive care nurses toward visits and open visiting policy. Intens. Care Med. 33 (6), 1060–1065.
Bhungalia, S., Kemp, C., 2002. (Asian) Indian health beliefs and practices related to the end of life. J. Hospice Palliative Nurs. 4 (1), 54–58.
Bijttebier, P., Delva, D., Vanoost, S., et al., 2000. Reliability and validity of the critical care family needs inventory in a Dutch-speaking Belgian sample. Heart Lung 29 (4), 278–286.
Biley, F.C., Millar, B.J., Wilson, A.M., 1992. Issues in intensive care visiting. Intens. Crit. Care Nurs. 9, 75–81.
Birkmeyer, J.D., Birkmeyer, C.M., Wennberg, D.E., Young, M., 2000. Leapfrog Patient Safety Standards: The Potential Benefits of Universal Adoption. Leapfrog Group, Washington, DC.
Blackmore, E., 1996a. A study to investigate the needs of relatives of patients on a cardiothoracic ICU, following routine cardiac surgery. Nurs. Crit. Care 1 (6), 268–277.
Blackmore, E., 1996b. The needs of relatives during the patient's stay in intensive care following routine cardiac surgery. Nurs. Crit. Care 1 (5), 230–236.
Blenkin, H., Deary, I., Sadler, A., Agius, R., 1995. Stress in NHS consultants. Br. Med. J. 310, 534.
Bohrer, T., Koller, M., Neubert, T., et al., 2002. How do general surgery patients experience the intensive care unit? Results of a prospective observational study. Der Chirurg 73 (5), 443–450.
Bonny, H.L., 1978. The Role of Taped Music Program in the Guided Imagery in Music (GIM) Process. Baltimore: ICM Press (per Updike, 1990).
Boocock, M., Weyman, A., McIlory, R., 2006. Bedside safety rails. Ergonomics 49 (7), 631–650.
Bovenzi, M., Collareta, A., 1984. Noise levels in a hospital. Ind. Health 22, 75–82.
Bowker Staff, 2003. Ulrich's Periodicals Directory. R. R. Bowker, New Providence, NJ.
Boyle, D.K., Kochinda, C., 2004. Enhancing collaborative communication of nurse and physician leadership in two intensive care units. J. Nurs. Adm. 34 (2), 60–70.
Brannon, L., Feist, J., 1997. Health Psychology: An Introduction to Behavior and Health. Wadsworth, Belmont, CA.
Brannon, L., Feist, J., 2000. Hea th Psychology: An Introduction to Behavior and Health, sixth ed. Wadsworth, Belmont, CA.
Brannon, P., Brady, A., Gailey, A., 1990. Visitation in the CCU: from rule to contracts. Nurs. Manage. 21 (2), 64.
Breslow, M.J., Rosenfeld, B.A., Doerfler, M., et al., 2004. Effect of a multiple-site intensive care unit telemedicine program on clinical and economic outcomes: an alternative paradigm for intensivist staffing. Crit. Care Med. 32 (1), 31–38.
Breu, C., Dracup, K., 1978. Helping the spouses of critically ill patients. Am. J. Nurs. 78 (1), 50–53.
Brickhill, C.E., 1995. ICU for the '90s. Nurs. Manage. 26 (1), 44–48.
Briggs, D., 1991. Preventing ICU psychosis. Nurs. Times 87 (19), 30–31.

Brummett Jr., B.H., Babyak, M.A., Barefoot, J.C., Bosworth, H.B., Clapp-Channing, N.E., Siegler, I.C., Williams, Jr., R.B., Mark, D.B., 1998. Social support and hostility as predictors of depressive symptoms in cardiac patients one month after hospitalization: a prospective study. Psychosom. Med. 60 (6), 707–713.

Buchanan, R., 1995. Wicked problems in design thinking. In: Margolin, V., Buchanan, R. (Eds.) The Idea of Design. MIT Press, Cambridge, MA, pp. 3–20.

Buddeberg-Fischer, B., Klaghofer, R., Stamm, M., et al., 2008. Work stress and reduced health in young physicians: prospective evidence from Swiss residents. Int. Arch. Occup. Environ. Health 82, 31–38.

Buemi, M., Allegra, A., Grasso, F., Mondio, G., 1995. Noise pollution in an intensive care unit for nephrology and dialysis. Nephrol. Dial. Transpl. 10 (12), 2235–2239.

Buerhaus, P.I., Staiger, D.O., Auerbach, I., 2002. Implications of an aging registered nurse workforce. J. Am. Med. Assoc. 283 (22), 2948–2954.

Buick, P., 2008. Commentary by Paula Buick. Payette Architects, Boston, MA.

Bullock-Loughran, P., 1982. Territoriality in critical care. Focus AACN 9 (5), 19–21.

Burleson, C.W., Burleson, S.W., 1987. Guide to the Texas Medical Center. University of Texas Press, Austin, TX.

Burnett, J., Hamilton, D., 1992. Case study: A room in the garden—Nature as a stimulus to recovery. In: Hamilton, D.K. (Ed.), Unit 2000: Patient Beds for the Future. Watkins Carter Hamilton Architects, Houston, TX.

Burr, G., 1998. Contextualizing critical care family needs through triangulation: An Australian study. Intens. Crit. Care Nurs. 14 (4), 161–169.

Burrington, M., 1999. Can Private Rooms be Justified in Today's Healthcare Market? The Center for Innovation in Health Facilities, Houston, TX.

Busch-Vishniac, I., West, J., Barnhill, C., et al., 2005. Noise levels in Johns Hopkins Hospital. J. Acoust. Soc. Am. 118 (6), 3639–3645.

Buβ, B., Friesdorf, W., 2007. Ergonomics: noise and alarms in health care. In: Carayon, P. (Ed.), Handbook of Human Factors and Ergonomics in Health Care and Patient Safety. Lawrence Erlbaum, Mahwah, NJ.

Byers, J.F., Smyth, K.A., 1997. Effect of a music intervention on noise annoyance, heart rate, and blood pressure in cardiac surgery patients. Am. J. Crit. Care 6 (3), 183–191.

Cadenhead, C. 2005. Square Footage Allocations in ICUs. Paper presented at the Soc. Crit. Care Med. Annual Congress. Phoenix, AZ, January.

Caine, R.M., 1991. Incorporating CARE into caring for families in crisis. AACN Clin. Issues Crit. Care Nurs. 2 (2), 236–241.

Caldwell, T., Weiner, M.F., 1981. Stresses and coping in ICU nursing. Gen. Hosp. Psychiatry 3, 119–127.

Cama, R., 2009. Evidence-Based Healthcare Design. Wiley & Sons, New York.

Campbell, E.S., Fournier, G.M., 1993. Certificate-of-need deregulation and indigent hospital care. J. Health Polit. Policy and Law 18 (4), 905–925.

Caplan, R., 1994. Stress, anxiety, and depression in hospital consultants, general practitioners, and senior health service managers. Br. Med. J. 309, 1261–1263.

Carlisle, C., 2000. Spatial Preferences of the Maternity Patient. Texas A&M University, College Station, TX. Unpublished M.Arch. thesis.

Carpenter, D., 2004. Behind the boom: what's driving hospital construction? Health Facil. Manage. 17 (3), 8–12.

Carpenter, D., 2006. The boom goes on: technology and consumer demands keep driving construction and renovation. Health Facil. Manage. 19 (2), 31–36.

Carpenter, D., March 2008. Hospital construction roars right along. Hosp. Health Netw. 82 (3), 40–44.

Carpenter, D., Hoppszallern, S., 2009. Boom or going bust? Credit and financial crisis make for uncertain hospital construction outlook. Health Facil. Manage. 22 (2), 11–18.

Casscells, S.W., Kurmel, T., Ponataski, E., 2009. Creating healing environments in support of the U.S. Military: a commitment to quality through the built environment. Health Environ. Res. Des. 2 (2), 134–145.

Cassem, N.H., Hackett, T.P., 1975. Stress on the nurse and therapist in the intensive-care unit and the coronary-care unit. Heart Lung 4 (2), 252–259.
Cassidy, R., 2003. Positive prognosis: architects and contractors are teaming with nurses, doctors, and administrators to build hospitals that demonstrably improve patient care. Build. Des. Constr. 44 (2), 32.
Cawood, C., 1993. Nursing units and common staffing problems. In: Hamilton, D.K. (Ed.), UNIT 2000: Patient Beds for the Future. Watkins Carter Hamilton Architects, Bellaire, TX, pp. 102–109.
Cazoria, C., Cravoisy, A., Gibot, S., et al., 2007. Patients' perception of their experience in the intensive care unit. Presse Méd. 36 (2), 211–216.
Centers for Disease Control, . Guidelines for hand hygiene in health-care settings, October 25, 2002. Morb. Mortal. Wkly Rep. 51, RR-16.
Chalfin, D.B., 1999. Assessing the cost-effectiveness of emerging therapies in the ICU. Semin. Respir. Crit. Care Med. 20 (3), 263–270.
Chambrin, M.C., 2001. Alarms in the intensive care unit: how can the number of false alarms be reduced? Crit. Care 5 (4), 184–188.
Chan, H., 2004. Sharing death and dying: advance directives, autonomy and the family. Bioethics 18 (2), 87–103.
Chang, E.M., Bidewell, J.W., Huntington, A.D., et al., 2007. A survey of role stress, coping and health in Australian and New Zealand hospital nurses. Int. J. Nurs. Stud. 44, 1354–1362.
Chang, E.M., Daly, J., Hancock, K.M., et al., 2006. The relationships among workplace stressors, coping methods, demographic characteristics and health in Australian nurses. J. Prof. Nurs. 22 (1), 30–38.
Charbon, G.A., Livingston, H.M., 1949. Planning recovery room for adequate care. Hospitals 23, 35–38.
Chartier, L., Coutu-Wakulczyk, G., 1989. Families in the ICU: their needs and anxiety level. Intens. Care Nurs. 5, 11–18.
Chaudhury, H., Mahmood, A., Valente, M., 2004. Nurses' perceptions of single versus multi-occupancy rooms in acute care environments: an exploratory comparative assessment. Simon Frasier University, Vancouver.
Chaudhury, H., Mahmood, A., Valente, M., 2005. Advantages and disadvantages of single-versus-multiple occupancy rooms in acute care environments. Environ. Behav. 37 (6), 760–786.
Chaudhury, H., Mahmood, A., Valente, M., 2006. Nurses' perception of single-occupancy versus multi-occupancy rooms in acute care environments: an exploratory comparative assessment. Appl. Nurs. Res. 19 (3), 118–125.
Chavez, C.W., Faber, L., 1987. Effect of an education-orientation program on family members who visit their significant other in the intensive care unit. Heart Lung 16 (1), 92–99.
Cherns, A., 1976. The principles of sociotechnical design. Hum. Relat. 29, 783–792.
Chesla, C.A., 1996. Reconciling technologic and family care in critical-care nursing. J. Nurs. Sch. 28 (3), 199–203.
Chesla, C.A., Stannard, D., 1997. Breakdown in the nursing care of families in the ICU. Am. J. Crit. Care 6 (1), 64–71.
Chlan, L., Engeland, W., Anthony, A., Guttormson, J., 2007. Influence of music on the stress response in patients receiving mechanical ventilatory support: a pilot study. Am. J. Crit. Care 16 (2), 141–145.
Christensen, M., 2007. Noise levels in a general intensive care unit: a descriptive study. Brit. Assoc. Crit. Care Nurs. 12 (4), 188–197.
Clarke, S.P., Sloane, D., Aiken, L.H., 2002. Effects of hospital staffing and organizational climate on needlestick injuries to nurses. Am. J. Public Health 92 (7), 1115–1119.
Clipson, C.W., Wehrer, J., 1973. Planning for Cardiac Care. The Health Administration Press 138–139.
Coile, R.C., 1998. Millennium Management: Better, Faster Cheaper Strategies for Managing 21st Century Healthcare Organizations. Health Administration Press, Ann Arbor, MI.
Coile, R.C., 2002. Futurescan 2002: Healthcare Environmental Outlook 2002–2006. Health Administration Press, Chicago, Chicago, IL.
Coile, R.C., 2003. Futurescan 2003: A Forecast of Healthcare Trends 2003–2007. Health Administration Press, Chicago, IL.

Collins, B.J., Deverill, C.E., Taylor, L., Oates, K., 1980. A survey of the use and abuse of bedpan macerators. Nurs. Times 76 (9 Suppl. 13), 4–6.

Conly, J., Johnston, L., 2001. The impact of health care restructuring on nosocomial infections and transmission of antimicrobial resistant organisms. Can. J. Infect. Dis. 12 (5), 271–274.

Conway, J., Johnson, B., Edgman-Levitan, S., et al., 2006. Partnering with Patients and Families to Design a Patient- and Family-Centered Health Care System. Institute for Family-Centered Care, Bethesda, MD.

Coomber, S., Todd, C., Park, G., et al., 2002. Stress in UK intensive care unit doctors. Brit. J. Anaesth. 89, 873–881.

Cooper Marcus, C., 1999. Acute care general hospitals: typology of outdoor spaces. In: Cooper Marcus, C., Barnes, M. (Eds.) Healing Gardens: Therapeutic Benefits and Design Recommendations. John Wiley and Sons, New York.

Cooper Marcus, C., Barnes, M., 1995. Gardens in Health Care Facilities: Uses, Therapeutic Benefits, and Design Considerations. The Center for Health Design, Martinez, CA.

Coron, D., 1994. What if anything does your unit do to reduce noise levels in the ICU? Crit. Care Nurs. 14 (6), 88.

Coughlan, A., 1994. Music therapy in ICU. Nurs. Times 90 (17), 35.

Coulter, M.A., 1989. The needs of family members of patients in intensive care units. Intens. Care Nurs. 5, 4–10.

Coulter, S., January 6, 1997. Redesign not downsize. Online J. Issues Nurs. 2 (1) Manuscript, 5.

Cowdery, A.E., 1994. Fighting for Life: American Military Medicine in World War II. The Free Press, New York, NY.

Cox, A., Groves, P., 1990. Hospitals and Health-Care Facilities. Butterworth Architecture, London.

Coye, M., 2007. How technology will reshape critical care. Hosp. Health Netw. 81 (5), 9.

Craft, M.J., Cohen, M.Z., Titler, M., DeHamer, M., 1993. Experiences in children of critically ill parents: a tie of emotional disruption and need for support. Crit. Care Nurs. Q. 16 (3), 64–71.

Cropp, A.J., Woods, L.A., Raney, D., Bredle, D.L., 1994. Name that tone: the proliferation of alarms in the intensive care unit. Chest 105 (4), 1217–1230.

Curtis, T., 1999. "Climbing the walls" ICU psychosis: Myth or reality? Nurs. Crit. Care 4 (1), 18–21.

Daley, L., 1984. The perceived immediate needs of families with relatives in the intensive care setting. Heart Lung 13 (3), 231–237.

Daly, K., Kleinpell, R.M., Lawinger, S., Casey, G., 1994. The effect of two nursing interventions on families of ICU patients. Clin. Nurs. Res. 3 (4), 414–422.

Darvas, J.A., Hawkins, L.G., 2002. What makes a good intensive care unit: a nursing perspective. Aust. Crit. Care 15 (2), 77–82.

Davies, J.M., 1986. Visiting acutely ill patients: a literature review. Intens. Care Nurs. 2, 163–165.

Davis-Martin, S., 1994. Perceived needs of families of long-term critical care patients: a brief report. Heart Lung 23 (6), 515–518.

Davis-Rollans, C., Cunningham, S.G., 1987. Physiologic responses of coronary care patients to selected music. Heart Lung 16 (4), 370–378.

Dayton, D., 1994. What, if anything, does your unit do to reduce noise levels in the ICU? Crit. Care Nurs. 14 (6), 89.

Dean, B., 1998. Reflections on technology: increasing the science but diminishing the art of nursing. Accid. Emerg. Nurs. 6 (4), 200–206.

Degner, L.F., Gow, C.M., Thompson, L.A., 1991. Critical nursing behaviors in care for the dying. Cancer Nurs. 14 (5), 246–253.

Diaz, J.R., 2000. Brief history of ICU design. In: Hamilton, D.K. (Ed.), ICU 2010 ICU Design for the Future. Center for Innovation in Health Facilities, Houston, pp. 143–152.

Diette, G., Lechtzin, N., Haponik, E., et al., 2003. Distraction therapy with nature sights and sounds reduces pain during flexible bronchoscopy: a complementary approach to routine analgesia. Chest 123 (3), 941–948.

Dilani, A., 2001. Design & Health – The Therapeutic Benefits of Design. Svensk Byggtjänst, Stockholm AB.

Dinh, A., Kemp, C., Rasbridge, L., 2000. Culture and the end of life: vietnamese health beliefs and practices related to the end of life. J. Hospice Palliat. Nurs. 2 (3), 111–117.
Divatia, J., 2006. Delirium in the ICU. Indian J. Crit. Care Med. 10 (4), 215–218.
Dobb, G.J., 1998. Critical care medicine in the Western Pacific region. ANN. Acad. Med. 27 (3), 381–386.
Dochin, Y., Seagull, F.J., 2002. The hostile environment of the intensive care unit. Curr. Opin. Crit. Care 8, 316–320.
Dossey, B., 1993. Guiding critical care nurses on the body-mind-spirit journey. Crit. Care Nurs. 13 (4), 105–111.
Douglas, S., Daly, B.J., Rudy, E.B., et al., 1996. Survival experience of chronically critically ill patients. Nurs. Res. 45 (2), 73–77.
Dracup, K., 1993. Helping patients and families cope. Crit. Care Nurs. 13, 3–9.
Dracup, K., Bryan-Brown, C.W., 1992. An open door policy in ICU. Am. J. Crit. Care 1 (2), 16–18.
Duffy, T.M., Florell, J.M., 1990. Intensive care units. J. Health Care Inter. Des. 2, 167–179.
Dunkel, J., Eisendrath, S., 1983. Families in the intensive care unit: their effect on staff. Heart Lung 12 (3), 258–261.
Dunn, C., Sleep, J., Collett, D., 1995. Sensing an improvement: an experimental study to evaluate the use of aromatherapy, massage, and periods of rest in an intensive care unit. J. Adv. Nurs. 21 (1), 34–40.
Durham, J., Hayward, C., 1996. Facility design strategies for operational restructuring. J. Healthcare Des. VIII, 85–89.
Dyer, O., 2007. Simple precautionary measures can reduce numbers of falls in hospital. Br. Med. J. 334, 447.
Easton, C., Mackenzie, F., 1988. Sensory-perceptual alterations: delirium in the intensive care unit. Heart Lung 17 (3), 229–237.
Edwards, S.C., 1998. An anthropological interpretation of nurses' and patients' perception of the use of space and touch. J. Adv. Nurs. 28 (4), 809–817.
Ehrenfeld, M., 1991. Social correlates of satisfaction and stress among Israeli nurses within intensive coronary care units (I, C.C.U.s). Int. J. Nurs. Stud. 28 (1), 39–45.
Eisendrath, S.J., Dunkel, J., 1979. Psychological issues in intensive care unit staff. Heart Lung 8 (4), 751–758.
Eisendrath, S.J., Link, N., Matthay, M., 1986. Intensive care unit: how stressful for physicians? Crit. Care Med. 14 (2), 95–98.
Elliott, D., 1992. A review of nursing strategies to reduce patient anxiety in coronary care, Part 2. Aust. Crit. Care 5 (3), 10–16.
Elliott, D., 1994. The effects of music and muscle relaxation on patient anxiety in a coronary care unit. Heart Lung 23 (1), 27–35.
Elliott, F.C., 2004. The Birth of the Texas Medical Center: A Personal Account. Texas A&M Press, College Station, TX.
Elpern, E.H., Patterson, P.A., Gloskey, D., Bone, R.C., 1992. Patients' preferences for intensive care. Crit. Care Med. 20 (1), 43–47.
Engli, M., Kirsivali-Farmer, K., 1993. Needs of family members of critically ill patients with and without acute brain injury. J. Neurosci. Nurs. 25 (2), 78–85.
Engström, Å., Söderberg, S., 2004. The experiences of partners of critically ill persons in an intensive care unit. Intensive Crit. Care Nurs. 20, 299–308.
Environmental Protection Agency, 1974. Information on Levels of Environmental Noise Requisite to Protect Health and Welfare with Adequate Margin of Safety (Publication No. 550/9-74-004). U.S. Government Printing Office, Washington, DC Condensed version "Protective Noise Levels" provided on http://www.batnet.com/askmar/Noise/EPA%20Levels/Contents.html.
Environmental Protection Agency (EPA), 1978. Noise: A Health Problem. U.S. EPA, Washington, DC.
Eriksson, T., Bergbom, I., 2007. Visits to intensive care unit patients – frequency, duration and impact on outcome. Nurs. Crit. Care 12 (1), 20–26.
Esberger, K.K., 1982. Staking a claim: steps patients take to establish their own territory, and how to help them. Geriatr. Nurs. 3 (4), 246–247.

Esser, A.H., Chamberlain, A.S., Chapple, E.D., Kline, N.S., 1965. Territoriality of patients on a research ward. In: Wortis, J. (Ed.), Recent Advances in Biological Psychiatry. Plenum Press, New York.
Estabrooks, C.A., 1989. Touch: a nursing strategy in the intensive care unit. Heart Lung 18 (4), 392–401.
Evanoff, B., Wolf, L., Aton, E., et al., 2003. Reduction in injury rates in nursing personnel through introduction of mechanical lifts in the workplace. Am. J. Ind. Med. 44, 451–457.
Evans, G.W., Cohen, S., 1987. Environmental stress. In: Stokols, D., Altman, I. (Eds.) Handbook of Environmental Psychology, vol. 1. John Wiley, New York.
Evans, H.L., Shaffer, M.M., Hughes., et al., 2003. Contact isolation in surgical patients: a barrier to care? Surgery 134 (2), 180–188.
Facility Guidelines Institute, 2006. Guidelines for Design and Construction of Health Care Facilities. American Institute of Architects, Washington, DC.
Fairman, J., Lynaugh, J.E., 1998. Critical Care Nursing: A History. University of Pennsylvania Press, Philadelphia, PA.
Falk, S.A., Woods, N.F., 1973. Hospital noise—levels and potential health hazards. N. Engl. J. Med. 289 (15), 774–781.
Fenner, E., Michels, G., 2003. Scl-90-R scoring of stress after myocardial infarction. Med. Klin. 98 (1), 7–12.
Field, M.J., Grigsby, J., 2002. Telemedicine and remote patient monitoring. JAMA 288 (4), 423–425.
Firth-Cozens, J., 1998. Individual and organizational predictors of depression in general practitioners. Br. J. Gen. Pract. 48, 1647–1651.
Fischer, J.E., Calame, A., Dettling, A.C., et al., 2000. Experience and endocrine stress responses in neonatal and pediatric critical care nurses and physicians. Crit. Care Med. 28 (9), 3281–3288.
Fong, D., 2006. Evidence-based lighting design. Healthc. Des. 6 (5), 50–53.
Forchuk, C., Dorsay, J., 1995. Hildegard Peplau meets family systems nursing: Innovation in theory-based practice. J. Adv. Nurs. 21 (1), 110–115.
Fornes, V.J., Gallego, C.G., Barcelo, O.M., et al., 1994. Causal and emotional factors related to work stress in ICU nursing staff: The importance of accurate measurement. Intensive Crit. Care Nurs. 10 (1), 41–50.
Forrester, D.A., Murphy, P.A., Price, D.M., Monaghan, J.F., 1990. Critical care family needs: Nurse-family member confederate pairs. Heart Lung 19, 655–661.
Foss, K.R., Tenholder, M.F., 1993. Expectations and needs of persons with family members in an intensive care unit as opposed to a general ward. South. Med. J. 86 (4), 380–384.
Fournier, M., 1995. L'amenagement des aires d'attente dans les unites de soins infensifs pur adultes [The design of family waiting rooms in intensive care units for adults]. Unpublished master's thesis, Laval University, Quebec, Canada.
Frampton, S., Gilpin, L., Charmel, P., 2003. Putting Patients First: Designing and Practicing Patient-Centered Care. Jossey-Bass, New York.
Franklin, J., Doelp, A., 1980. Shocktrauma. St. Martin's Press, New York, NY.
Freichels, T.A., 1991. Needs of family members of patients in the intensive care unit over time. Crit. Care Nurs. Q. 14 (3), 16–29.
Freiherr von Manteuffel, K., 1998. An introduction to grounded theory. Retrieved December 24, 2001 from ,http://www.geocities.com/ResearchTriangle/Lab/1491/gnm-gtm.en.html/>.
Freitas, K., Kimura, M., Ferreira, K., 2007. Family members' needs at intensive care units: Comparative analysis between a public and private hospital. Rev. Latinoam. Enferm. 15 (1), 84–92.
Fridh, I., Forsberg, A., Bergbom, I., 2007. Family presence and environmental factors at the time of a patient's death in an ICU. Acta Anaesthesiol. Scand. 51, 395–401.
Fumagalli, S., Boncinelli, L., Lo Nostro, A., et al., 2006. Reduced cardiocirculatory complications with unrestrictive visiting policy in an intensive care unit: results from a pilot, randomized trial. Circulation 113 (7), 946–952.
Furukawa, M.M., 1996. Meeting the needs of the dying patient's family. Crit. Care Nurs. 16 (1), 51–57.
Gaba, D.M., 2004. The future vision of simulation in health care. Qual. Saf. Health Care 13 (Suppl 1), i2–i10.

Gabor, J., Cooper, A., Hanly, P., 2001. Sleep disruption in the intensive care unit. Curr. Opin. Crit. Care 7 (1), 21–27.
Gallant, D., Lanning, K., 2001. Streamlining Patient Care Processes through Flexible Room and Equipment Design. Crit. Care Nurs. Q. 24 (3), 59–76.
Garrouste-Orgeas, M., Philippart, F., Timsit, J.F., et al., 2008. Perception of a 24-hour visiting policy in the intensive care unit. Crit. Care Med. 36 (1), 30–35.
Gast, P., Baker, C., 1989. The CCU patient: anxiety and annoyance to noise. Crit. Care Nurs. Q. 12 (3), 39–54.
Gaw-Ens, B., 1994. Informational support for families immediately after CABG surgery. Crit. Care Nurs. 14 (1), 41–50.
Gearon, C.J., 2002. Planetree: 25 years older. H&HN: Hosp. Health Netw. 76 (10), 41.
Gelling, L., 1999. Causes of ICU psychosis: The environmental factors. Nurs. Crit. Care 4 (1), 22–26.
Gibbons, C., Geller, S., Glatz, E., 1998. Biomedical equipment in the neonatal intensive care unit: Is it a stressor? J. Prenat. Neonatal Nurs. 12 (3), 67–73.
Gieras, I., Ebben, S., 2007. Advancing patient safety through human factors engineering. Med. Des. Technol. 11 (2), 30.
Gifford, R., 1987. Environmental Psychology: Principles and Practice. Allyn and Bacon, Boston.
Girard, T.D., Shintani, A.K., Jackson, J.C., et al., 2007. Risk factors for post-traumatic stress disorder symptoms following critical illness requiring mechanical ventilation: a prospective cohort study. Crit. Care 11, R28.
Glaser, B.G., 1978. Theoretical Sensitivity. Sociology Press, Mill Valley, CA.
Glaser, B.G., Strauss, A.L., 1967. The Discovery of Grounded Theory: Strategies for Qualitative Research. Aldine, Chicago, IL.
Golden, R., Gaynes, B., Ekstrom, D., et al., 2005. The efficacy of light therapy in the treatment of mood disorders: a review and meta-analysis of the evidence. Am. J. Psychiatry 162, 656–662.
Good, M., 1995. A comparison of the effects of jaw relaxation and music on postoperative pain. Nurs. Res. 44 (1), 52–57.
Goodfellow, A., Varnam, R., Rees, D., Shelly, M.P., 1997. Staff stress on the intensive care unit: a comparison of doctors and nurses. Anaesthesia 52, 1037–1041.
Gournic, G.L., 1982. Families' needs and perceptions of the coronary care environment. In: Noble, A. (Ed.), The ICU Environment. Reston Publishing, Reston, VA.
Granger, C.E., George, C., Shelly, M.P., 1995. The management of bereavement on intensive care units. Intensive Care Med. 21, 429–436.
Gurses, A., Carayon, P., 2007. Performance obstacles of intensive care nurses. Nurs. Res. 56 (3), 185–194.
Guzzetta, C.E., 1988. Unitary person assessment tool: easing problems with nursing diagnoses. Focus Crit. Care 15 (2), 12–24.
Guzzetta, C.E., 1989. Effects of relaxation and music therapy on patients in a coronary care unit with presumptive acute myocardial infarction. Heart Lung 18, 609–616.
Guzzanti, E., 2006. The hospital of the future: origins, evolution and perspectives. Recenti Prog. Med. 97 (11), 594–603.
Haas, J.S., Cook, E.F., Puopolo, A.L., et al., 2002. Is the professional satisfaction of general internists associated with patient satisfaction? J. Gen. Intern. Med. 15, 122–128.
Hackman, R.J., Oldham, G.R., 1980. Work Redesign. Addison-Wesley, Reading, MA.
Hafsteindottir, T.B., 1996. Patients' experiences of communication during the respirator treatment period. Intensive Crit. Care Nurs. 12 (5), 261–271.
Hagland, M.R., 1995. Nurse-patient communication in intensive care: a low priority. Intensive Crit. Care Nurs. 11 (2), 111–115.
Hairon, N., 2007. Using a range of interventions to prevent falls in hospital. Nurs. Times 103 (9), 23–24.
Hall, D.S., 1997. Communication: something to point to. Crit. Care Nurs. 17 (5), 104.
Hall, E.T., 1963. The Hidden Dimension. Doubleday, New York.
Hall-Lord, M.L., Larsson, G., Steen, B., 1998. Pain and distress among elderly intensive care unit patients: Comparison of patients' experiences and nurses' assessments. Heart Lung 27 (2), 123–132.

Halm, M.A., 1990. Effects of support groups on anxiety of family members during critical illness. Heart Lung 19 (1), 62–71.
Halm, M.A., 1991. Strategies for developing a family support group. Focus Crit. Care 18 (6), 444–459.
Halm, M.A., Alpen, M.A., 1993. The impact of technology on patients and families. Nurs. Clin. North Am. 28 (2), 443–457.
Halm, M.A., Titler, M.G., 1990. A visitation in the CCU: from "rules" to contracts. Nurs. Manage. 5, 25–37.
Halm, M.A., Titler, M.G., Kleiber, C., et al., 1993. Behavioral responses of family members during critical illness. Clin. Nurse Res. 2 (4), 414–437.
Halpern, N.A., Pastores, S.M., Price, J.B., Alicea, M., 1999. Hearing loss in critical care: An unappreciated phenomenon. Crit. Care Med. 27 (1), 211–219.
Hamill-Ruth, R.J., Ruth, R.A., Googer, K., et al., 1998. Use of otoacoustic emissions to screen for hearing loss in critically ill patients. Audiology 37, 344–352.
Hamilton, D.K., 1999. Design for flexibility in critical care. New Horizons, J. Soc. Crit. Care Med. 7 (2), 205–217.
Hamilton, D.K. (Ed.), 2000. ICU 2010: ICU Design for the Future, A Critical Care Design Symposium. Center for Innovation in Health Facilties, Houston, TX.
Hamilton, D.K., 2003a. The four levels of evidence-based practice. Healthc. Des. 3 (11), 18–26.
Hamilton, D.K., 2003b. Design of Patient Units and Organizational Performance: Two Case Studies. Unpublished master's thesis, Pepperdine University, Malibu.
Hamilton, D.K., 2004a. A better building. Hosp. Health Netw. Online site: www.hospitalconnect.com/hhn-mag, March 12.
Hamilton, D.K., 2004b. Certification for evidence-based projects: a proposal for comparing evidence-based healthcare designs. Healthc. Des. 4 (5), 38–40.
Hamilton, D.K., 2004c. Hypothesis and measurement: essential steps for evidence-based design. Healthc. Des. 4 (3), 43–46.
Hamilton, D.K., 2005a. A progress report on certification for evidence-based design. Healthc. Des. 5 (9), 12–13.
Hamilton, D.K., 2005b. Evidence-based design and the art of healing. In: Wagenaar, C. (Ed.), The Architecture of Hospitals. NAI Publications, Rotterdam.
Hamilton, D.K., 2006. Evidence-based design supports evidence-based medicine in the ICU. ICU Manage. J. (Belgium) 6 (3), 31.
Hamilton, D.K., Orr, R.D., 2006. Cultural transformation and design. In: Marberry, S. (Ed.), Improving Healthcare with Better Building Design. Health Administration Press, Chicago, IL, pp. 145–160.
Hamilton, D.K., Watkins, D.H., 2009. Evidence-Based Design for Multiple Building Types. Wiley & Sons, New York, NY.
Hamilton, D.K., Orr, R.D., Raboin, W.E., 2008. Organizational transformation: a model for joint optimization of culture change and evidence-based design. Health Environ. Res. Des. 1 (3), 40–60.
Hamner, H.B., 1990. Visitation policies in the ICU: a time for change. Crit. Care Nurs. 10 (1), 48–53.
Hansell, H.N., 1984. The behavioral effects of noise on man: the patient with "intensive care unit psychosis." Heart Lung 13 (1), 59–65.
Hanson, C.W., Aranda, M., 1999. Impact of intensivists and ICU teams on patient outcomes. J. Intensive Care Med. 14 (6), 254–261.
Hanson, R.B., Sayers, B., 1995. Work and Role Redesign: Tools and Techniques for Health Care Setting. American Hospital Publishing, Chicago, IL.
Haraden, C., Resar, R., 2004. Patient flow in hospitals: Understanding and controlling it better. Front. Health Serv. Manage. 20 (4), 3–15.
Hardicre, J., 2003. Meeting the needs of families of patients in intensive care units. Nurs. Times 99 (27), 26–27.
Hargest, T.S., 1978. Quiet please! for patients' sake. Hospitals 52 (14), 115.
Harvey, A.M., 1974. Neurosurgical genius – walter edward dandy. Johns Hopkins Med. J. 135, 358–368.

Harvey, C., Dixon, M., Padberg, N., 1995. Support group for families of trauma patients: a unique approach. Crit. Care Nurs. 15 (4), 59–63.

Harvey, M.A., Ninos, N.P., Adler, D.C., et al., 1993. Results of the consensus conference on fostering more human critical care: Creating a healing environment. AACN Clin. Issues Crit. Care Nurs. 4 (3), 484–549.

Harvey, M., 2000. Nursing roles and staffing models. In: Hamilton, K. (Ed.), ICU 2010: ICU Design for the Future. Center for Innovation in Health Facilities, Houston, pp. 6–18.

Hay, D., Oken, D., 1972. The psychological stresses of intensive care unit nursing. Psychosom. Med. 34 (2), 109–118.

Heitz, L., Symreng, T., Scamman, F.L., 1992. Effect of music therapy in the postanesthesia care unit: A nursing intervention. J. Post Anesth. Nurs. 7 (1), 22–31.

Helton, M.C., 1980. The correlation between sleep and sleep deprivation and the ICU syndrome. Heart Lung 9 (3), 464–468.

Hendee, W.R., 2002. Oncologic Imaging, second ed. WB Saunders, Philadelphia, PA.

Hendrich, A., 2003. Case study: the impact of acuity adaptable rooms on future designs, bottlenecks and hospital capacity. Impact Conference, Atlanta, GA.

Hendrich, A., 2006. Inpatient falls: lessons from the field. Patient Saf. Qual. Healthc. From http://www.psqh.com/mayjun06/falls.html. May/June.

Hendrich, A., Bender, P.S., Nyhuis, A., 2003. Validation of the hendrich II fall risk model: a large concurrent case/control study of hospitalized patients. Appl. Nurs. Res. 16 (1), 9–21.

Hendrich, A., Fay, J., Sorrells, A.K., 2004. Effects of acuity-adaptable rooms on flow of patients and delivery of care. Am. J. Crit. Care 13 (1).

Hendrich, A., Nyhuis, A., Kippenbrock, T., Soja, M.E., 1995. Hospital falls: development of a predictive model for clinical practice. Appl. Nurs. Res. 8 (3), 129–139.

Henneman, E.A., Cardin, S., 1992. Need for information. Interventions for practice. Crit. Care Nurs. Clin. North Am. 4 (4), 615–621.

Henneman, E.A., McKenzie, J.G., Dewa, C.S., 1992. An evaluation of interventions for meeting the information needs of families of critically ill patients. Am. J. Crit. Care 1 (3), 85–93.

Henry, L.L., 1995. Music therapy: A nursing intervention for the control of pain and anxiety in the ICU: A review of the research literature. Dimens. Crit. Care Nurs. 14 (6), 295–304.

Hepworth, J., Hendrickson, S., Lopez, J., 1994. Time series analysis of psychological response during ICU visitation. West. J. Nurs. Res. 16, 704–717.

Heulat, B.J., 2003. Healing Environments: Design for Body, Mind & Spirit. Medezyn, Alexandria, VA.

Hewitt, J., 2002. Psycho-affective disorder in intensive care units: a review. J. Clin. Nurs. 11 (5), 575–584.

Heyland, D.K., Rocker, G.M., O'Callaghan., et al., 2003. Dying in the ICU: perspective of family members. Chest 124, 392–397.

Hickey, M., 1990. What are the needs of families of critically ill patients? A review of the literature since 1976. Heart Lung 19 (4), 401–415.

Hickey, M., Lewandowski, M., 1988. Critical care nurses' role with families: a descriptive study. Heart Lung 17 (6 pt. 1), 670–676.

Hignett, S., 2007. Physical ergonomics in healthcare. Chapter 20. In: Carayon, P. (Ed.), Handbook of human factors and ergonomics in healthcare and patient safety. Lawrence Erlbaum Associates Inc, New Jersey, pp. 309–321.

Hilberman, M., 1975. The evolution of intensive care units. Crit. Care Med. 3 (4), 159–165.

Hilton, B., 1976. Quantity and quality of patients' sleep and sleep-disturbing factors in a respiratory intensive care unit. J. Adv. Nurs. 1 (6), 453–468.

Hilton, B., 1985. Noise in acute patient care areas. Res. Nurse Health 8 (3), 283–291.

Hilton, B., 1987. The hospital racket: How noisy is your unit? Am. J. Nurs. 87 (1), 59–61.

Hoffman, H., Patterson, D., Carrougher, G., 2000. Use of virtual reality for adjunctive treatment of adult burn pain during physical therapy: a controlled study. Clin. J. Pain 16, 244–250.

Hollick, M., 2004. Sunlight and vitamin D for bone health and prevention of autoimmune diseases, cancers, and cardiovascular disease. Am. J. Clin. Nutr. 80 (6), 1678S–1688S.

Hopkins, A.G., 1994. The trauma nurse's role with families in crisis. Crit. Care Nurs. 14, 35–41.

Hopping, B.L., Sickbert, S.F., Ruth, J., 1992. A study of factors associated with CCU visiting policies. Crit. Care Nurs. 12, 8–15.

Horsburgh, C.R., 1997. Current issues: hospital design qualities to facilitate healing. J. Health Care Des. 9, 89–92.

Horton, S., 1995. Support for bereaved relatives in ICU. Prof. Nurse 10 (9), 568–570.

Hudak, C.M., Gallo, B.M., Morton, P.G. (Eds.), 1998. Critical Care Nursing: A Holistic Approach. Lippincott, Philadelphia.

Hudson, G.R., 1993. Empathy and technology in the coronary care unit. Intensive Crit. Care Nurs. 9 (1), 55–61.

Hudson, P., 2003. Applying the lessons of high risk industries to health care. Qual. Saf. Health Care 12 (Suppl 1), 7i–12i.

Humphreys, H., Johnson, E.M., Warnock, D.W., 1991. An outbreak of aspergillosis in a general ITU. J. Hosp. Infect. 18 (3), 167–177.

Hupcey, J.E., 1998. Establishing the nurse-family relationship in the intensive care unit. West. J. Nurs. Res. 20 (2), 180–194.

Hupcey, J.E., 1999. Looking out for the patient and ourselves—the process of family integration into the ICU. J. Clin. Nurs. 8, 253–262.

Institute of Medicine, 2000. To Err is Human: Building a Safer Health System. National Academy Press, Washington, DC.

Institute of Medicine, 2001. Crossing the Quality Chasm: A New Health System for the 21st Century. National Academy Press, Washington, DC.

Intensive Care Society, 2003. Evolution of Intensive Care in the UK. Intensive Care Society, London.

Ireland, S.R., Warren, Y., Herringer, L., 1992. Anxiety and color saturation preference. Percept. Mot. Skills 75 (2), 545–546.

Jacono, J., Hicks, G., Antonioni, C., et al., 1990. Comparison of perceived needs of family members between registered nurses and family members of critically ill patients in intensive care and neonatal intensive care units. Heart Lung 19 (1), 68–72.

James, W.P., Tatton-Brown, W., 1986. Hospitals: Design and Development. The Architectural Press, London.

Jarvis, P., 1999. The Practitioner-Researcher: Developing Theory from Practice. Jossey-Bass, San Francisco, CA.

Jastremski, C.A., 1998. Caring for the families of those who die in the critical care unit. Crit. Care Med. 26 (7), 1150–1151.

Johansson, I., Fridlund, B., Hildingh, C., 2004. Coping strategies of relatives when an adult next-of-kin is recovering at home following critical illness. Intensive Crit. Care Nurs. 20, 281–291.

Johnson, A.P., Pearson, A., Duckworth, G., 2005. Surveillance and epidemiology of MRSA bacteraemia in the UK. J. Antimicrob. Chemother. 56 (3), 455–462.

Johnson, D., Wilson, M., Cavanaugh, B., et al., 1998. Measuring the ability to meet family needs in an intensive care unit. Crit. Care Med. 26 (2), 266–271.

Johnson, J.J., Frank, D.I., 1995. Effectiveness of a telephone intervention in reducing anxiety of families of patients in an intensive care unit. Appl. Nurs. Res. 8 (1), 42–43.

Johnson, M.N., 1979. Anxiety/stress and the effects on disclosure between nurses and patients. Adv. Nurs. Sci. 1 (4), 1–20.

Johnston, K., Rohaly-Davis, J., 1996. An introduction to music therapy: helping the oncology patient in the ICU. Crit. Care Nurse Q. 18 (4), 54–60.

Joint Commission on Accreditation of Healthcare Organizations, 1994. Framework for Improving Performance: From Principles to Practice. JCAHO, Oakbrook Terrace, IL.

Joint Commission on Accreditation of Healthcare Organizations, 2004. Improving Care in the ICU. JCAHO, Oakbrook Terrace, IL.

Jones, B.R., 2006. A smart solution to the worker shortage. Hosp. Health Netw. From http://www.hhnmag.com/hhnmag_app/jsp/articledisplay.jsp?dcrpath 5 HHNMAG/PubsNewsArticle/data/060131HHN_Online_Jones&domain 5 HHNMAG.

Jones, C., Skirrow, P., Griffiths, R., et al., 2004. Post-traumatic stress disorder-related symptoms in relatives of patients following intensive care. Intensive Care Med. 30, 456–460.

Joseph, A., Fritz, L., 2006. Ceiling lifts reduce patient handling injuries. Healthc. Des. 6, 10–13.

Joseph, A., Hamilton, D.K., 2008. The pebble projects: coordinated evidence-based case studies. Build. Res. Inf. 36 (2), 129–145.

Joseph, A., Rashid, M., 2007. The architecture of safety. Curr. Opin. Crit. Care 13, 714–719.

Justic, M., 2000. Does ICU psychosis really exist? Crit. Care Nurs. 20 (3), 28–37.

Kahn, D.M., Cook, T.E., Carlisle, C.C., et al., 1998. Identification and modification of environmental noise in an ICU setting. Chest 114 (2), 535–540.

Kam, P.C.A., Kam, A.C., Thompson, J.F., 1994. Noise pollution in the anaesthetic and intensive care environment. Anaesthesia 49 (11), 982–986.

Kaplan, R., Kaplan, S., 1989. The Experience of Nature: A Psychological Perspective. Cambridge Press, New York.

Kelly, K., 1995. Health Care Work Redesign. Series on Nursing Administration, 7. Sage Publications, Thousand Oaks, CA.

Kemp, C., 2000. Culture and the end of life: series introduction. J. Hosp. Palliat. Nurs. 2 (3), 109–110.

Kemp, C., 2001. Culture and the end of life: Hispanic cultures. J. Hosp. Palliat. Nurs. 3 (1), 29–34.

Kemp, C., Rasrbridge, L.A., 2001. Culture and the end of life: East African Cultures: Part I. Somali. J. Hosp. Palliat. Nurs. 3 (2), 59–61.

Keovilay, L., Rasbridge, L., Kemp, C., 2000. Culture and the end of life: Cambodian and Laotian health beliefs and practices related to the end of life. J. Hosp. Palliat. Nurs. 2 (4), 143–151.

Kerr, J.A., 1982. An overview of theory and research related to space use in hospitals. West. J. Nurs. Res. 4 (4), 395–405.

Kim, D., 2001. Specialized Knowledge Roles and the Professional Status of Healthcare Architects, Unpublished doctoral dissertation, Texas A&M University, College Station, TX.

Kirchoff, K.T., Pugh, E., Calame, R.M., Reynolds, N., 1993. Nurses' beliefs and attitudes toward visiting in adult critical care settings. Am. J. Crit. Care 2 (3), 238–245.

Kjerulff, K.H., Pillar, B., Mills, M.E., Lanigan, J., 1992. Technology anxiety as a potential mediating factor in response to medical technology. J. Med. Syst. 16 (1), 7–13.

Kleiber, C., Halm, M., Titler, M., et al., 1994. Emotional responses of family members during a critical care hospitalization. Am. J. Crit. Care 3 (1), 70–76.

Kleinpell, R., 2008. Visiting hours in intensive care unit: more evidence that open visitation is beneficial. Crit. Care Med. 36 (1), 334–335.

Kleinpell, R.M., Powers, M., 1992. Needs of family members of intensive care unit patients. Appl. Nurs. Res. 5 (91), 2–8.

Kleman, M., Bickert, A., Karpinski, A., et al., 1993. Physiologic responses of coronary care patients to visiting. J. Cardiovasc. Nurs. 7 (3), 52–62.

Knapp, C., 2006. Bronson Methodist Hospital: journey to excellence in quality and safety. Jt. Comm. J. Qual. Patient. Saf. 32 (10), 556–563.

Knauth, P., Hornberger, S., 2003. Preventive and compensatory measures for shift workers. Occup. Med. 53 (2), 109–116.

Knutsson, S., 2007. Custodians' viewpoints and experiences from their child's visit to an ill or injured nearest being cared for at an adult intensive care unit. J. Clin. Nurs. 16 (2), 362–371.

Knutsson, S., Bergbom, I., 2007. Nurses' and physicians' view points regarding children visiting/not visiting adult ICUs. Nurs. Crit. Care 12 (2), 6473.

Kohn, L.T., Corrigan, J.M., Donaldson, M.S., 2000. To Err is Human: Building a Safer Health System. National Academy Press, Washington, DC.

Konrad, T.R., Williams, E.S., Linzer, M., et al., 1999. Measuring physician job satisfaction in a changing workplace and a challenging environment. Med. Care 37 (11), 1174–1182.

Kouri, D., 2002. Is Regionalization Working? Can. Health Care Manag.

Kornecki, L., 1994. An Rx for hospital safety: watch your back. Saf. Health 149, 56–60.

Krizner, K., 2008. Clinicians improve patient outcomes with remote communication. Manag. Healthc. Exec. 18 (1), 21.

Krumberger, J.M., 1996. Culture—an inextricable component of care. Crit. Care Nurs. 16 (3), 118.

Laguardia, C., Katz, B., Katz, L.S. (Eds.), 2003. Magazines for Libraries. R. R. Bowker, New Providence, NJ.

Lam, P., Beaulieu, M., 2004. Experiences of families in the neurological ICU: a "Bedside Phenomenon". J. Neurosci. Nurs. 36 (3), 142–155.

Landon, B.E., Reschovsky, J., Blumenthal, D., 2003. Changes in career satisfaction among primary care and specialist physicians, 1997–2001. J. Am. Med. Assoc. 289, 442–449.

Langley, G.J., Nolan, K.M., Nolan, T.W., et al., 1996. The Improvement Guide: A Practical Approach to Enhancing Organizational Performance. Jossey-Bass, San Francisco, CA.

Larson, J.A., 1997. Healthcare Redesign Tools and Techniques. Quality Resources, New York, NY.

Lasater, K.L., Grisanti, D.J., 1975. Postcardiotomy psychosis: indications and interventions. Heart Lung 4 (5), 724–729.

Latour, J., 2007. Families in the ICU: do we truly consider their needs, experiences and satisfaction? Nurs. Crit. Care 12 (4), 173–174.

Latour-Perez, J., Gutierrez-Vicen, T., Reig-Ferrer, A., Ribera-Domene, D., 1994. Construction and validation of an index of psychosocial adjustment in intensive care without interviewing the patient. Med. Clin. 102 (8), 290–293.

Lave, J.R., Lave, L.B., 1974. The Hospital Construction Act: An Evaluation of the Hill-Burton Program, 1948–1973. American Enterprise Institute for Public Policy Research, Washington, DC.

Lawton, M.P., Nahemow, L., 1973. Ecology and the ageing process. In: Eisdorfer, C., Lawton, M. (Eds.) The Psychology of Adult Development and Aging. American Psychological Association, Washington, DC, pp.

Lazarus, R.S., 1993. From psychological stress to the emotions: a history of changing outlooks. Annu. Rev. Psychol. 44, 1–21.

Lazure, L.L.A., 1997. Strategies to increase patient control of visiting. Dimens. Crit. Care Nurs. 16 (1), 11–19.

Lazure, L.L., Baun, M.M., 1995. Increasing patient control of family visiting in the coronary care unit. Am. J. Crit. Care 4 (2), 157–164.

Lee, F., 2004. If Disney Ran your Hospital: 9½ Things you Would do Differently. Second River Healthcare Press, Bozeman, MT.

Lee, B.K., Ellenbecker, M.J., Moure-Ersaso, R., 2003. Alternatives for treatment and disposal cost reduction of regulated medical wastes. Waste Manag. 24 (2), 143–151.

Lee, D., Chan, A., Wong, S., et al., 2004. Can visual distraction decrease the dose of patient controlled sedation required during colonoscopy? A prospective randomized controlled trial. Endoscopy 36, 197–201.

Lee, L.Y., Lau, Y.L., 2003. Immediate needs of adult family members of adult intensive care patients in Hong Kong. J. Clin. Nurs. 12, 490–500.

Lee, M., 2007. Visiting hours policies in New England intensive care units: strategies for improvement. Crit. Care Med. 35 (2), 497–501.

Leong, J., Sirio, C., Rotondi, A.J., 2005. eICU program favorably affects clinical and economic outcomes. Crit. Care 9 (5), E22.

Leske, J.S., 1986. Needs of relatives of critically ill patients: a follow up. Heart Lung 15 (2), 189–193.

Leske, J.S., 1992a. Comparison ratings of needs? importance after critical illness from family members with varied demographic characteristics. Crit. Care Nurs. Clin. North. Am. 4 (4), 607–613.

Leske, J.S., 1992b. Needs of adult family members after critical illness. Crit. Care Nurs. Clin. North. Am. 4 (4), 587–596.

Leske, J.S., 1998. Treatment for family members in crisis after critical injury. AACN Clin. Issues 9 (1), 129–139.
Levetown, M., 1998. Palliative care in the intensive care unit. New Horiz. 6, 383–397.
Levin, D.J., 2008. Defining evidence-based design. Healthc. Des. 8 (8), 8.
Levy, M., 2007. A view from the other side. Crit. Care Med. 35 (2), 603–604.
Lewandowski, L.A., 1992. Needs of children during the critical illness of a parent or sibling. Crit. Care Nurs. Clin. North. Am. 4 (4), 573–585.
Lilly, M., 2008. A personal reflection: family survival in the pediatric intensive care unit. Dimens. Crit. Care Nurs. 27 (4), 157–159.
Lincoln, Y.S., Guba, E.G., 1985. Naturalistic Inquiry. Sage Publications, Newbury, CA.
Lipowski, J., 1990. Delirium: Acute Confusional States. Oxford University Press, New York, NY.
Llenore, E., Ogle, K.R., 1999. Nurse-patient communication in the intensive care unit: a review of the literature. Aust. Crit. Care 12 (4), 142–145.
Long, C.O., Greeneich, D.S., 1994. Family satisfaction techniques: meeting family expectations. Dimens. Crit. Care Nurs. 13 (2), 104–111.
Lopez-Fagin, L., 1995. Critical care family needs inventory. A cognitive research utilization approach. Crit. Care Nurs. 15 (4), 21–26.
Lovern, E., 2002. Wave of the future: leapfrog's release of hospital information sets off swell of activity. Mod. Healthc. 32 (3), 4–6.
Lu, H., While, A.E., Barriball, K., 2005. Job satisfaction among nurses: a literature review. Int. J. Nurs. Stud. 42 (2), 211–227.
Lu, H., While, A.E., Barriball, K.L., 2007. Job satisfaction and its related factors: a questionnaire survey of hospital nurses in Mainland China. Int. J. Nurs. Stud. 44, 574–588.
Lumsdon, K., 1993. Baby boomers grow up. Hosp. Health Netw./AHA 67 (18).
Lusk, B., Lash, A.A., 2005. The stress response, psychoneuroimmunology, and stress among ICU patients. Dimens. Crit. Care Nurs. 24 (1), 25–31.
Lynn-McHale, D.J., Bellinger, A., 1988. Needs? satisfaction levels of family members of critical care patients and accuracy of nurses' perceptions. Heart Lung 17, 447–453.
Madigan, C.K., Donaghue, D.D., Carpenter, H.V., 1999. Development of a family liaison model during operative procedures. MCN. Am. J. Matern. Child Nurs. 24 (4), 185–189.
Malacrida, R., Bettelini, C.M., Degrate, A., et al., 1998. Reasons for dissatisfaction: a survey of relatives of intensive care patients who died. Crit. Care Med. 26 (7), 1187–1193.
Malenbaum, S., Keefe, F.J., de C. Williams, A.C., et al., 2008. Pain in its environmental context: implications for designing environments to enhance pain control. Pain 134, 241–244.
Malkin, J., 1992. Hospital Interior Architecture: Creating Healing Environments for Special Patient Populations. Van Nostrand Reinhart, New York, NY.
Malkin, J., 2000. Healing environments and family amenities. In: Hamilton, D.K. (Ed.), ICU 2010. Center for Innovation in Health Facilities, Houston, TX pp. .
Malkin, J., 2003. The business case for creating a healing environment. Hospital Engineering & Facilities Management, The Center for Health Design.
Malkin, J., 2008. A Visual Reference for Evidence-Based Design. The Center for Health Design, Concord, CA.
Malone, M., 2002a. Presentation to the Board of the Center for Health Design, Phoenix, AZ, April, 2002.
Malone, M., November 9, 2002b. Personal Communication about Press, Ganey Survey Methods, Houston.
Maloney, J.P., 1982. Job stress and its consequences on a group of intensive care and non–intensive care nurses. Adv. Nurs. Sci. 4 (2), 31–42.
Mann, R.E., 1992. Preserving humanity in an age of technology. Intensive Crit. Care Nurs. 8 (1), 54–59.
MAPEI, 2006. The Basics of Green Building and LEED. MAPEI Corporation.
Marberry, S., 1996. Most use research information. Aesclepius. 5 (1), 2.
Marberry, S., Zagon, L., 1995. The Power of Color. John Wiley, New York, NY.

Marfell, J.A., Garcia, J.S., 1995. Contracted visiting hours in the coronary care unit: a patient-centered quality improvement project. Nurs. Clin. North. Am. 30 (1), 87–96.
Massura, E.K., 1982. The view from both sides of intensive care. Focus AACN 9 (4), 3–5.
Mather, H.G., Morgan, D.C., Pearson, N.G., et al., 1976. Myocardial infarction: a comparison between home and hospital care for patients. Br. Med. J. 1 (6015), 925–929.
Mattke, S., Matorell, F., 2005. Recruitment and retention of a High-Quality Healthcare Workforce. Rand Health, 1–14.
McCaffrey, R., 2008. Music listening: its effects in creating a healing environment. J. Psychosoc. Nurs. Ment. Health. Serv. 46 (10), 39–44.
McClement, S.E., Degner, L.F., 1995. Expert nursing behaviors in care of the dying adult in the intensive care unit. Heart Lung 24 (5), 408–419.
McGhee, K., Dziuban, C., 1993. Visual preferences of preschool children for abstract and realistic paintings. Percept. Mot. Skills. 76 (1), 155–158.
McGuire, B.E., Basten, C.J., Ryan, C.J., Gallagher, J., 2000. Intensive care unit syndrome: a dangerous misnomer. Arch. Intern. Med. 160 (7), 906–909.
McKahan, D., Hamilton, D.K., 2006. How the ICONS have fared. American Society of Healthcare Engineering Planning, Design, and Construction Conference. San Diego, February 27, 2006.
McKinney, A.A., Deeny, P., 2002. Leaving the intensive care unit: a phenomenological study of the patient's experience. Intensive Crit. Care Nurs. 18 (6), 320–331.
McLaughlin, A., McLaughlin, B., Elliott, J., Campalani, G., 1996. Noise levels in a cardiac surgical intensive care unit: a preliminary study conducted in secret. Intensive Crit. Care Nurs. 12 (4), 226–230.
McMurray, J.E., Linzer, M., Konrad, T.R., et al., 2000. The worklives of women physicians. J. Gen. Intern. Med. 15, 372–380.
McNeese-Smith, D.K., 1997. The influence of manager behavior on nurses' job satisfaction, productivity, and commitment. J. Nurs. Adm. 27 (9), 47–55.
Mealer, M., Shelton, A., Berg, B., et al., 2006. Increased prevalence of post traumatic stress disorder symptoms in critical care nurses. Am. J. Respir. Crit. Care Med. 175 (7), 693–697.
Medland, J.J., Ferrans, C.E., 1998. Effectiveness of a structured communication program for family members of patients in an ICU. Am. J. Crit. Care 7 (1), 24–29.
Melamed, S., Bruhis, S., 1996. The effects of chronic industrial noise exposure on urinary cortisol, fatigue and irritability. J. Occup. Environ. Med. 38 (3), 253–256.
Mendonca, D., Warren, N.A., 1998. Perceived and unmet needs of critical care family members. Crit. Care Nurs. Q. 21 (1), 58–67.
Mendyka, E., 1993. The dying patient in the intensive care unit: assisting the family in crisis. AACN Clin. Issues Crit. Care Nurs. 4 (3), 550–557.
Menegazzi, J., Paris, P., Kersteen, C., et al., 1991. A randomized, controlled trial of the use of music during laceration repair. Ann. Emerg. Med. 20 (4), 348–350.
Meredith, C., Edworthy, J., 1995. Are there too many alarms in the intensive care unit? An overview of the problems. J. Adv. Nurs. 21 (1), 15–20.
Merriam-Webster., 2005. The Merriam-Webster Dictionary. Merriam-Webster, Springfield, MA.
Meuser, P., Shirmer, C., 2006. New Hospital Buildings in Germany, Vol. 1: General Hospitals and Health Centres. DOM Publishers, Berlin.
Meyer, T.J., Eveloff, S.E., Bauer, M.S., et al., 1994. Adverse environmental conditions in the respiratory and medical ICU settings. Chest 105 (4), 1211–1216.
Meyer-Falcke, A., Rack, R., Eichwede, F., Jansing, P., 1994. How noisy are anaesthesia and intensive care medicine? Quantification of the patients' stress. Eur. J. Anaesthesiol. 11 (5), 407–411.
Millar, B., 1989. Critical support in critical care. Nurs. Times 19 (85), 31–32.
Miller, A., Hickman, L., Lemasters, G., 1992. A distraction technique for control of burn pain. J. Burn. Care Rehabil. 13, 576–581.
Minckley, B.B., 1968. A study of noise and its relationship to patient discomfort in the recovery room. Nurs. Res. 17, 247.

Misak, C., 2005. ICU psychosis and patient autonomy: some thoughts from the inside. J Med Philos 30, 411–430.

Mitchell, M., Courtney, M., 2004. Reducing family members' anxiety and uncertainty in illness around transfer from intensive care: an intervention study. Intensive Crit. Care Nurs. 20, 223–231.

Mitka, M., Michael, E., DeBakey, M.D., 2005. Father of Modern Cardiovascular Surgery. J. Am. Med. Assoc. 293, 913–918.

Mohl, P.C., Denny, N.R., Mote, T.A., Coldwater, C., 1982. Hospital unit stressors affect on nurses: Primary task vs. social factors. Psychosomatics 23 (4), 366–374.

Mohta, M., Sethi, A.K., Tyagi, A., Mohta, A., 2003. Psychological care in trauma patients. Injury 34 (1), 17–25.

Molter, N.C., 1976. The Identification of the Needs of and their Importance to Relatives of Critically Ill Patients, Unpublished master's thesis, Emory University, Atlanta, GA.

Molter, N.C., 1994. Families are not visitors in the critical care unit. Dimens. Crit. Care Nurs. 13 (1), 2–3.

Mongiardi, F., Payman, B.C., Hawthorn, P.J., 1987. The needs of relatives of patients admitted to the coronary care unit. Intensive Care Nurs. 3, 67–70.

Monk, T., 2004. Hospital Builders. Wiley-Academy, Chichester, UK.

Moodie, D.S., 2003. Regionalization of pediatric cardiac services. Prog. Pediatr. Cardiol. 18 (1), 55–58.

Moore, M.M., Nguyen, D., Nolan, S.P., et al., 1998. Interventions to reduce decibel levels on patient care units. Am. Surg. 64 (9), 894–899.

Morris, R., 1998. Personal Communication with a Healthcare Engineer, Houston, April 23.

Morrison, I., 2000. Health Care in the New Millenium: Vision, Values, and Leadership. Jossey-Bass, San Francisco, CA.

Morrison, W., Haas, E., Shaffner, D., et al., 2002. Noise, stress and annoyance in a pediatric intensive care unit. Crit. Care Med. 31 (1), 113–119.

Morrissey, J., 2003. A matter of safety: leapfrog to announce collaboration with CMS. Mod. Healthc. 33 (6), 17.

Morse, D.J.M., 1997. Preventing Patient Falls. Sage Publications Inc, Thousands Oaks, CA.

Moseley, M.J., Jones, A.M., 1991. Contracting for visitation with families. Dimens. Crit. Care Nurs. 10 (6), 364–371.

Mulligan, M.E., George, W. ., Rolfe, R.D., Finegold, S.M., 1980. Epidemiological aspects of *Clostridium difficile*-induced diarrhea and colitis. Am. J. Clin. Nutr. 33 (Suppl. 11), 2533–2538.

Murphy, P.A., Forrester, D.A., Price, D.M., Monaghan, J.F., 1992. Empathy of intensive care nurses and critical care family needs assessment. Heart Lung 21 (1), 25–30.

Murray, A., Montgomery, J.E., Chang, H., et al., 2001. Doctor discontent: a comparison of physician satisfaction in different delivery system settings, 1986 and 1997. J. Gen. Intern. Med. 16, 451–459.

Myhren, H., Ekeberg, Ø., Langen, I., Stokland, O., 2004. Emotional strain, communication, and satisfaction of family members in the intensive care unit compared with expectations of the medical staff: experience from a Norwegian University Hospital. Intensive Care Med. 30, 1791–1798.

National Fire Protection Association, 2009. NFPA 101: Life Safety Code. NFPA, Quincy, MA.

National Institute for Standards and Technology. 2002. Frequently Asked Questions about the Malcolm Baldrige National Quality Award. www.nist.gov/public_affairs/factsheet/baldfaqs.htm/>

Nelson, A., Baptiste, A., Matz, M., 2007. Evidence-based interventions for patient care ergonomics. In: Carayon, P. (Ed.), Handbook of Human Factors and Ergonomics in Health Care and Patient Safety. Lawrence Erlbaum, Mahwah, NJ pp

Nelson, J., Meier, D., 1999. Palliative care in the intensive care unit: Part I. J. Intensive. Care Med. 14, 130–139.

Nelson, J., Meier, D., Oei, E., et al., 2001. Self-reported symptom experience of critically ill cancer patients receiving intensive care. Crit. Care Med. 29 (2), 277–282.

Neuhof, H., Klapp, B.F., Gerlach, O., et al., 1980. The effects of "relaxing music" on patients, doctors and nursing staff of a medical intensive care unit. Dtsch. Med. Wochenschr. 105 (16), 556–560.

Nickl-Weller, C., Nickl, H., 2007. Hospital Architecture. Verlagshaus Braun, Berlin.

Nicholson, A.C., Titler, M., Montgomery, L.A., et al., 1993. Effects of child visitation in adult critical care units: a pilot study. Heart Lung 22 (1), 36–45.

Nilsson, U., Rawal, N., Unosson, M., 2003. A comparison of intra-operative or post-operative exposure to music – a controlled trial of the effects on postoperative pain. Anaesthesia 58 (7), 699–703.

Nightingale, F., 1859. Notes on Hospitals. John W. Parker and Sons, London.

Nightingale, F., 1863. Notes on Hospitals, third edn. Longmans, Green and Co., London.

Nixon, R.L., Jaramillo, F., 2003. Impact of practice arrangements on physicians' satisfaction. Hosp. Top. 81 (4), 19–25.

Noble, M., 1979. Communicating in the ICU: therapeutic or disturbing? Nurs. Outlook 27 (3), 195–198.

Noble, M., 1982. Staff communication: An unexpected finding. In: Nobel, M. (Ed.), The ICU Environment: Directions for Nursing. Reston Publishing, Reston, VA pp.

Norris, L.O., Grove, S.K., 1986. Investigation of selected psychosocial needs of family members of critically ill adult patients. Heart Lung 15 (2), 194–199.

Novaes, M.A., Knobel, E., Bork, A.M., et al., 1999. Stressors in the ICU: perception of the patient, relatives, and healthcare team. Intensive Care Med. 25 (12), 1421–1426.

O'Brien-Pallas, L., Shamian, J., Thomson, D., et al., 2004. Work-Related Disability in Canadian Nurses. J. Nurs. Sch. 36 (4), 352–357.

Ognibene, F.P., 2000. Resistant strains, isolation, and infection control. In: Hamilton, D.K. (Ed.), ICU 2010: ICU Design for the Future. Center for Innovation in Health Facilities, Houston, pp. 102–111.

O'Keefe, S.T., Lavan, J.N., 1996. Predicting delirium in elderly patients: development and validation of a risk-stratification mode. Age Ageing 25, 317–321.

O'Malley, P., Anderson, B., Siewe, S., et al., 1991. Critical care nurse perceptions of family needs. Heart Lung 20 (2), 189–201.

Onen, S., Alloui, A., Gross, A., et al., 2001. The effects of total sleep deprivation, selective sleep interruption and sleep recovery on pain tolerance thresholds in health subjects. J. Sleep. Res. 10, 35–42.

Orr, R., 1989. Healthcare environments for healing. J. Health. Care Inter. Des. 1, 71–76.

Orr, R., 1992. The Planetree Philosophy. J. Health Care Des. 4, 29–34.

Oschner, A.J., 1950. Recovery rooms contribute to better patient care. Hospitals 24, 50.

O'Sullivan, R.J., 1991. A musical road to recovery: music intensive care. Intensive Care Nurse 7 (3), 160–163.

Ott, J.N., 2000. Health and Light: The Effects of Natural and Artificial Light on Man and Other Living Things. Ariel Press, New York, NY.

Oyarzun, M.C.Z., 1996. Informacion a los familiares de pacientes ingresados en una Unidad de Cuidados Intensivos. Enferm. Intensiva 7 (1), 147–151.

Paparrigopoulos, T., Melissaki, A., Efthymiou, A., et al., 2006. Short-term psychological impact on family members of intensive care unit patients. J. Psychosom. Res. 61 (5), 719–722.

Park, J., 2007. Environmental Color for Pediatric Patient Room Design, Unpublished doctoral dissertation, Texas A&M University, College Station, TX.

Parmenter, E., 2001. Health Care Cost: What is it? Where is it headed? Why is it so high? What can be done about it? Benefit Planning Consultants, Inc.

Partonen, T., Lonnqvist, J., 2000. Bright light improves vitality and alleviates distress in healthy people. J. Affect. Disord. 57, 55–61.

Patel, C.T., 1996. Hope-inspiring strategies of spouses of critically ill adults. J. Holist. Nurs. 14 (1), 44–65.

Patrick, P.K., 1979. Burnout: job hazard for health workers. Hospitals 53 (22), 87–88, 90.

Peña, W.M., Parshall, S.A., 2001. Problem Seekingi, fourth ed. John Wiley & Sons, New York, NY.

Pennock, B.E., Crawshaw, L., Maher, T., et al., 1994. Distressful events in the ICU as perceived by patients recovering from coronary artery bypass surgery. Heart & Lung 23, 323–327.

Peolsi, P., Solca, M., Ravagnan, I., et al., 1996. Effects of heat and moisture exchangers on minute ventilation, ventilatory drive, and work of breathing during pressure-support ventilation in acute respiratory failure. Crit. Care Med. 24 (7), 1184–1188.

Perez de Ciriza, A., Otamendi, S., Ezenarro, A., Asiain, M.C., 1996. Factors causing stress in patients in intensive care units. Enferm. Intensiva 7 (3), 95–103.

Pérez-San Gregorio, M.A., Blanco-Picabia, A., Murillo-Cabezas, F., et al., 1992. Psychological problems in the family members of gravely traumatized patients admitted into an intensive care unit. Intensive Care Med. 18 (5), 278–281.

Perras, B., Meier, M., Dodt, C., 2007. Light and darkness fail to regulate melatonin release in critically ill humans. Intensive Care Med. 33 (11), 1954–1958.

Pettigrew, J., 1990. Intensive nursing care: the ministry of presence. Crit. Care Nurs. Clin. North. Am. 2 (3), 503–508.

Piazza, D., 1983. A nursing intervention and the Cognitive Functioning of Family Members of Critically Ill Patients. Unpublished doctoral dissertation, University of Alabama, Tuscaloosa, AL.

Picker Institute, 1999. Health Care Design Action Kit. Picker Institute, Boston, MA.

Piemme, J.A., 1982. Burnout in critical care nursing. In: Noble, M.A. (Ed.), The ICU Environment. Reston, Reston, VA pp.

Pierce, L.N.B., 2001. Patient safety and production pressure: ICU nursing perspective. Anesth. Patient Saf. Found. Newslet. Spring From; http://www.apsf.org/resource_centernewsletter/2001/spring/12ICU%20RN.htm.

Pittman, M.A., 2006. A worldwide crisis. Hosp. Health Network DOI.

Placek, M.Y., 1977. Territoriality and the patient's life space. Va. Nurse Q. 45 (1), 17–22.

Press, I., 2002. Patient Satisfaction: Defining, Measuring, and Improving the Experience of Care. Health Administration Press, Ann Arbor, MI.

Price, D.M., Forrester, D.A., Murphy, P.A., Monaghan, J.R., 1991. Critical care family needs in an urban teaching medical center. Heart & Lung 20 (2), 183–188.

Proctor, M.L., Pastore, J., Gerstle, J.T., Langer, J.C., 2003. Incidence of medical error and adverse outcomes on a pediatric general surgery service. J. Pediatr. Surg. 38 (9), 1361–1365.

Quan, X., 2005. Handwashing Compliance in Three ICU Settings. Presentation at Health Industry Advisory Council, Texas A&M University, College Station, November. 2005

Quinio, P., Savry, C., Deghelt, A., et al., 2002. A multicenter survey of visiting policies in French intensive care units. Intensive Care Med. 28, 1389–1394.

Radl, F., 2000. Materials management – keeping the patient at the heart of supply delivery. In: Hamilton, D.K. (Ed.), ICU 2010: ICU Design for the Future. Center for Innovation in Health Facilities, Houston, pp. 284–292.

Raffensberger, D., 1988. An intensive care unit that really cares. Nursing 18 (1), 64A, 64D.

Rainey, T., 2000. Clinical context: treatment protocols, physician roles and intensivist-lead teams. In: Hamilton, D.K. (Ed.), ICU 2010 ICU Design for the Future. Center for Innovation in Health Facilities, Houston, pp. 28–35.

Rainey, T.G., Kabcenell, A., Berwick, D.M., Roessner, J., 1998. Reducing Costs and Improving Outcomes in Adult Intensive Care. Institute for Healthcare Improvement, Boston.

Ramirez, A.J., Graham, J., 1996. Mental health of hospital consultants: the effects of stress and satisfaction at work. Lancet 347 (9003), 724–729.

Ramsey, P.W., 1986. Bringing a patient through ICU psychosis. Regist. Nurse 49 (9), 42–45.

Ramsey, P., Cathelyn, J., 2000. Restricted versus open ICUs. Nurs. Manage. 31 (1), 42–44.

Rattray, J., Johnston, M., Wildsmith, J.A., 2004. The intensive care experience: development of the ICE questionnaire. J. Adv. Nurs. 47 (1), 64–73.

Ray, M.A., 1987. Technological caring: a new model in critical care. Dimens. Crit. Care Nurs. 6 (3), 166–173.

Redding, J.S., Hargest, T.S., Minsky, S.H., 1977. How noisy is intensive care? Crit. Care Med. 5 (6), 275–276.

Reiling, J., 2004. Facility design focused on patient safety. Front. Health Serv. Manage. 21 (1), 41–46.

Reiling, J., 2005. Creating a culture of patient safety through innovative hospital design. In: Advances in Patient Safety: From Research to Implementation. Volume 2. Concepts and Methodology. Agency for Healthcare Research and Quality, Rockville, MD.

Reiling, J., Chernos, S., 2007. Human factors in hospital safety design. In: Carayon, P. (Ed.), Handbook of Human Factors and Ergonomics in Health Care and Patient Safety. Lawrence Erlbaum, Mahway, NJ. pp.

Reiling, J., Breckbill, C., Murphy, M., et al., 2003. Facility designing around patient safety and its effect on nursing. Nurs. Econ. 21 (3), 143–147.

Reilly, P., 2002. Leaders of the pack: solucient's annual list of the nation's 100 Top Hospitals features organizations that take excellence several steps further. Mod. Healthc. December 9, 28–35.

Retsas, A., Pinikahana, J., 2008. Manual handling activities and injuries among nurses: an Australian hospital study. J. Adv. Nurs. 31 (4), 875–883.

Richards, K., Nagel, C., Markie, M., et al., 2003. Use of complementary and alternative therapies to promote sleep in critically ill patients. Crit. Care Nurs. Clin. North Am. 15 (3), 329–340.

Richards, T., Johnson, J., Sparks, A., Emerson, H., 2007. The effect of music therapy, patients' perception and manifestation of pain, anxiety, and patient satisfaction. Medsurg Nurs. 16 (1), 7–14.

Roberts, B., Rickard, C., Rajbhandari, D., Reynolds, P., 2007. Factual memories of ICU: recall at two years post-discharge and comparison with delirium status during ICU admission – a multicentre cohort study. J. Clin. Nurs. 16 (9), 1669–1677.

Rogers, C.D., 1983. Needs of relatives of cardiac surgery patients during the critical care phase. Focus Crit. Care 10 (5), 50–55.

Rosen, I.M., Bellini, L.M., Shea, J.A., 2004. Sleep behaviors and attitudes among internal medicine housestaff in a U.S. university-based residency program. Acad. Med. 79 (5), 407–416.

Rouse, W., 1985. On better mousetraps and basic research: getting the applied world to the laboratory door. IEEE Trans. Syst. Man Cybern. 15 (1), 2–8.

Routhieaux, R.L., Tansik, D.A., 1997. The benefits of music in hospital waiting rooms. Health Care Superv. 16 (2), 31–40.

Rubin, H.R., Owens, A.J., Golden, G., 1998. Status Report: An Investigation to Determine Whether the Built Environment Affects Patients' Medical Outcomes. The Center for Health Design, Martinez, CA.

Rudy, E.B., Daly, B.J., Douglas, S., et al., 1995. Patient outcomes for the chronically critically ill: special care unit versus intensive care unit. Nurs. Res. 44 (6), 324–331.

Rukholm, E.E., Bailey, P.H., Coutu-Wakulczyk, G., 1992. Anxiety and family needs of the relatives of cardiac medical-surgical ICU patients. Canadian J. Cardiovasc. Nurs. 2 (4), 15–22.

Rukholm, E.E., Bailey, P., Coutu-Wakulczyk, G., Bailey, W.B., 1991. Needs and anxiety levels in relatives of intensive care unit patients. J. Adv. Nurs. 16, 920–928.

Runy, L.A., 2002. The dynamics of satisfaction. Hosp. Health Netw. November, 57–62.

Russek, L.G.S., Schwartz, G.E.R., 1998. Reducing stress in the intensive care unit: integrating mind-body values with modern technology. Adv. Mind Body Med. 14, 43–73.

Russell, S., 1999. An exploratory study of patients' perceptions, memories, and experiences of an intensive care unit. J. Adv. Nurs. 29 (4), 783–791.

Ryherd, E., Persson Waye, K., Ljungkvist, L., 2008. Characterizing noise and perceived work environment in a neurological intensive care unit. J. Acoust. Soc. Am. 123 (2), 747–756.

Sackett, D.L., Rosenberg, W.M.C., Muir Gray, J.A., et al., 1996. Evidence-based medicine: what it is and what it isn't. Br. Med. J. 312, 71–72.

Salyer, J., Stuart, B.J., 1985. Nurse-patient interaction in the intensive care unit. Heart & Lung 14 (1), 20–24.

Santa Maria-Punongbayan, L., 1982. Perceived intrusions into territorial and personal space as anxiety-producing factors to hospitalized patients: implications to nursing. Philipp. J. Nurs. 52 (2), 26–28.

Särkämö, T., Tervaniemi, M., Laitinen, S., et al., 2008. Music listening enhances cognitive recovery and mood after middle cerebral artery stroke. Brain 131, 866–867.

Sawada, N.O., Correia, F.A., Mendes, I.A., Coleta, J.A., 1996. Personal and territorial space of the patients: a nursing ethics question. Med. Law 15 (2), 261–270.

Sawatzky, J.A., 1996. Stress in critical care nurses: actual and perceived. Heart & Lung 25 (5), 409–417.

Scalise, D., 2001. Who's rating you? Hosp. Health Netw. December, 36–40.

Schein, E.H., 1992. Organizational Culture & Leadership. From ,http://www.tnellen.com/ted/tc/schein.html/>.
Schelling, G., 2002. Effects of stress hormones on traumatic memory formation and the development of post traumatic stress disorder in critically ill patients. Neurobiol. Learn. Mem. 78 (3), 596–609.
Schinner, K.M., Chisholm, A.H., Grap, M.J., et al., 1995. Effects of auditory stimuli on intracranial pressure and cerebral perfusion pressure in traumatic brain injury. J. Neurosci. Nurs. 27 (6), 348–354.
Schulte, D., Burrell, L., Gueldner, S., et al., 1993. Pilot study of the relationship between heart rate and ectopy and unrestricted vs. restricted visiting hours in the coronary care unit. Am. J. Crit. Care 2, 134–146.
Schwartz, W.B., 2000. Life Without Disease: The Pursuit of Medical Utopia. University of California Press.
Scullion, P.A., 1994. Personal cost, caring, and communication: an analysis of communication between relatives and intensive care nurses. Intensive Crit. Care Nurs. 10 (1), 64–70.
Selye, H., 1956. What is stress? Metab. Clin. Exp. 5 (5), 525–530.
Shepley, M., 1996a. Can research be done in private practice? Three healthcare facility case studies. Proceedings of the Architectural Research Center Consortium, 155–158.
Shepley, M., 1996b. Healthcare facility lifeline: Integrating research into the design process. Proceedings of the 1996 International Conference on Health Facility Planning Design and Construction, American Hospital Association/American Society for Hospital Engineering, Chicago, 561–568.
Shepley, M., 1997. A users' guide to healthcare design research. J. Center Health Des. IX, 9–12.
Shepley, M., 2005. The healthcare environment. In: Rollins, J. (Ed.), The Psychosocial Needs of Children Across the Healthcare Continuum. Aspen Publishers, Gaithersburg, MD pp.
Shepley, M., 2006. Evidence-based design and architecture. In: Wagenaar, C. (Ed.), The Architecture of Hospitals Rotterdam. NAI Publishers, The Netherlands pp.
Shepley, M., 2006. The role of positive distraction in neonatal intensive care unit settings. Am. J. Perinatol. 26, S37–S43.
Shepley, M., Davies, K., 2003. AIDS nursing unit configuration and its relationship to noise and nurse walking behavior. AIA Acad. J. 6 <http://www.aia.org/aah_journal_archivelist.>
Shepley, M., Quan, X., 2003. Health design research literature review: 1998–2002. Unpublished paper, Texas A&M University, College Station, TX.
Shepley, M., Fournier, M., McDougal, K., 1998. Healthcare Environments for Children and their Families. Kendall-Hunt, Dubuque.
Shertzer, K., Keck, J., 2001. Music in the PACU environment. J. Perinanesth. Nur. 16 (2), 90–102.
Shi, S.F., Munjas, B.A., Wan, T.T., et al., 2003. The effects of preparatory sensory information on ICU patients. J. Med. Syst. 27 (2), 191–204.
Shirani, K.Z., et al., 1986. Effects of environment on infection in burn patients. Arch. Surg. 121, 31–36.
Shonkwiler, M.A., 1985. Sibling visits in the pediatric intensive care unit. Crit. Care Q. 8 (1), 67–72.
Shortell, S.M., Kaluzny, A.D., 2000. Health Care Management: Organization Design and Behavior, fourth ed. Thompson Delmar, Albany, NY.
Shugerman, R., Linzer, M., Nelson, K., et al., 2001. Pediatric generalists and subspecialists: Determinants of career satisfaction. Pediatrics 108 (3) From <http://www.pediatrics.org/cgi/content/full/108/3/e40>.
Siegel, D.M., 1987. The high cost of medical technology: Getting at the heart of the matter. Med. Care 25 (10), 979–987.
Simon, S., Phillips, K., Badaamenti, S., et al., 1997. Current practices regarding visitation policies in critical care units. Am. J. Crit. Care 6 (3), 210–217.
Simpson, T., 1989. Needs and concerns of families of critically ill adults. Focus Crit. Care 16, 388–397.
Simpson, T., 1991. Critical care patients' perceptions of visits. Heart & Lung 20, 681–688.
Simpson, T., 1993. Visit preferences of middle-aged vs. older critically ill patients. Am. J. Crit. Care 2 (4), 339–345.
Simpson, T., 1996. Implementation and evaluation of a liberalized visiting policy. Am. J. Crit. Care 5 (6), 420–426.

Simpson, T., Shaver, J., 1990. Cardiovascular responses to family visits in coronary care patients. Heart & Lung 19, 344–351.

Snoby, P., 2005. Practice alert: Family presence during CPR and invasive procedures. J. Radiol. Nurs. 24 (3), 49–51.

Snyder-Halpern, R., 1985. The effect of critical care unit noise on patient sleep cycles. Crit. Care Q. 7 (4), 41–51.

Society of Critical Care Medicine, 1995. Guidelines for intensive care unit design. Crit. Care Med. 23 (3), 582–588.

Sommer, R., 1969. Personal Space. Prentice-Hall, Englewood Cliffs, NJ.

Song, R., Daly, B.J., Rudy, E.B., et al., 1997. Nurses' job satisfaction, absenteeism, and turnover after implementing a special care unit practice model. Res. Nurs. Health 20 (5), 443–452.

Sosnowski, C., Ustik, M., 1994. Early intervention: coma stimulation in the intensive care unit. J. Neurosci. Nurs. 26 (6), 336–341.

Spatt, L., Ganas, E., Hying, S., et al., 1986. Informational needs of families of intensive care patients. Qual. Rev. Bull. 12 (1), 16–21.

Spear, M., 1997. Designing the universal patient care room. J. Healthc. Des. IX, 81–83.

Spencer, L., 1994. How do nurses deal with their own grief when a patient dies on an intensive care unit, and what help can be given to enable them to overcome their grief effectively. J. Adv. Nurs. 19 (6), 1141–1150.

Spittler, K.L., 2006. Family presence during CPR and invasive procedures. Pulm. Rev. 11 (3).

Spoth, R., Konewko, P., 1987. Intensive care staff stressors and life event changes across multiple settings and work units. Heart & Lung 16 (3), 278–284.

Stanchina, M., Abu-Hijleh, M., Chaudhry, B., et al., 2005. The influence of white noise on sleep in subjects exposed to ICU noise. Sleep Med. 6, 423–428.

Stanton, D.J., 1991. The psychological impact of intensive therapy: the role of nurses. Intensive Care Nurs. 7 (4), 230–235.

Steckel, C.M., King, R.P., 1996. Therapeutic touch in the coronary care unit. J. Cardiovasc. Nurs. 10 (3), 50–54.

Steenkamp, W.C., van der Merwe, A.E., 1998. The psychosocial functioning of nurses in a burn unit. Burns 24 (3), 253–258.

Stern, P.N., 1995. Grounded Theory methodology: its uses and processes. In: Glazer, B.G. (Ed.), Grounded Theory 1984–1994. Sociology Press, Mill Valley, CA. pp.

Stichler, J.F., 2007. Using evidence-based design to improve outcomes. J. Nurs. Adm. 37 (1), 1–4.

Stillwell, S.B., 1984. Importance of visiting needs as perceived by family members of patients in the intensive care unit. Heart & Lung 13 (3), 238–242.

Stockdale, L.L., Hughes, J.P., 1988. Critical care unit visiting policies: a survey. Focus Crit. Care 15 (6), 45–48.

Stroud, R., 1997. The effects of technology on relatives in critical care environments. Nurse Crit. Care 2 (6), 272–275.

Suchetka, M., 1994. What, if anything, does your unit do to reduce noise levels in the ICU? Crit. Care Nurs. 14 (6), 89.

Sussex, J., 2001. The Economics of the Private Finance Initiative in the NHS. Office of Health Economics, London.

Swaiss, I.G., Badran, I., 2004. Discomfort, awareness, and recall in the intensive care—still a problem? Middle East J. Anesthesiol. 17 (5), 951–958.

Tai, D.Y.H, Ng, K.S., 2001. Intensive care medicine in Singapore: challenges in a New Era. Ann. Acad. of Med. Singapore 30 (3), 6.

Takman, C., Severinsson, E., 2006. A description of healthcare provider's perceptions of the needs of significnat others in intensive care units in Norway and Sweden. Intensive Crit. Care Nurs. 22 (4), 228–238.

Tanimoto, S., Takayanagi, K., Yokota, H., Yamamoto, Y., 1999. The psychological and physiological effects of an intensive-care unit environment on healthy individuals. Clin. Perform. Qual. Health Care 7 (2), 77–82.

Thompson, C.A., 2006. Michigan hospital captures national quality award. Am. J. Health Syst. Pharm. 63 (3), 198–206.

Thompson, D.R., Clemmer, T.P., Applefeld, J.J., et al., 1994. Regionalization of critical care medicine: task force report of the american college of critical care medicine. Crit. Care Med. 22 (8), 1308–1313.

Thomson, R., 2008. St John's hospital saves staff time with wireless access to patient data. Comput. Weekly April 29, 42.

Thompson, R., Boyle, D., Teel, C., et al., 1999. A qualitative analysis of family member needs and concerns in the population of patients with burns. J. Burn Care Rehabil. 20, 487–496.

Tiernan, P.J., 1994. Independent nursing interventions: relaxation and guided imagery in critical care. Crit. Care Nurs. 14 (5), 47–51.

Titler, M.G., Cohen, M.Z., Craft, M.J., 1991. Impact of adult critical care hospitalization: perceptions of patients, spouses, children and nurses. Heart & Lung 20 (2), 174–182.

Tonges, M.C., 1993. Work redesign: theory, approaches, and lessons. In: McDonagh, K.J. (Ed.), Patient-Centered Hospital Care. Health Administration Press, Ann Arbor, MI. pp.

Topf, M., 1984. A framework for research on aversive physical aspects of the environment. Res. Nurs. Health 7 (1), 35–42.

Topf, M., 1988. Noise-induced occupational stress and health in critical care nurses. Hosp. Top. 66 (1), 30–34.

Topf, M., 1992. Effects of personal control over hospital noise on sleep. Res. Nurs. Health 15 (1), 19–28.

Topf, M., 2000. Hospital noise pollution: an environmental stress model to guide research and clinical interventions. J. Adv. Nurs. 31 (3), 520–528.

Topf, M., Davis, J.E., 1993. Critical care unit noise and rapid eye movement (REM) sleep. Heart & Lung 22 (3), 252–258.

Topf, M., Dillon, E., 1988. Noise-induced stress as a predictor of burnout in critical care nurses. Heart & Lung 17 (5), 567–574.

Topf, M., Bookman, M., Arand, D., 1996. Effects of critical care unit noise on the subjective quality of sleep. J. Adv. Nurs. 24, 545–551.

Trinkoff, A.M., Brady, B., Nielsen, K., 2003. Workplace prevention and musculoskeletal injuries in nurses. J. Nurs. Adm. 33 (3), 153–158.

Tse, M., Ng, J., Chung, J., Wong, T., 2002. The effect of visual stimuli on pain threshold and tolerance. J. Clin. Nurs. 11, 264–269.

Tsiou, C., Eftymiatos, D., Theodossopoulou, E., et al., 1998. Noise sources and levels in the Evgenidion Hospital intensive care unit. Intensive Care Med. 24, 845–847.

Turnock, C., 1991. Communicating with patients in ICU. Nurs. Stand. 5 (15/16), 38–40.

Twibell, R.S., 1998. Family coping during critical illness. Dimens. Crit. Care Nurs. 17 (2), 100–113.

Ulrich, R., 1984. View through a window may influence recovery from surgery. Science 224, 420–421.

Ulrich, R., 1986. Effects of hospital environments on patient well-being. Research Report from Department of Psychiatry and Behavioral Medicine 9 (55) Trondheim, Norway: Department of Psychiatry and Behavioral Medicine, University of Trondheim.

Ulrich, R., 1991. Effects of interior design on wellness: theory and recent scientific research. J. Healthc. Des. 3, 97–109.

Ulrich, R., 1997. A theory of supportive design for healthcare facilities. J Healthc. Des. IX, 3–7.

Ulrich, R., 1999. Effects of gardens on health outcomes: theory and research. In: Cooper Marcus, C., Barnes, M. (Eds.) Healing Gardens: Therapeutic Benefits and Design Recommendations. John Wiley and Sons, New York. pp.

Ulrich, R., 2000. Environmental research and critical care, In: Hamilton, D.K. (Ed.), ICU 2010. Center for Innovation in Health Facilities, Houston, TX. pp.

Ulrich, R., 2001. Effects of healthcare environmental design on medical outcomes. In: Dilani, A. (Ed.), Design and Health—The Therapeutic Benefits of Design. Proceedings of the Second International Conference on Design & Health, 2000, Svenskbyggtjanst, Stockholm, pp.

Ulrich, R., 2006. Essay: evidence-based health-care architecture. Lancet 368, 538–539.

Ulrich, R., Lundén, O., 1993. Effects of nature and abstract pictures on patients recovering from heart surgery. Abstract of a Poster Presentation at the First International Congress of Behavioral Medicine, Uppsala, Sweden, June 27–30.

Ulrich, R.S., Wilson, P., 2006. Evidence-based design. Public Serv. Rev. Health (UK) 8, 24–25.

Ulrich, R.S., Zhu, X., 2007. Medical complications of intra-hospital patient transports: implications for architectural design and research. Health Environ. Res. Des. J. 1 (1), 31–43.

Ulrich, R., Quan, X., Zimring, C., et al., 2004. The Role of the Physical Environment in the Hospital of the 21st Century: A Once-in-a-Lifetime Opportunity. The Center for Health Design, Concord, CA.

Ulrich, R.S., Zimring, C.M., Zhu, X., et al., 2008. A review of the research literature on evidence-based health care design. Health Environ. Res. Des. J. 1 (3), 61–125.

Updike, P., 1990. Music therapy results for ICU patients. Dimens. Crit. Care Nurs. 9 (1), 39–45.

van den Berg, E., 2005. Health Impacts of Healing Environments. From www.thearchitectureofhospitals.org/>.

Varnam, D.C. (). Famlies in the ED: helpful or harmful? Nurs. Spectr. 5.

Varon, J., Fromm, R., 2002. Handbook of Practical Critical Care Medicine. Springer, New York, NY.

Verdecchia, P., Staessen, J.A., et al., 2002. Properly defining white coat hypertension. Eur. Heart J. 23 (2), 106–109.

Verderber, S., 1986. Dimensions of person-window transactions in the hospital environment. Environ. Behav. 18, 450–466.

Verity, S., 1996. Communicating with sedated ventilated patients in intensive care: focusing on the use of touch. Intensive Crit. Care Nurs. 12 (6), 354–358.

Vieira, E.R., Miller, L., 2008. Facing the challenge of patient transfers: using ceiling lifts in healthcare facilities. Health Environ. Res. Des. J. 2 (1), 6–16.

Viets, E., 2009. Lessons from evidence-based medicine: what healthcare designers can learn from the medical field. Health Environ. Res. Des. J. 2 (2), 73–87.

Villaire, M., 1993. Cathie guzzetta and barbara dossey: guiding critical care nurses on the body-mind-spirit journey. Crit. Care Nurs. 13 (4), 105–111.

Vincent, J.L., 1997. Communication in the ICU. Intensive Care Med. 23 (10), 1093–1098.

Vincent, J.L., Thijs, L., Cerny, V., 1997. Critical care in Europe. Crit. Care Clin. 13 (2), 45–54.

Virtanen, P., Oksanen, T., Kivimaki, M., et al., 2008. Work stress and health in primary health care physicians and hospital physicians. Occup. Environ. Med. 65, 364–366.

Wagner, J.T., Higdon, T.L., 1996. Spiritual issues and bioethics in the intensive care unit: the role of the chaplain. Crit. Care Clin. 12 (1), 15–27.

Walch, J., Rabin, B., Day, R., et al., 2005. The effect of sunlight on post operative analgesic medication use: a prospective study of patients undergoing spinal surgery. Psychosoma. Med. 67, 156–163.

Walder, B., Francioli, D., Meyer, J.J., et al., 2000. Effects of guidelines implementation in a surgical intensive care unit to control nighttime light and noise levels. Crit. Care Med. 28, 2242–2247.

Wall, R., Curtis, J., Cooke, C., Engelberg, R., 2007. Family satisfaction in the ICU: differences between families of survivors and nonsurvivors. Chest 132 (5), 1425–1433.

Walters, A.J., 1994. A hermeneutic study of the concept of "focusing" in critical care nursing practice. J. Nurs. Inq. 1, 23–30.

Warren, N., 1993. Perceived needs of the family members in the critical care waiting room. Crit. Care Nurs. Q. 16 (3), 56–63.

Watson, L.A., 1989. A Description of Nursing Intervention Designed to Meet Family Needs of Critically Ill Patients. Unpublished doctoral dissertation, University of Alabama, Birmingham, AL.

Weber, W., 2001. Paris' Pompidou hospital plagued by setbacks. Lancet 357 (9250), 130. 13.

Weber, R.J., Oszko, M.A., Bolender, B.J., Grysiak, D.L., 1985. The intensive care unit syndrome: causes, treatment, and prevention. Drug Intell. Clin. Pharm. 19 (1), 13–20.

Weiner, S.J., Schwartz, A., Yudkowsky, R., et al., 2007. Evaluating physician performance at individualizing care: a pilot study tracking contextual errors in medical decision making. Med. Decis. Making 27, 726–734.

Werdal, L., 2000. Case study: griffin hospital, derby connecticut. In: Hamilton, D.K. (Ed.), ICU 2010: ICU Design for the Future. Center for Innovation in Health Facilities, Houston. pp.

Wessels, L., Verweij, M., 2002. Developments in Healthcare Building in the Netherlands Seen in a European Perspective. Netherlands Board for Hospital Facilities.

Westball, C., 1994. What, if anything, does your unit do to reduce noise levels in the ICU? Crit. Care Nurs. 14 (6), 88–89.

Wetterneck, T.B., Linzer, M., McMurray, J.E., et al., 2002. Worklife and satisfaction of general internists. Arch. of Intern. Med. 162, 649–656.

White, D., Tonkin, J., 1991. Registered nurse stress in intensive care units—an Australian perspective. Intensive Care Nurs. 7 (1), 45–52.

White, J.M., 1992. Music therapy: an intervention to reduce anxiety in the myocardial infarction patient. Clin Nurse Spec. 5, 58–63.

White, J.M., 1999. Effects of relaxing music on cardiac autonomic balance and anxiety after acute myocardial infarction. Am. J. Crit. Care 8 (4), 220–230.

White, R.D., 2004. Lighting design in the neonatal intensive care unit: practical applications of scientific principles. Clin. Perinatol. 31 (2), 323–330.

Wilcox, M.H., Cunniffe, J.G., Trundle, C., Redpath, C., 1996. Financial burden of hospital-acquired Clostridium difficile infection. J. Hosp. Infect. 34 (1), 23–30.

Wilkins, A.L., Ouchi, W.G., 1983. Efficient cultures: exploring the relationship between culture and organizational performance. Adm. Sci. Q. 28 (3), 468–481.

Wilkins, A.J., Nimmo-Smith, I., Slater, A.I., Bedocs, L., 1989. Fluorescent lighting, headaches and eyestrain. Light. Res. Technol. 21 (1), 11–18.

Williamson, J.W., 1992. The effects of ocean sounds on sleep after coronary artery bypass graft surgery. Am. J. Crit. Care 1 (1), 91–97.

Wilson, K.H., Frederick, J., 1996. Clostridium difficil—contaminating the environment around a bedpan washing unit in a Veterans Hospital. Unpublished study.

Wise, M.G., 1998. Psychosocial interventions with patients and families by the healthcare team in critical care. New Horiz. 6 (4), 344–353.

Witte, D., Grobbee, D., Bots, M., Hoes, A., 2005. A meta-analysis of excess cardiac mortality on Monday. Eur. J. Epidmiology 20 (5), 401–406.

Wolitzky, K., Fivush, R., Zimand, E., et al., 2005. Effectiveness of virtual reality distraction during a painful medical procedure in pediatric oncology patients. Psychol. Health 6, 817–824.

Wooley, N., 1990. Crisis theory: a paradigm of effective intervention with families of critically ill people. J. Adv. Nurs. 15, 1402–1408.

Wynne, R., 2004. Ten Australian ICU nurses' perceptions of organizational restructuring. Aust. Crit. Care 17 (1), 16–24.

Wysocki, B., 2002. Doctor prescribes quality control for medicine's ills. Wall St. J. May 30.

Yamada, N., Martin-Iverson, M., Daimon, K., et al., 1995. Clinical and chronobiological effects of light therapy on nonseasonal affective disorders. Biol. Psychiatry 37, 866–873.

Yeoman, B., Paisley, L., 2005. Out, out, brown spot; or, ceiling tile alternatives. NAEB J., 16–17.

Yoshiya, I., Baik, S.W., 1997. Critical care in Japan and Korea. the market of excellence. Crit. Care Clin. 13 (2), 67–85.

Yox, S.B., 2004. An interview with ANA president Barbara Blakeney. Medscape Nurs. 6 (1).

Zazpe, C., Margall, M.A., Otano, C., et al., 1997. Meeting needs of family members of critically ill patients in a Spanish intensive care unit. Intensive Crit. Care Nurs. 13 (1), 12–16.

Zimmerman, L.M., Pierson, M.A., Marker, J., 1988. Effects of music on patient anxiety in coronary care units. Heart & Lung 17 (5), 560–566.

Zimmerman, L., Nieveen, J., Barnason, S., Schmaderer, M., 1996. The effects of music interventions on postoperative pain and sleep in coronary artery bypass graft (CABG) patients. Sch. Inq. Nurs. Pract. 10 (2), 153–170.

Zimmerman, L.M., et al., 1988. Effects of music on patient anxiety in coronary care units. Heart & Lung 17, 560–566.

Zimring, C., 1981. Stress and the designed environment. J. Soc. Issues 37 (1), 145–171.

Index

Knowledge-based design, 236–237

CPSIA information can be obtained at www.ICGtesting.com
Printed in the USA
LVOW02s0008240715

447425LV00005B/15/P

9 780750 665308